SpringerWienNewYork

Acta Neurochirurgica
Supplements

Editor: H.-J. Steiger

Intraoperative Imaging

Edited by

M. Necmettin Pamir, Volker Seifert, Talat Kırış

Acta Neurochirurgica

Supplement 109

SpringerWienNewYork

M. Necmettin Pamir
Professor and Chairman, Department of Neurosurgery, Acibadem University, School of Medicine, Inonu Cad, Okur Sok 20, 34742 Kozytagi, Istanbul, Turkey

Volker Seifert
Univ. Klinikum Frankfurt, Zentrum Neurologie und Neurochirurgie, Klinik für Neurochirurgie, Schleusenweg 2-16, 60528 Frankfurt, Haus 95, Germany

Talat Kırış
University of Istanbul, School of Medicine, Dept. Neurosurgery, 34390 Capa, Istanbul, Turkey

Printed in Germany
SpringerWienNewYork is part of Springer Science+Business Media
springer.at

Typesetting: SPI, Pondichery, India

Printed on acid-free and chlorine-free bleached paper
SPIN: 12744831

Library of Congress Control Number: 2010935184

With 117 (partly coloured) Figures

ISSN 0065-1419
ISBN 978-3-211-99650-8 e-ISBN 978-3-211-99651-5
DOI: 10.1007/978-3-211-99651-5
SpringerWienNewYork

Preface

In the pursuit of the goal of continuous improvement in surgical results, intraoperative imaging technologies have taken an ever-increasing role in the daily practice of neurosurgeons. To adapt available imaging technologies to the operating room a considerable amount of effort has been focused on the subject. Most centers have taken individual and independent approaches on the subject and an ever-diversifying field of "intraoperative imaging" has been created. In an initiative of coordinating and symbiotically integrating these novel technologies, the international "Intraoperative Imaging Society" has been formed. After the second international meeting of the society, this book is aimed to bring together both the essence and details of the current status.

The initial drive for intraoperative imaging in neurosurgery came from the demands of neurooncology. Accumulating evidence over the years has indicated that a more complete resection of brain tumors was associated with a lower incidence of recurrences and longer survival. This led to a search for techniques and technologies to improve the extent of surgical resections. Stereotactic techniques have led to the development of Neuronavigation as a means to define brain anatomy during surgery and to guide surgical interventions. The technology was welcomed with much enthusiasm as it provided precise stereotactic definition of both the brain anatomy and the boundaries of intracranial lesions. However, neuronavigation was based on preoperatively acquired images and the brain shift caused by the surgical intervention severely affected the accuracy and therefore the dependability of this technology. Meanwhile several different technologies of intraoperative imaging were under development. Ultrasonography (U/S), computed tomography (CT) and MRI are currently the most prominent of these techniques. Initial designs were tested in the clinic and most were replaced by never designs to accommodate clinical needs and to compensate for the shortcomings. The financial burden of these sophisticated intraoperative imaging technologies was also a serious consideration and had an important influence on equipment and facility designs. Intraoperative imaging technology certainly did not stay confined to the field of neurooncology. Neurovascular, pediatric, functional and spine surgery had different needs and these were fulfilled by development of even more diversified technologies.

The increasing attention and interest on intraoperative imaging also necessitated international interaction and collaboration and the Intraoperative Imaging Society was formed in 2007. The first Annual Meeting of the Intra-operative Imaging Society was held at the Hyatt Regency Resort, Spa and Casino in Lake Tahoe-Nevada in 2008. After this very successful meeting, the second meeting was held in Istanbul-Turkey from June 14 to 17, 2009. This book brings together highlights from this second meeting of the Intraoperative Imaging Society. The first section of the book gives an overview of the emergence and development of the intraoperative imaging technology and it gives a glimpse on where the technology is heading. Among all technologies, intraoperative MRI has received most of the attention due to immense technical potential of this modality. Various new technologies have been developed in the last decade and this led to very diverse designs. Therefore, we have divided this section into parts discussing low, high and ultra-high field designs. The second, third and fourth sections provide separate reports on each system. After reading these chapters the reader should have a general idea on intraoperative MRI technology and know the pros and cons of each design. The sections on CT and Ultrasonography are followed by a section with reports from the most prominent centers which have attempted integrating different imaging technologies. The last one is a diverse section bringing together ancillary techniques as well as reports on intraoperative robotic technology.

We believe that this book will provide an up-to date and comprehensive general overview of the current intraoperative imaging technology as well as detailed discussions on individual techniques and clinical results.

Istanbul, Turkey M.N. Pamir, T. Kırış
Frankfurt, Germany V. Seifert
March 2010

Contents

History- Development- Prospects of Intraoperative Imaging

From Vision to Reality: The Origins of Intraoperative MR Imaging

Peter Black, Ferenc A. Jolesz, and Khalid Medani

Abstract Intraoperative MR imaging has become one of the most important concepts in present day neurosurgery. The brain shift problem with navigation, the need for assessment of the degree of resection and the need for detection of early postoperative complications were the three most important motives that drove the development of this technology. The GE Signa System with the "double donut" design was the world's first intraoperative MRI. From 1995 to 2007 more than 1,000 neurosurgical cases were performed with the system. The system was used by several different specialties and in neurosurgery it was most useful for complete resection of low-grade gliomas, identification and resection of small or deep metastases or cavernomas, recurrent pituitary adenomas, cystic tumors, biopsies in critical areas and surgery in recurrent GBM cases. Main superiorities of the system were the ability to scan without patient movement to get image updates, the ability to do posterior fossa cases and other difficult patient positioning, the easiness of operation using intravenous sedation anesthesia and the flexibility of the system to be used as platform for new diagnostic and therapeutic modalities.

Keywords GE Signa · Intraoperative MR · MRI · Navigation

Abbreviations

BWH Brigham and Women's Hospital
CSF CerebroSpinal Fluid
fMRI Functional MRI
GBM Glioblastoma Multiforme
MEG Magnetoencephalography
MR(I) Magnetic Resonance(Imaging)
MRT Magnetic Resonance Tomography
NIH National Institute of Health
OR Operation Room

P. Black (✉) and K. Medani
Department of Neurosurgery, Brigham and Women's Hospital, Harvard Medical School, Boston, MA, USA
e-mail: peterblackwfns@gmail.com

F.A. Jolesz
Department of Radiology, Brigham and Women's Hospital, Harvard Medical School, Boston, MA, USA

Introduction

The Beginning

Intraoperative MR imaging has become one of the most important concepts in present day neurosurgery. Many factors led to the emergence of intraoperative MRI; the most important were:

(1) Brain shift (*movement of the brain relative to the cranium between the time of scanning and surgery*). One of the main reasons for developing intraoperative imaging was the shift of cortical brain structures during surgery because of loss of CSF, shrinkage of brain tissue, and resection of the lesion. These changes make it difficult to navigate accurately with preoperatively acquired images. This was particularly important for biopsies of cystic lesions, for resection of deep lesions or those with cysts or near the ventricles. Intraoperative MR can accurately estimate changes to the brain which occur during surgery, a property which is lacking in navigation systems using preoperatively acquired images [1–6].
(2) Assessing the degree of resection during surgery. Achieving greater tumor resection was another reason for developing the intraoperative MR. Residual tumor can be detected using this modality and can be removed without a return to the operating room. This turned out to be particularly important for pediatric tumors, gliomas and pituitary adenomas.
(3) Evaluating intraoperative complications. Intraoperative MR also has the capability to recognize acute intraoperative changes such as hemorrhage, infarct, and edema. These complications may be treated immediately, avoiding long-term disability.

The GE Signa System was the world's first intraoperative MRI. It used a novel "double donut" design in which the magnetic field was between two open magnets (Fig. 1). The main contributors to the system were Ferenc Jolesz and then Ron Kikinis and Richard Schwartz of the BWH Dept of Radiology, Peter Black and Eben Alexander, III of Neurosurgery, Marvin Fried from the Ear, Nose, and Throat Department, Mory Blumenthal from General Electric, BWH Biomedical Engineering, Maureen Hanley of nursing, Linda Aglio and George Topoulos of the anesthesia staff, and the hospital administration.

An important feature the system was a collaborative arrangement between the BWH and Children's Hospital. Drs. Mark Rockoff and Sulpiciano Soriano were particularly important in this. On Wednesday each week the system became an outpost of the Children's Hospital next door. The nursing and anesthesia staff were all from Children's; the patient was cared for preoperatively and postoperatively at Children's Hospital.

As the years developed, Dr. Fried left the BWH and ENT applications diminished. Radiation oncology under Dr. Anthony Amico became an important application, using the magnet for real time dosimetry for prostate cancer brachytherapy. For most of the life of the magnet, neurosurgery and radiation oncology shared its use.

The magnet arrived at BWH in 1993. The components included the magnet, console, anesthesia machines and monitors. The Midas REX drill system, operating microscope and CAVITRON ultrasonic device were developed over the next few years with particular help from neurosurgical fellows. In 1995, we performed the first brain tumor craniotomy using the intraoperative MR [1].

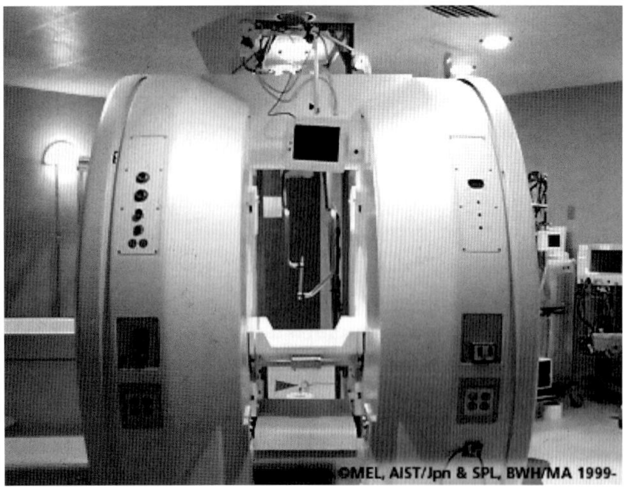

Fig. 1 The GE Signa intraoperative MRI

The GE Signa MRT System

In the GE 0.5 tesla Signa system, surgery is done directly in the MRI scanner. All instruments must be non-ferromagnetic. The device also acts as a powerful navigation system using software called slicer [7, 8]. Neurosurgical MRT fellows included: Tom Moriarty, Claudia Martin, Andrew Danks, Kate Drummond, Vivek Mehta, Arya Nabavi, David Walker, Lorenzo Bello, Dennis Oh, Elizabeth Claus., Juan Ortega, and Andrew Morokoff. They were instrumental in developing the instrument and its applications.

The slicer was a unique feature of our system developed by the Surgical Planning Lab (SPL), an immensely talented and powerful post-processing MR laboratory group led by Ron Kikinis. With the slicer, the MRI itself became a navigation system so no additional fiducials or registration was needed.

An example of a case operated using the GE Signa intraoperative MR is presented in Fig. 2: a 21-year-old woman came from Europe with intractable seizures of the right leg and hand with speech arrest. The MRI showed a tumor in the medial aspect of her left motor cortex (Fig. 2). Surgery was successfully performed to resect her gangliocytoma using the intraoperative MR. The images taken during the surgery show how the tumor was totally resected and the brain returned to normal (Fig. 3). The patient was discharged from the hospital two days after surgery with no deficit. One week after surgery, she was ready to go back to her home and has been seizure-free for the four years following surgery.

Besides its real-time updates during surgery and its strong navigation system, other advantages of the GE Signa system included:

1. The joy of working with a great team.
2. The little risk of ferro-magnetic instrumental injury because everything was screened before entering the room.
3. The ability to scan without patient movement to get updates.
4. The ability to do posterior fossa cases and other positioning which is difficult for regular navigation systems.
5. The ready ability to operate on patients using intravenous sedation anesthesia. For low grade gliomas, the combination of intraoperative navigation and intravenous sedation anesthetic with brain mapping gave an accuracy and safety not possible with other systems and ideal for the patient.
6. The ability to use the scanner as a platform for new diagnostic and therapeutic modalities such as scanning with a patient upright to look at disc disease and use of laser hyperthermia for noninvasive ablation of a target.

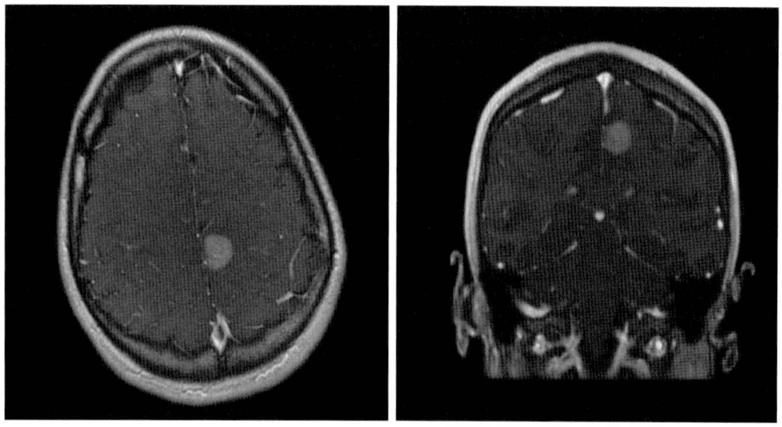

Fig. 2 21-year-old female with a gangliocytoma, before surgery

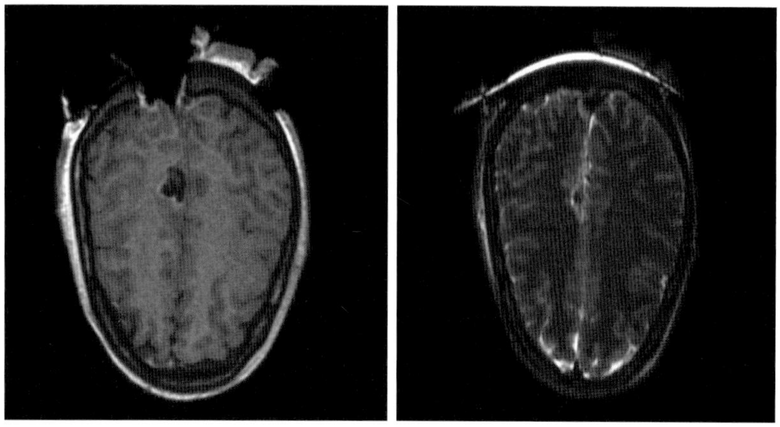

Fig. 3 21-year-old female with a gangliocytoma during surgery, using the GE Signa intraoperative MR. The lesion is localized with the slicer in the coronal and sagittal planes; it is removed (lower left) and the bone is replaced without difficulty. She had no postoperative deficit despite the proximity of the lesion to primary sensory and motor cortex

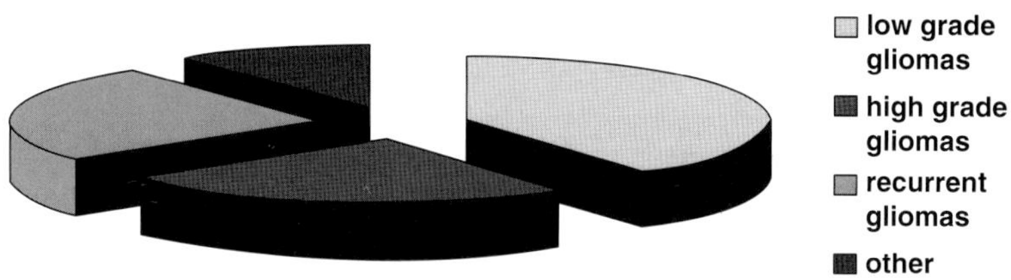

Fig. 4 Tumor types in 900 cases at BWH using the GE Signa intraoperative MRI

Disadvantages of the system included:

1. A modest restriction on positioning to get the "sweet spot" for imaging.
2. Early on, limitation of instrumentation because of the requirement for non-ferromagnetic tools.
3. Relatively low field strength compared with some other systems.

Uses of Our System

More than 1,000 neurosurgical cases were done in the Signa MRT system from 1995 to 2007. They included more than 800 craniotomies, 120 biopsies and 80 other procedures (cyst drainage, transsphenoidal procedures, etc). The majority of tumors were low-grade gliomas (50%); high-grade gliomas (24%), recurrent glioblastomas (26%), and other (10%) (Fig. 4).

Forty percent of the low-grade gliomas were done with mapping and intravenous sedation anesthesia. In 38% of cases, unexpected tumor was identified on intraoperative repeat imaging. The Cincinnati, Erlangen, and Boston experience confirmed that 40–50% of cases showed residual tumor that could be removed [9, 10]. The complication rate was only 5%, even in eloquent cortex, and the intraoperative imaging predicted postoperative imaging very well.

In recurrent gliomas, intraoperative MR significantly helped in resection of such tumors where the anatomical landmarks have been lost (Fig. 5). Intraoperative MR is

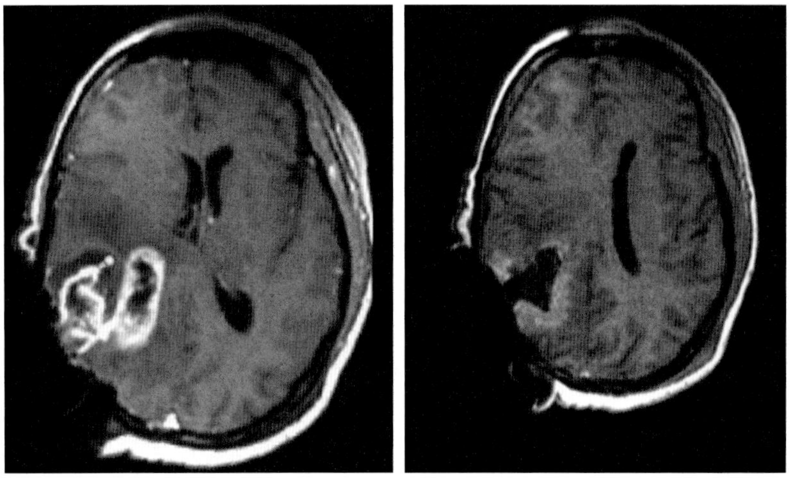

Fig. 5 Pre and post-operative recurrent glioblastoma, using the GE Signa intraoperative MRI

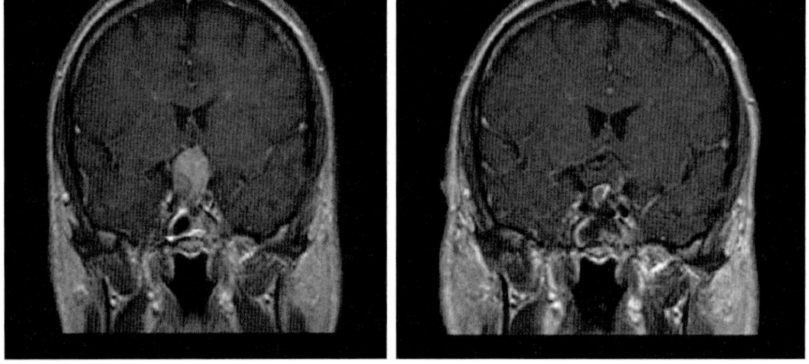

Fig. 6 Pre- and post-operative recurrent pituitary adenoma, using the GE Signa intraoperative MRI

also very useful in recurrent pituitary adenomas again demonstrating residual tumor otherwise unresected [11] (Fig. 6).

We concluded that intraoperative MR was important for complete resection of low-grade gliomas, identification and resection of small or deep metastases or cavernomas, recurrent pituitary adenomas, cystic tumors, biopsies in critical areas and recurrent GBM [11–17].

Accomplishments

Many improvements in patient care resulted from the use of the intraoperative MRI at the BWH; they include: improvement of the degree of resection of all tumors, shortening the duration of hospital stay, and reduction in the postoperative complication rate.

The unit was also extremely important in grant funding, including large NIH grants for post-processing of images, applications of intraoperative imaging, and new therapeutic approaches. These grants included program projects, national centers of excellence, RO-1's, and foundation grants.

The Future

In the near future, Intraoperative MR can be a broad base for different advance imaging techniques such as fMRI, MEG, MR Spectroscopy, as well as new therapeutic modalities such as laser hyperthermia for lesion destruction, focused ultrasonic surgery of tumors, robotic neurosurgery and, the new Advanced Multimodality Image Guided Operating (AMIGO) Suite at BWH [7, 18]. These topics will be covered by Dr. Jolesz's paper in this volume.

Perhaps the most important task, however, is the creation of class-one evidence for the usefulness of intraoperative imaging and the development of other applications including spinal and functional neurosurgery.

Conclusion

The early days of intraoperative MR imaging were pioneering, exciting, and visionary. Particularly important were the teams developed, the concept of the power of this modality, and the stimulation of the next generation to move the field forward. The creation of the intraoperative imaging society is an important step in consolidating this field and it will be exciting to see how this develops.

Conflict of interest statement Dr. Jolesz has received consultant fees from General Electric, who pioneered this system.

References

1. Black PM, Moriarty T, Alexander ER, Stieg P, Woodard EJ, Gleason PL, Martin CH, Kikinis R, Schwartz RB, Jolesz FA (1997) Development and implementation of intraoperative magnetic resonance imaging and its neurosurgical applications. Neurosurgery 41:831–842, discussion 842–845
2. Hata N, Nabavi A, Wells WMR, Warfield SK, Kikinis R, Black PM, Jolesz FA (2000) Three-dimensional optical flow method for measurement of volumetric brain deformation from intraoperative MR images. J Comput Assist Tomogr 24:531–538
3. Hill DL, Maurer CRJ, Maciunas RJ, Barwise JA, Fitzpatrick JM, Wang MY (1998) Measurement of intraoperative brain surface deformation under a craniotomy. Neurosurgery 43:514–526, discussion 527–528
4. Nabavi A, Black PM, Gering DT, Westin CF, Mehta V, Pergolizzi RSJ, Ferrant M, Warfield SK, Hata N, Schwartz RB, Wells WMR, Kikinis R, Jolesz FA (2001) Serial intraoperative magnetic resonance imaging of brain shift. Neurosurgery 48:787–797, discussion 797–798
5. Nimsky C, Ganslandt O, Hastreiter P, Fahlbusch R (2001) Intraoperative compensation for brain shift. Surg Neurol 56:357–364, discussion 364–365
6. Reinges MH, Nguyen HH, Krings T, Hutter BO, Rohde V, Gilsbach JM (2004) Course of brain shift during microsurgical resection of supratentorial cerebral lesions: limits of conventional neuronavigation. Acta Neurochir (Wien) 146:369–377, discussion 377
7. Black PM (2003) Current and future developments in intraoperative imaging: MRI. In: Apuzzo MLJ (ed) The operating room for the 21st century. AANS, Park Ridge, pp 45–51
8. Hinks RS, Bronskill MJ, Kucharczyk W, Bernstein M, Collick BD, Henkelman RM (1998) MR systems for image-guided therapy. J Magn Reson Imaging 8:19–25
9. Darakchiev BJ, Tew JMJ, Bohinski RJ, Warnick RE (2005) Adaptation of a standard low-field (0.3-T) system to the operating room: focus on pituitary adenomas. Neurosurg Clin N Am 16:155–164
10. von Keller B, Nimsky C, Ganslandt O, Fahlbusch R (2004) Intraoperative MRI in 62 patients with pituitary adenoma. Deutsche Gesellschaft für Neurochirurgie. Ungarische Gesellschaft für Neurochirurgie. 55. Jahrestagung der Deutschen Gesellschaft für Neurochirurgie e.V. (DGNC), 1. Joint Meeting mit der Ungarischen Gesellschaft für Neurochirurgie. Köln, 25.-28.04.2004. Düsseldorf, Köln: German Medical Science DocMO.01.05
11. Martin CH, Schwartz R, Jolesz F, Black PM (1999) Transsphenoidal resection of pituitary adenomas in an intraoperative MRI unit. Pituitary 2:155–162
12. Lacroix M, Abi-Said D, Fourney DR, Gokaslan ZL, Shi W, DeMonte F, Lang FF, McCutcheon IE, Hassenbusch SJ, Holland E, Hess K, Michael C, Miller D, Sawaya R (2001) A multivariate analysis of 416 patients with glioblastoma multiforme: prognosis, extent of resection, and survival. J Neurosurg 95:190–198
13. Lagerwaard FJ, Levendag PC, Nowak PJ, Eijkenboom WM, Hanssens PE, Schmitz PI (1999) Identification of prognostic factors in patients with brain metastases: a review of 1292 patients. Int J Radiat Oncol Biol Phys 43:795–803
14. Moriarty TM, Quinones-Hinojosa A, Larson PS, Alexander ER, Gleason PL, Schwartz RB, Jolesz FA, Black PM (2000) Frameless stereotactic neurosurgery using intraoperative magnetic resonance imaging: stereotactic brain biopsy. Neurosurgery 47:1138–1145, discussion 1145–1146
15. Pollack IF, Claassen D, al-Shboul Q, Janosky JE, Deutsch M (1995) Low-grade gliomas of the cerebral hemispheres in children: an analysis of 71 cases. J Neurosurg 82:536–547
16. Schwartz RB, Hsu L, Black PM, Alexander ER, Wong TZ, Klufas RA, Moriarty T, Martin C, Isbister HG, Cahill CD, Spaulding SA, Kanan AR, Jolesz FA (1998) Evaluation of intracranial cysts by intraoperative MR. J Magn Reson Imaging 8:807–813
17. Schwartz RB, Hsu L, Wong TZ, Kacher DF, Zamani AA, Black PM, Alexander ER, Stieg PE, Moriarty TM, Martin CA, Kikinis R, Jolesz FA (1999) Intraoperative MR imaging guidance for intracranial neurosurgery: experience with the first 200 cases. Radiology 211:477–488
18. Hynynen K, Vykhodtseva NI, Chung AH, Sorrentino V, Colucci V, Jolesz FA (1997) Thermal effects of focused ultrasound on the brain: determination with MR imaging. Radiology 204: 247–253

Development of Intraoperative MRI: A Personal Journey

Rudolf Fahlbusch

Abstract The initial attempts at intraoperative image guidance and imaging dates back to early 1980s. Since then Neuronavigation and intraoperative imaging technologies were developed in parallel. This works aims at summarizing the developments and giving an insider's view into the beginning stage of these technologies. The successes and obstacles encountered in the first few decades are relayed from the angle of one of the initial developers.

Keywords Intraoperative MR · MRI · Navigation

Dreams in my neurosurgical life were focussed on continous improvement of surgical results and I was convinced that this could be achived by early or real time testing. In the seventies I introduced endocrinological methods to predict early outcome of pituitary surgery. In the eighties neurophysiological monitoring for brainstem- and cerebellopontine angle (CPA) tumors improved functional surgical results. In the nineties computer – and engineering sciences were incorporated in surgical planning and surgical manoeuvres, in order to obtain a safer and more accurate brain tumor surgery. From the very beginning neuronavigation and intraoperative MRI were – from my point of view – two parallel developments, supporting each other. This shall be illustrated by my personal experience. Certainly this is not a systematic complete presentation of all efforts in this field.

There are moments for decisions in our professional lives, which can be regarded as destiny, maybe a favourable opportunity, prepared already in our inner development. Such an event happened to me in January 1992, when Peter Heilbrunn, at that time Chairman of the Department of Neurosurgery University of Utah in Salt Lake City, and main organiser of the Lende Winter Meeting, invited me to his winter house in Snowbird. When he asked Robert Spetzler and myself for a visit of his bedroom we could not understand immediately, which machine Peter was going to introduce to us there. Some days later, in his computer-laboratory, which came out to be the first one in neurosurgery up to my knowledge, he presented to me the first prototype of a pointer related neuro-navigation system. When I asked him to provide me with the first commercial navigation system in Europe, this happened to us in Erlangen in 1993. Peter Heilbrunn's pilot-system ("machine vision") was later commercialized as the Stealth System by Surgical Navigation company, directed by Kurd Smith, who helped intensively and frequently to integrate the system in our OR. It was *Richard Buchholz* from St. Louis, who completed the device, introducing also special LEDS (This navigation system was distributed later by Sofamor-Danek and latest by Medtronics). It was at a much earlier opportunity in the middle of the seventies when I would have had the chance to realize the significance of an early mechanical navigation system, I overlooked it a long while, after its principles were presented to us by Eiju *Watanabe, when he* was a research fellow in Erlangen, coming from Tokyo University. Retrospectively I was not completely convinced about the practical use of this-at that time – not so accurate system. Nevertheless we used it for a while in traumatology cases. Watanabe's cooperation with his teacher Kintomo *Takakura* was published in 1987 [1]. Today he is regarded as the "father" of the modern neuro-navigator.

Other pioneers in this field of intraoperative imaging were Patrick Kelly with "volumetric stereotaxy" in 1979 [2], Schlöndorff, a German ENT-professor with "computer assisted surgery" in 1986 [3] and Alim-Louis Benabid, who constructed a stereotactic robot for performing biopsies and positioning of deep seated electrodes in 1987 [4]. Together with Christian Saint Rose he had also developed a neuronavigation system (see below). With the beginning of the nineties the former neurosurgeon and later radiologist Frank Jolesz founded together with the radiologist and computer scientist Ron Kikinis the first Surgical Planning Lab in Boston. In 1995 Kazuhiru Hongo introduced navigated micromanipulation onto the way of robotics. As early as

R. Fahlbusch
International Neuroscience Institute Hannover, Hannover, Germany
e-mail: fahlbusch@ini-hannover.de

DOI 10.1007/978-3-211-99651-5_2,

1991 Dade Lundsford introduced intraoperative CT (ioCT) in Pittsburgh, but gave it up due to minor resolution for imaging of brain tumors.

The following experiences shall illustrate how close developments in neuronavigation and intraoperative MRI were running parallel and, supported each other. In the beginning of the nineties a technical engineer from Zeiss company, Mr Marcovic, stayed with us in our operating room in Erlangen as a guest (observer) After some days he asked me, how far I would be interested to see the MR-images no longer in the traditional way on the screen at the wall, but within the eyepieces of the microscope. I was fully convinced by this principle, when Mr. Marcovic and Mr. Luber demonstrated me the first pilot microscope in the Zeiss laboratories later in Tuttlingen, which could offer projection of MR images into the eyepiece of the microscope for the use of navigation. Furthermore I could discover, that this Zeiss MKM was not only a tool for neuro-navigation, but offered also robotic potential. Its movement from the stand-by position to the point of view position in the operating field could be ordered by voice. In my eyes this was the birthday of microscope-guided navigation. So far we were working with pointer-guided systems for example with the Stealth navigation system. Some months later I visited the Siemens development laboratories in Erlangen and became aware of a newly developed open MRI. The 0.2 T machine offered not only an acceptable resolution for diagnosis, but could document manoeuvers in orthopaedic surgery, in a way of combined imaging and navigation, showing nearly on line movements of instruments.

It was during the Meeting of the "International Pituitary Neurosurgeons Society" in Bamberg, at the opportunity of a social evening event in a beer cellar, when I asked my colleagues, if they have heard also that someone in United States is going to introduce MRI in the operating room. I was so much surprised that my table neighbour Peter Black said, "Yes, it is me".

It was only a question of time when I went to see the first equipment for ioMRI, the 0.5 T Signa SP (Double donut), in Boston. This was a development of GE in cooperation and on demand of Frank Jolesz and Peter Black, probably as a result of their experiences they had gained in their Surgical Navigation Planning Lab: the problem of brain shift. After an intensive preparation time of more then 2 years-including safety aspects for patients and medical staff being in or close to a magnetic field for a longer time- the first operation a brain biopsy was performed in June 1995-the first trepanation was performed in January 1996.Peter Black had invited me to demonstrate a biopsy for a brain tumor in fall 1995, I could observe ENT doctors using a copper-endoscope for surgery of the paranasal sinuses. It was obvious that this continuously running magnetic field tolerated within its field strength only MR compatible equipment, starting with surgical instruments ending with machines for anaesthesiology, positioned close by. A narrow working area for the neurosurgeon was the price for receiving online MRI data. The neurosurgeons could use this permanent image information during their resection of a brain tumor, which allowed them to follow and compensate the brain shift for navigation for the first time. I was fascinated too by the Surgiscope, a highly sophisticated navigation system, developed originally by Alim-Louis Benabid and Christian Saint Rose, pioneers in neuronavigation, Saint Rose had demonstrated convincingly its accuracy to me during a resection of a pediatric glioma in Paris. Later it came out that Electa company, the distributer of the Surgiscope, and the distributor of the first open low field MRI (Magnetom) Siemens had no common "Schnittstelle" – this was for me the end of a potential realisation.

Our wish to realise an intraperative MRI system together with navigation in Erlangen was favoured by the fact, that the former director of Siemens Medical Solution, Dr. Grassman became Director of Zeiss, Tuttlingen and that he was followed by Prof Reinhardt, with whom we cooperated before with some projects of MRI visualisation of pituitary tumors and surrounding arteries (MR angiography.)

One year after our common decision, induced by Mr Schöck, the chancellor of Erlangen University, our new OR suite with the 0.2 T open MRI and the Zeiss MKM (Figs. 1 and 2), could be realised together with the neurosurgeon Ralf *Steinmeier*. We were able to perform our first operation in March 1996-accompanied by a lot of worries. Would everything run really well during the transport of our patient with an open trepanation after a brain tumor resection from his position on the operating table, into the gantry of the MR scanner, then docking this table to the MR machine, which took this over as examination table-and the same procedure backwards? What about sterility during this prolonged surgery? How would the images look like, would the resolution of images be sufficient, how intensive would artefacts influence the results? For pituitary surgery

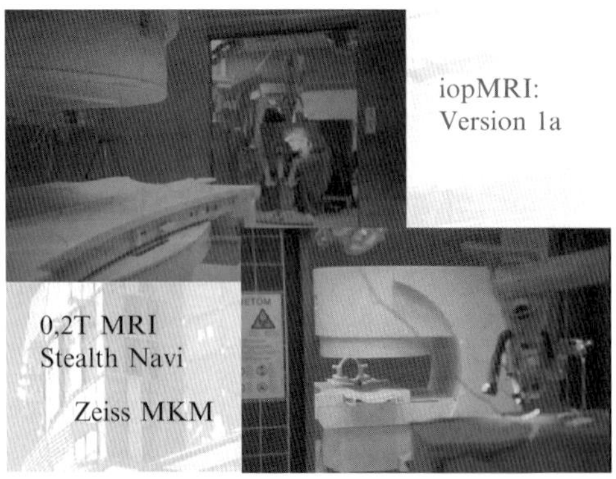

Fig. 1 The original, initial ioMRI (open Magnetom (version 1a) in Erlangen. *Above*: view from the room with the Magnetom Open into the OR room. *Below*: view from the OR with Zeiss MKM and Stealth station to the MRI room

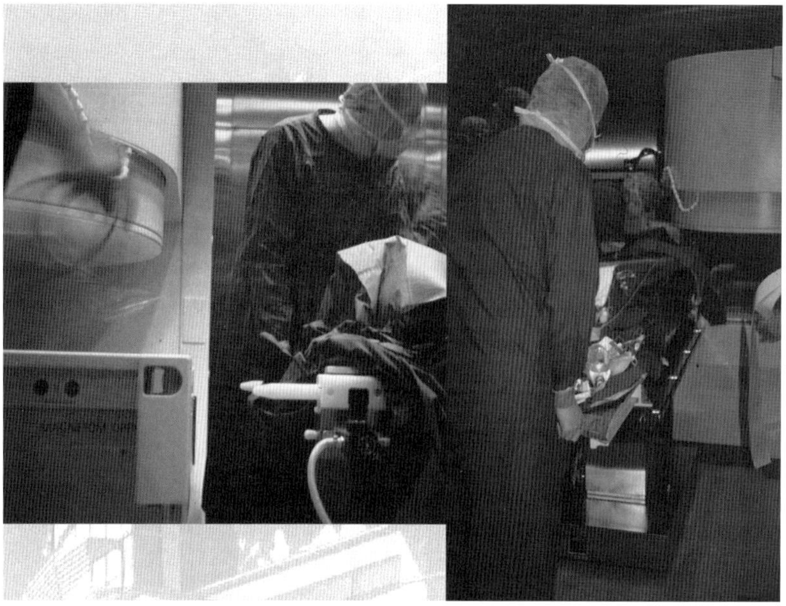

Fig. 2 Docking manoeuvre of the OR table with the MR scanner (version 1a)

we learned to avoid drilling artefacts by using porcelain coated drills instead of stainless steel drills and to insert a small wax plate at the sellar floor after tumor resection to separate the intrasellar space from the sphenoid sinus, with its bleeding artefacts during data acquisition.

From the very beginning of developing intraoperative MRI there existed different options and concepts for its realisation, which could not be tested in an experimental way before:

A continuous magnetic field for on line imaging with surgery within the magnetic field.

A magnet separate from the operating field, where the advantages of microscope navigation could be used. Another concept decision was related to the field strength: low field vs high field: This concept as well as the concept of the relation of the patient's to the magnet position is till today in discussion: Shall the patient be transported into the gantry of the magnet or the magnet to the patient. We used pointer related navigation and microscope guided navigation as well. At the beginning it was necessary to have two different rooms, one room for the surgical procedure, including navigation and the other room for MR control. Both were connected to each other, but could be separated by a shielded door. This had the advantage that the MR room could be used during surgery also for examinations of other patients (a concept in ioMRI systems, which is still used today for commercial reasons.) At that time we could not perform surgery and MRI examinations in one common room. Tests have demonstrated that there was no compatibility of equipment. 1995 and 1996 in parallel the Heidelberg group of neurosurgeons (Stefan Kunze, Christian Wirtz, Volker Tronnier) had developed "our" concept too, they introduced compatible coils as well as a special operating table. Where their operating room was large and the MRI room small it was the other way around in our concept. This was an unforeseen advantage, since we could work later on with the newly introduced Zeiss NC4 closer to the MR gantry, within the room with the Magnet, some tests have demonstrated before compatibility of the equipment (Fig. 3, version 1b). From now on we could operate on the diagnostic MRI table which was connected with a special compatible head holding device, the time for major transportation seemed to be passed away. We also found out that we could work without any compatibility problems outside and at the so called 5 Gauss line (Fig. 4).

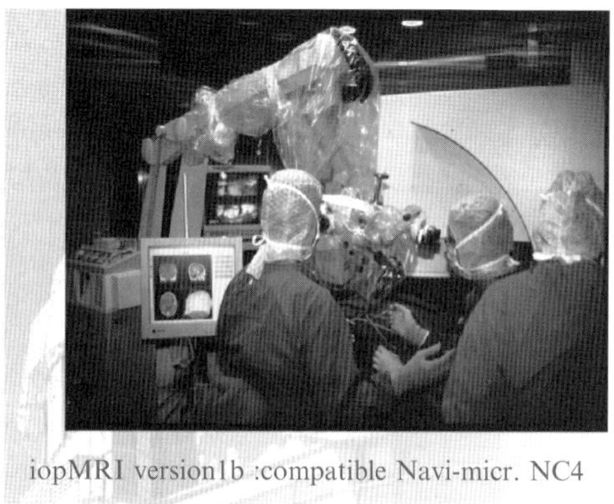

Fig. 3 ioMRI (version 1b) integration of the compatible navigation microscope Zeiss NC4 close to the modified diagnostic and therapeutic operation table

Chronologically the introduction of a high field strength MRI, the 1.5 T(Philips) was just following the developments of low field MRI systems in Boston, Erlangen and Heidelberg

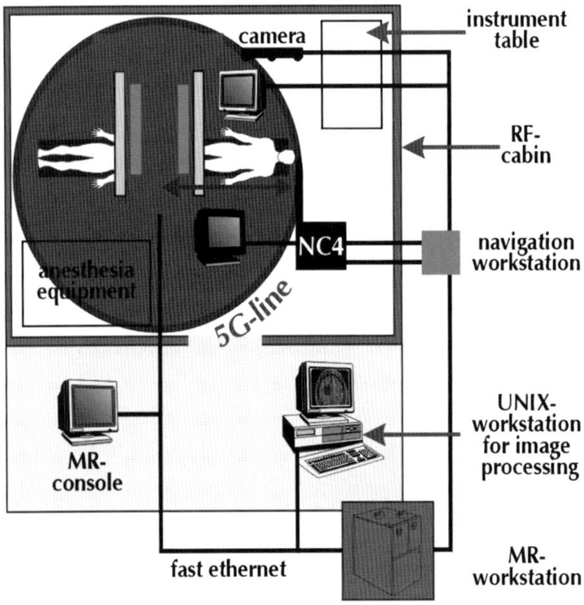

Fig. 4 Head position and surgery at the s.c 5 Gauss line, the safety border for safe surgery (version 1b)

of in 1997. The radiologist Charles Truwitt, together with the neurosurgeon Walter Hall gained their first experiences with biopsies ,later with trepanations at the University of Minneapolis. However they were unable to introduce navigation at the beginning. Initially biopsies were taken close to the gantry of the MRI on the specially equipped diagnostic table, later on the trepanations had to be performed depart from the gantry and the table had to be transported some meters from a more distant place for surgery. In contrast to this concept of patient to the magnet Garnette Sutherland developed a system for magnet to the patient (1.5 T MRI, IMRIS) in Calgary, Canada in 1996.

In contrast to these efforts of early installation of high field magnets the development of low field system continued, stimulated by the attraction of lower costs and earlier availability. On one hand John Koivokangas installed an open 0.36 T MRI (Philips) in Oulu, Finland in 1996/1997, following the concept patient to the magnet. A similar device was introduced by Ronald E. Warnick and John Tew with the 0.3 T MRI, produced by Hitachi company and was later used by Kintomo Takakura and Tomokatsu Hori in Tokio. The first an ultra low field MRI system in a magnet to patient system was developed in Israel and introduced to patients by Moshe Hadani in Tel Aviv and by Peter Carmel and Michael Schulder in Newark: the Odin Pole Star N10 had a field strength of 0.12 T in 2000, the N15 version a field strength of 0.15 T.The transportable magnet is positioned below the operating ,when not needed and can be swinged upwards to the head, when intraoperative maneuvers shall be controlled. Till today the discussion about the value of a "useable resolution" of the low field images, stands in discussion with the more convincing images, gained by high field systems.

The real breakthrough in the use of intraoperative MRI happened from our point of view, when we were able to combine functional navigation with high field 1.5 T MRI in Erlangen (Fig. 5 and 6). After intensive planning and developments together with Christopher Nimsky and the industrial companies we could integrate the Siemens 1.5.T MRI Sonata and the BrainLab Vecor Vision sky system navigation (Vilsmaier, Ehrke, Kraft) in our new concept. This included also an integrated head coil for automatic registration intraoperatively. Functional MRI, using tools of MEG (Kober, Grummich) and the Bold effect of MRI (together with Oliver Ganslandt) allowed accurate localisation of eloquent areas such as sensor, motor, speech area (Broca and Wernicke). Functional and morphological data could be segmented, used for intraoperative navigation and could be upgraded after intraoperative MRI control. With the version of a rotating table the patient's transport was solved, we could work at the 5 Gauss line with normal instrumentation. Even epilepsy surgery with EEG and ECG detections was successfully performed (Michael Buchfelder, Johann Romstöck). An experimental test documented that even the use of a robotic system close to the operating able was also tolerated. The advantages of high field strength for quicker acquisition time and improved anatomical, imaging became obvious: the intraoperative resolution quality was the same, even superior, to the preop one, we came to the statement that there is a necessity to incorporate functional imaging and visualisation into Ors, since about 30–40% of resectable brain tumors (pituitary adenomas and gliomas for example), are overlooked or not visible initially and can be resected safely, which can be documented immediately. The other high field strength advantages are functional imaging which allowed us also to complement cortical mapping with DTI-tractography (*Christopher Nimsky*) and to introduce Proton spectroscopy with *Ganslandt* and the physicists Moser and Stadlbauer from Vienna a potential for higher cytoreduction. Meanwhile it became obvious that there was no need for more then one, maximal three intraoperative MRI controls, which made the permanent online detecting of date unnecessary. The first ioMRI system, the double doughnut, was no longer promoted by its industrial company. With the availability of 3 T MRI for diagnostic purpose, with advantages for functional and metabolic imaging, there introduction in the OR was only a question of time. In 2005 and 2006 Necmettin Pamir (Siemens), Christian Raftopoulos (Philips) and Robert Spetzler (GE) started to installed these systems for therapeutic use.

In 2007 we opened the INI-BRAIN SUITE at the International Neuroscience Institute: the first Open (70 cm bore!) intraoperative high field MRI for therapeutic use (Fig. 7). For the first time I was convinced to plan "2 operating theatres in one room" simultaneously. The actual one for stable daily use on high quality level, the later one a 3 T, in case that the actual problems of 3 T MR will be solved: surface distortion, workflow with table transportation. Integration of ceiling mounted microscope Zeiss Pentero. Retrospectively the time from planning and decision for an MRI lasted 1 year for the 0.2 T version, nearly 3.5 year for the 1.5 T version in Erlangen and less then 2 year for the 1.5 version in Hannover. The walls of the OR are isolated in a way required for 3 T systems. The exchange from a 1.5 T to a new 3 T (Siemens Verio) would prolong the 5 Gauss line only approximately 20 cm (4.5–4.2 m distance) from the Gantry.

It happened in October 2004 in Dresden, at the opportunity of a joint meeting of the German Society and German Academy with the American Academy of Neurosurgeons that the necessity of ioMRI was accepted obviously in the international neurosurgical community. This was the definite result of a contemporary formal discussion between Spetzler and Fahlbusch in the topic *Controversies in Neurosurgery: Intraoperative MRI: Gimmick or Godsend.* Meanwhile about 150 ioMRI systems are installed world wide, dominated by low field systems. All systems have different advantages and disadvantages for:

1-image/quality benefit, 2-acquisition time, 3-imaging modalities workflow, and 4-costs

The scientific development of intraoperative imaging were accompanied by a number of meetings on local and international level. Since 1996/1997-on the US level – Peter Black ad GE initiated symposia and workshops – with GE users as well as guests using other equipments – in Boston and at the opportunity of Congresses of AANS, CNS and WFNS. In Europe symposia were organised organised by René L. Bernays (the later first president of the Intraoperative Imaging Society in Foundation) in Zürich, Switzerland and by Johannes Schramm (the later EANS president) in Seeheim Jugenheim, Germany as an EANS Symposium. In Germany the first symposium for navigation and intraoperative MRI was organised by Joachim Gilsbach, Aachen, fol-

a

b

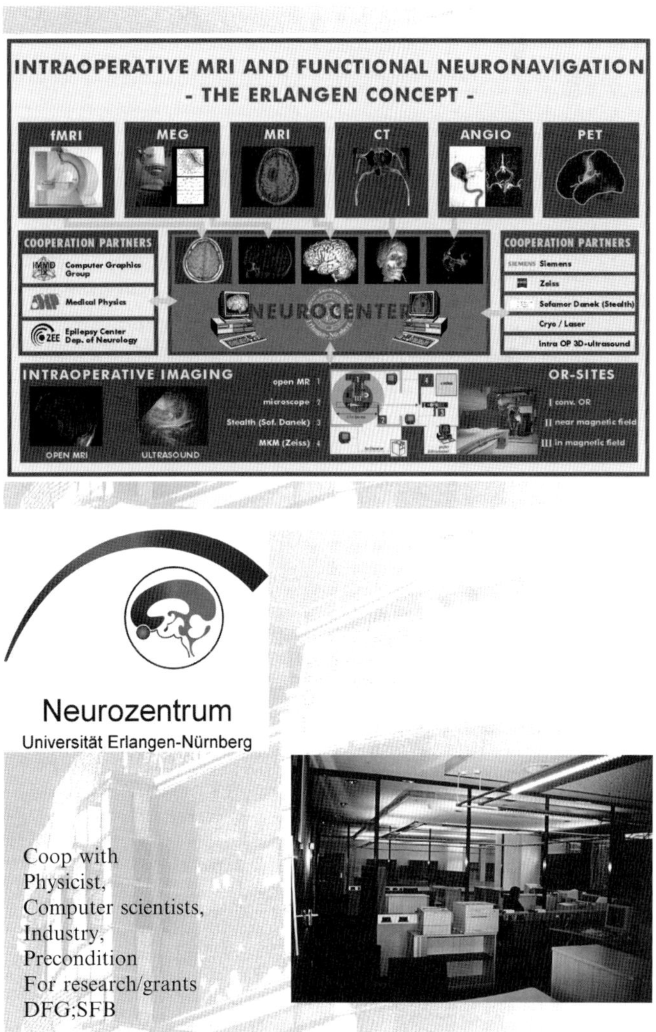

Fig. 5 (**a**) Concept of the interdisciplinary Neurocenter (1996) Intraoperative MRI and functional Neuronavigation – the Erlangen Concept – to centralise neurodata for fusion, post processing and finally surgery. (**b**) View into the interdisciplinary Neurocenter, opened 7/2000

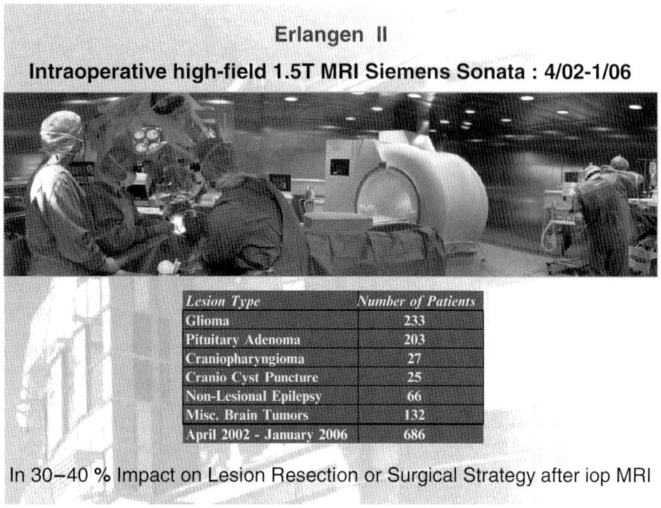

Lesion Type	Number of Patients
Glioma	233
Pituitary Adenoma	203
Craniopharyngioma	27
Cranio Cyst Puncture	25
Non-Lesional Epilepsy	66
Misc. Brain Tumors	132
April 2002 - January 2006	686

Fig. 6 IoMRI version 2: 1.5 T MRI Siemens Sonata with a rotating table and the Zeiss NC4 (later Pentero) BrainLab Vector Sky Navigation system in one room. First operation in February 2002

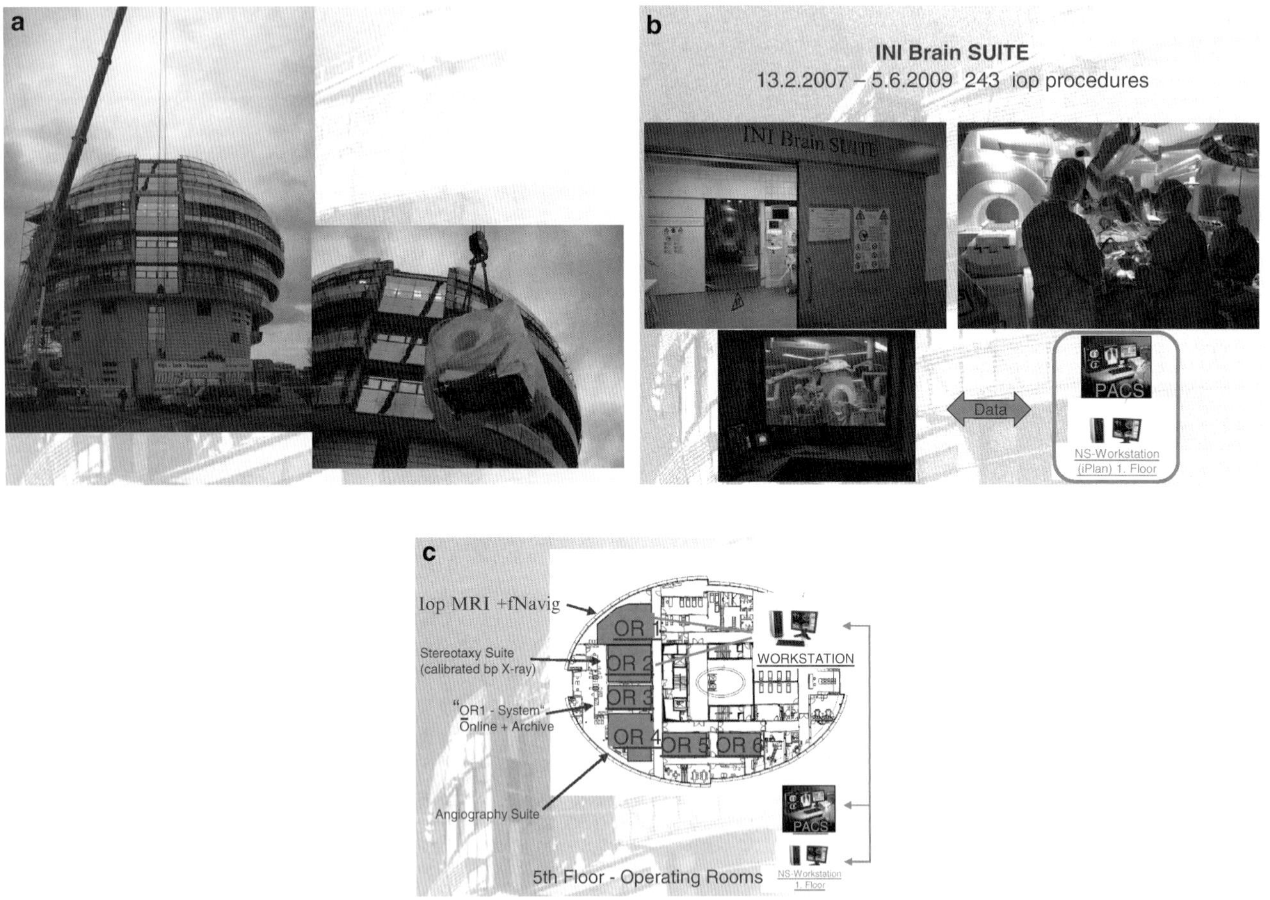

Fig. 7 (**a**) INI BrainSuite (version 3) Installation procedure of the MRI scanner at the INI Hannover. (**b**) View into INI BrainSuite. First operation 13.2.2007 Open 1.5 T MRI Siemens Espree with 70 cm Gantry with BrainLab Navigation and Zeiss NC4, later with a ceiling mounted Pentero. (**c**) Localisation of the BrainSuite within the OR tract on fifth floor. Structural engineering for construction stability was planned already with the construction of the INI building, finished in 7/2000

lowed by Rudolf Fahlbusch and Christopher Nimsky in Erlangen, Maximillian Mehdorn and Arya Nabavi in Kiel. At this time it became obvious that neurosurgeons had to cooperate and incorporate with engineering and computer scientists. In 1996 we planned the "Neurocenter" in the Head. Clinic Erlangen, which we could open in July 2000, were experts and users of all clinical neurodisciplines and computer scientists gathered neurodata for post-processing procedures, which could be used for patients' operation.(Led by the physicists Kober and Grummich, the computer scientist Hastreiter). Without this symbiotic input, research funding would not have been successful (Fig. 5a, b).

A round table with participants from clinical users such as neurosurgeons and radiologists, from industrial companies, university administration and ministeries of the government was established to work out concepts for MEDICAL PROCESS OPTIMIZING, this included also economic aspects. Generally open problems in image guided surgery are the reduction and concentration of image data, application accuracy, visualization from 2D to 3D improved, as well as model based safety corridors for surgical maneuvers. Further perspectives for intraoperative MRI scanning are the following: less cost intensive systems should be provided, and improvement of ergonomic integration into the OR environment and workflow – a vision would be a nearly invisible and nearly online flat or tabletop magnet-integration of therapeutic devices (e.g. smart intelligent instruments, thermoablation, focused ultrasound).

Within the next 10 years we can expect the following developments in MR technology: "a widespread shift to higher field systems (3 T), further improvement of coil technology, including further increase of channels, introduction of molecular MRI agents and combined modality methods" [5].

Meanwhile hybrid systems for io-imaging are installed, respectively in development: Mitsumori Matsumae, Tokai university, Japan, connected the OR to a CT and MR suite as well [6]. In Boston the planned AMIGO suite will connect the OR with 3 T MRi and a PET-CT. Meanwhile a commercial PET-MR is available (Werner Siemens Foundation, Radiology Tübingen, Germany) and will open further aspects of application.

The escalating resources in intraoperative imaging include also other imaging developments, the already established ultrasound technology and the newly developing optical imaging, such as optical coherence tomography and multiphoton excitation microscopy-working on a cellular level, which for itself or in combination with ioMRI underline the scientific efforts, which will allow the increasing establishment of this kind of adaptive tumor resection as a standard procedure.

The First Society for Computer and Robotic Assisted *Surgery* was founded in Leipzig, Germany in 2001. It was expected that this scientific community would support further development. Later on members of industrial companies organised user meetings. BrainLab 1007 in Houston and 2008 in Singapore, whereas Medtronic organised a previous meeting for the foundation of the International Imaging Society in Lake Tahoe in 2008, under the guidance of Moshe Hadani, Rene Bernays and Michael Schulder. In June 11–14 2009 the *Intraoperative Imaging Society* was definitely founded in Istanbul, where Necmettin Pamir, one of the initial pioneers of intraoperative 3 T-MRI, hosted the first official conference of this society.

Conflict of interest statement We declare that we have no conflict of interest.

Acknowledgement I especially would like to thank Christopher Nimsky for his fundamental work in this field, he as well as other quoted authors are contributors of this book.

References

1. Watanabe E, Watanabe T, Manaka S, Mayanagi Y, Takakura K (1987) Three-dimensional digitizer (neuronavigator): new equipment for computed tomography-guided stereotaxic surgery. Surg Neurol 27:543–547
2. Kelly PJ, Kall BA, Goerss S (1984) Transposition of volumetric information derived from computed tomography scanning into stereotactic space. Surg Neurol 21:465–471
3. Schlondorff G, Mosges R, Meyer-Ebrecht D, Krybus W, Adams L (1989) CAS (computer assisted surgery). A new procedure in head and neck surgery. HNO 37:187–190
4. Benabid AL, Cinquin P, Lavalle S, Le Bas JF, Demongeot J, de Rougemont J (1987) Computer-driven robot for stereotactic surgery connected to CT scan and magnetic resonance imaging. Technological design and preliminary results. Appl Neurophysiol 50:153–154
5. Blamire AM (2008) The technology of MRI – the next 10 years? Br J Radiol 81:601–617
6. Matsumae M, Koizumi J, Fukuyama H, Ishizaka H, Mizokami Y, Baba T, Atsumi H, Tsugu A, Oda S, Tanaka Y, Osada T, Imai M, Ishiguro T, Yamamoto M, Tominaga J, Shimoda M, Imai Y (2007) World's first magnetic resonance imaging/X-ray/operating room suite: a significant milestone in the improvement of neurosurgical diagnosis and treatment. J Neurosurg 107:266–273

Selected Readings

7. Black PM, Moriarty T, Alexander E 3rd, Stieg P, Woodard EJ, Gleason PL, Martin CH, Kikinis R, Schwartz RB, Jolesz FA (1997) Development and implementation of intraoperative magnetic resonance imaging and its neurosurgical application. Neurosurgery 41:831–842

8. Blamire AM (2008) The technology of MRI: the next 10 years. Br J Radiol 89:601–617
9. Buchholz R, MacNeil W, McDumont L (2004) The operating room of the future. Clin Neurosurg 51:228–237
10. Fahlbusch R, Samii A (2007) A review of cranial imaging techniques: potential and limitations. Clin Neurosurg 54:100–104
11. Steinmeier R, Fahlbusch R, Ganslandt O, Nimsky C, Buchfelder M, Kaus M, Heigl T, Lenz G, Kuth R, Huk W (1998) Intraoperative magnetic resonance imaging with the magnetom open scanner concepts, neurosurgical indications, and procedures: a preliminary report. Neurosurgery 43:739–747
12. Watanabe E, Watanabe T, Manaka S, Mayanagi Y, Takakura K (1987) Three dimensional Digitizer (Neuronavigator): new equipment for computed tomography-guided stereotactic surgery. Surg Neurol 27:543–547

Lows and Highs: 15 Years of Development in Intraoperative Magnetic Resonance Imaging

T. Schmidt, R. König, M. Hlavac, G. Antoniadis, and C.R. Wirtz

Abstract Intraoperative magnetic resonance imaging (ioMRI) during neurosurgical procedures was first implemented in 1995. In the following decade ioMRI and image guided surgery has evolved from an experimental stage into a safe and routinely clinically applied technique. The development of ioMRI has led to a variety of differently designed systems which can be basically classified in one- or two-room concepts and low- and high-field installations. Nowadays ioMRI allows neurosurgeons not only to increase the extent of tumor resection and to preserve eloquent areas or white matter tracts but it also provides physiological and biological data of the brain and tumor tissue. This article tries to give a comprehensive review of the milestones in the development of ioMRI and neuronavigation over the last 15 years and describes the personal experience in intraoperative low and high-field MRI.

Keywords Image-guided neurosurgery · Intraoperative magnetic resonance imaging · Low field–high field MRI · Neuronavigation

Introduction

The concept of image guided surgery has resulted in a strategic shift in MRI from diagnosis to treatment. Since the fundamental neurosurgical studies at several institutions [1–4] in the 1990s, intra-operative magnetic resonance imaging (ioMRI) and neuronavigation now enables neurosurgeons to increase radicality of tumor resection while preserving functionality. Numerous past and contemporary studies could demonstrate a statistically significant prolongation of survival time and improved postoperative performance after gross total resection [5–9]. Additionally in early postoperative MRI residual tumor could be detected particularly in supratentorial glioma in up to 70% of operations [5]. These results reveal an enormous discrepancy between the surgeons perception of resection extent and objective radicality. In this respect the implementation of neuronavigation has been associated with high expectations in regard to the increase of radicality. These expectations have been disappointing at least in part, presumably due to the intraoperative brain shift [10]. Consistently this data and the high sensitivity of MRI in detecting brain tumors generated a necessity that led to the integration of ioMRI. The ioMRI suite development has followed two general concepts. The first concept developed by the Black group is based on continuously refreshed images [1, 11] and was used to perform magnetic resonance imaging (MRI) during surgery using a dedicated MRI suite in which surgery took place within the magnet at a midfield strength of 0.5 T. It allowed the surgeon access to the patient during the imaging procedure through the 56-cm-wide gap of the open-bore and provided the surgeon with nearly real-time neuronavigation. The second alternative concept was to separate the place of surgery and imaging into a one- or two-room suite design. ioMRI was performed discontinuously during the surgical procedure by either transferring the patient to the MRI scanner or move the MRI to the patient [4, 12–17]. Although surgery has to be interrupted for imaging this suite design allows the neurosurgeon to use conventional surgical tools and therefore reduces the fringe field related restrictions. In the following decade the tremendous improvements in MRI technique directly found their way into the neurosurgical operation room. At present the ioMRI systems can be divided into low- or ultra-low-field installations [18–20] and high-field installations at 1.5 T or 3 T [12, 13, 15, 17, 21]. At least advanced imaging modalities such as diffusion tensor imaging and tractography could be successfully integrated to the microscope-based neuronavigation both for preoperative and intraoperative surgical planning [22–24]. However, cost constrains and

T. Schmidt (✉), R. König, M. Hlavac, G. Antoniadis, and C. Wirtz
Department of Neurosurgery, District Hospital Günzburg, University of Ulm, Ludwig Heilmeyer Straße 2, 89312 Günzburg, Germany
e-mail: thomas.e.schmidt@uni-ulm.de

the lack of studies that prove the superiority of high-field-systems in terms of progression-free-survival and longterm-survival have to be considered. Against the background of 15 year of intraoperative magnetic resonance imaging and neuronavigation this articles reviews the personal clinical and scientific experience at low-field and high-field ioMRI.

The Low-Field Experience at 0.2 T

In 1995 a low-field C-shaped resistive magnet (Magnetom Open, Siemens AG, Medical Solutions, Erlangen, Germany) with a lateral patient access of 240° was installed and modified for intraoperative use. In the "Heidelberg concept" the magnetic shielded cabin was installed adjacent to the neurosurgical operating room and connected by a RF-shielded sliding door. This setting allowed continued use of standard instruments for microsurgical procedures. The detailed description of the installation, the dedicated transport and positioning system, and the integrated modified headholder have been published previously [4, 25]. In 1996 we demonstrated that neuronavigation can be updated using ioMRI and that intraoperative re-registration was feasible with excellent accuracy [26, 27]. Until 2008 688 patients were examined intraoperatively, 541 for microsurgical operations, mainly for high-grade and low-grade gliomas, and 147 for interventional procedure like biopsies, cyst-aspirations or abscess-drainages. Image quality at low-field 0.2T ioMRI was good or acceptable in about 87.5% of the cases. However in 11.5% only bad image quality was achieved or imaging was not possible at all due to technical malfunction. In the systematic analysis of the intraoperative images we identified four types of surgically induced contrast enhancement representing a potential risk of misinterpretation of ioMRI [28]. Surgically diminished contrast enhancement in high-grade residual tumor that showed a strong contrast enhancement in the preoperative dataset could also be observed in some cases. For that reason consideration of the location, configuration and time course of contrast enhancement in ioMRI is mandatory to avoid confusion regarding the further surgical strategy. In a subgroup of 182 patients who underwent 192 microsurgical operations in 63.4% the surgical resection was continued due to the detection of residual tumor which could be significantly reduced subsequently [29]. The analysis of the survival data showed a significant increase in progression-free and overall survival. This could also be demonstrated for low-grade glioma in a recent retrospective study [30].

The High-Field Experience at 1.5 T

In September 2008 we began performing intraoperative high-field 1.5 T MR imaging at our institution. Until July 2009 a total of 75 patients underwent ioMRI in 76 microsurgical procedures. The mean age was 50 ± 17 years (range, 5–78 years). 41 patients were male (mean age 49 ± 16.7; range 5–78 years) and 34 female (mean age 51 ± 17.1; range 10–77 years).

The digitally integrated neurosurgical suite (BrainSUITE®, BrainLAB AG, Feldkirchen, Germany) combining ioMRI, neuronavigation and a comprehensive OR data management at our institution was workflow-optimized on a

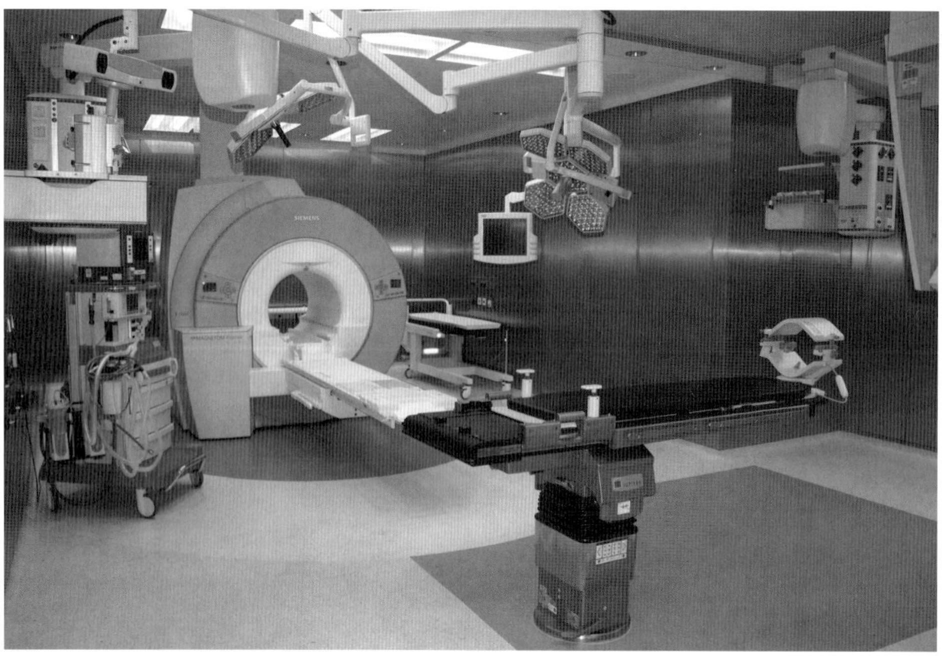

Fig. 1 BrainSUITE® ioMRI Miyabi with MRI Magnetom Espree 1.5T in the background. MR-compatible anesthesia equipment is on the left. The coloured floor coverings represent the laminar air flow field and fringe field distribution at 5mT and 50 mT. Photograph demonstrate the Miyabi bridgeboard transfer system in surgical position. In this position the patients body is completely outside the 5mT line and enables a 360° access to the patient. The 8-channel phased array head coil is adapted to the transfer shell

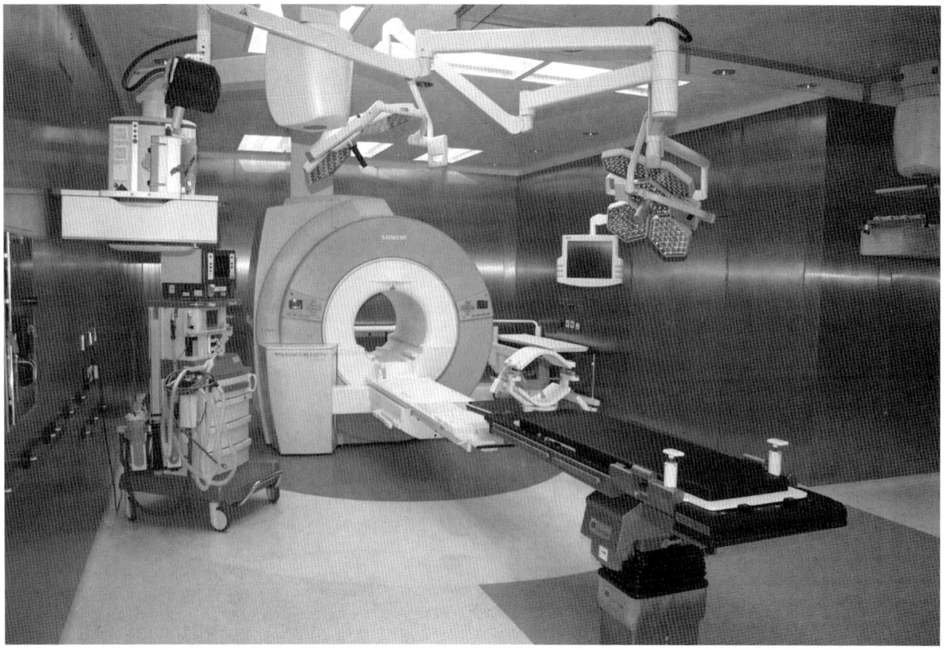

Fig. 2 Transfer position: Following a 90°-rotation from the surgery axis to the imaging axis the Miyabi table is ready for connection to the MR-tabletop. The integrated bridgeboard has been released and arrested previously. Now the shell and the patient can easily be moved to the MR-Scanner. The entire transfer procedure takes about 3 minutes

one room concept with an surface area of 64 m^2. This setup is functionally compartmentalized along two perpendicular axes in areas which are dedicated to the field of surgery, anesthesia and imaging. These axes are defined by the position of OR table related to the MR scanner (Figs. 1, 2). In surgical position the patients body is completely outside the 5 mT line and provides a 360° access to the patient. The ceiling flange of the ceiling-mounted microscope (OPMI Pentero C, Carl Zeiss Meditec AG, Jena, Germany) has been adjusted to attain a maximum coverage of the patient by the working range of the microscope. Neuronavigational components are the ceiling-mounted Vector Vision sky and the treatment planning software iPlan-Net (BrainLAB AG, Feldkirchen, Germany). The MR scanner (Magnetom Espree 1.5 T; Siemens AG, Medical Solutions, Erlangen, Germany) is characterized by its compact length of 125 cm and an body coil diameter of 70 cm. The gradient system has a maximum field strength of 33 mT/m and a maximum slew rate of 100 T/ms. The fringe field distribution is symbolized by coloured conductive floor coverings at the 5 mT (250 × 172 cm) and 50 mT lines (160 × 131 cm). Through the room control system all electrical devices can be centrally controlled. To bridge the distance between the MR isocenter and the table column of about 480 cm we chose the Miyabi bridgeboard transfer system (Trumpf Medical Systems, Saalfeld, Germany) with a weight limit of 160 kg which was worldwide unique to that time. The patient is positioned on the MR-compatible Miyabi-shell, which is locked by clamps to the tabletop during surgery, the head is fixed in the five-point holder of the 8-channel phased array coil (Noras MRI products GmbH, Hoechberg, Germany). To transfer the patient the integrated and retracted bridgeboard (length 60 cm) has to be released and connected to the MRI-tabletop. Then the shell can easily be moved to the imaging position. The entire procedure takes about 3 min in average in both directions and we encountered no transfer related complication. Intraoperative imaging protocol was determined by the underlying pathology (mean time 21 min). In glioma the standard protocol consists of isotropic 3D-MPRAGE, T2-TSE, T2-FLAIR and diffusion-weighted imaging, if indicated all available advanced imaging modalities and contrast administration can be added. Image quality was good or excellent in all cases. Microsurgical operation for 36 high-grade and 7 low-grade gliomas, 9 pituitary adenomas, 4 aneurysms, 2 medulloblastomas and 14 other were successfully completed. 4 patients were surgically treated for lesional or non-lesional epilepsy. The preliminary result of our ongoing workflow-analysis suggests a safe and efficient setup. The suite has been integrated into routine and runs on a daily basis.

Conclusions

High-field ioMRI at 1.5 T significantly reduces imaging time, increases anatomical resolution and provides imaging quality up to a standard that equals state of the art routine diagnostic imaging. Meanwhile ioMRI has entered a stage, where imaging objectives are far beyond the assessment of anatomy, pathology and extent of tumor resection. Recent development of advanced MR sequences enables quantitative and semi-quantitative measurement of cerebral blood volume and flow, water movement and the chemical composition of the tissue and therefore provides non-invasive insight in brain and tumour physiology and biology intraoperatively which definitely will open a new chapter of ioMRI.

Conflict of interest statement We declare that we have no conflict of interest.

References

1. Black PM, Moriarty T, Alexander E 3rd, Stieg P, Woodard EJ, Gleason PL, Martin CH, Kikinis R, Schwartz RB, Jolesz FA (1997) Development and implementation of intraoperative magnetic resonance imaging and its neurosurgical applications. Neurosurgery 41:831–842
2. Jolesz FA, Blumenfeld SM (1994) Interventional use of magnetic resonance imaging. Magn Reson Q 10:85–96
3. Schenck JF, Jolesz FA, Roemer PB, Cline HE, Lorensen WE, Kikinis R, Silverman SG, Hardy CJ, Barber WD, Laskaris ET et al (1995) Superconducting open-configuration MR imaging system for image-guided therapy. Radiology 195:805–814
4. Tronnier VM, Wirtz CR, Knauth M, Lenz G, Pastyr O, Bonsanto MM, Albert FK, Kuth R, Staubert A, Schlegel W, Sartor K, Kunze S (1997) Intraoperative diagnostic and interventional magnetic resonance imaging in neurosurgery. Neurosurgery 40:891–900
5. Albert FK, Forsting M, Sartor K, Adams HP, Kunze S (1994) Early postoperative magnetic resonance imaging after resection of malignant glioma: objective evaluation of residual tumor and its influence on regrowth and prognosis. Neurosurgery 34:45–60, discussion 60–41
6. Ammirati M, Vick N, Liao YL, Ciric I, Mikhael M (1987) Effect of the extent of surgical resection on survival and quality of life in patients with supratentorial glioblastomas and anaplastic astrocytomas. Neurosurgery 21:201–206
7. Ciric I, Ammirati M, Vick N, Mikhael M (1987) Supratentorial gliomas: surgical considerations and immediate postoperative results. Gross total resection versus partial resection. Neurosurgery 21:21–26
8. Stummer W, Pichlmeier U, Meinel T, Wiestler OD, Zanella F, Reulen HJ (2006) Fluorescence-guided surgery with 5-aminolevulinic acid for resection of malignant glioma: a randomised controlled multicentre phase III trial. Lancet Oncol 7:392–401
9. Stummer W, Reulen HJ, Meinel T, Pichlmeier U, Schumacher W, Tonn JC, Rohde V, Oppel F, Turowski B, Woiciechowsky C, Franz K, Pietsch T (2008) Extent of resection and survival in glioblastoma multiforme: identification of and adjustment for bias. Neurosurgery 62:564–576
10. Wirtz CR, Albert FK, Schwaderer M, Heuer C, Staubert A, Tronnier VM, Knauth M, Kunze S (2000) The benefit of neuronavigation for neurosurgery analyzed by its impact on glioblastoma surgery. Neurol Res 22:354–360
11. Kollias SS, Bernays R, Marugg RA, Romanowski B, Yonekawa Y, Valavanis A (1998) Target definition and trajectory optimization for interactive MR-guided biopsies of brain tumors in an open configuration MRI system. J Magn Reson Imaging 8:143–159
12. Hall WA, Galicich W, Bergman T, Truwit CL (2006) 3-Tesla intraoperative MR imaging for neurosurgery. J Neurooncol 77:297–303
13. Jankovski A, Francotte F, Vaz G, Fomekong E, Duprez T, Van Boven M, Docquier MA, Hermoye L, Cosnard G, Raftopoulos C (2008) Intraoperative magnetic resonance imaging at 3-T using a dual independent operating room-magnetic resonance imaging suite: development, feasibility, safety, and preliminary experience. Neurosurgery 63:412–424
14. Nimsky C, Ganslandt O, von Keller B, Fahlbusch R (2003) Preliminary experience in glioma surgery with intraoperative high-field MRI. Acta Neurochir Suppl 88:21–29
15. Pamir MN, Peker S, Ozek MM, Dincer A (2006) Intraoperative MR imaging: preliminary results with 3 tesla MR system. Acta Neurochir Suppl 98:97–100
16. Schulder M, Salas S, Brimacombe M, Fine P, Catrambone J, Maniker AH, Carmel PW (2006) Cranial surgery with an expanded compact intraoperative magnetic resonance imager. Technical note. J Neurosurg 104:611–617
17. Sutherland GR, Kaibara T, Louw D, Hoult DI, Tomanek B, Saunders J (1999) A mobile high-field magnetic resonance system for neurosurgery. J Neurosurg 91:804–813
18. Kanner AA, Vogelbaum MA, Mayberg MR, Weisenberger JP, Barnett GH (2002) Intracranial navigation by using low-field intraoperative magnetic resonance imaging: preliminary experience. J Neurosurg 97:1115–1124
19. Schulder M (2009) Intracranial surgery with a compact, low-field-strength magnetic resonance imager. Top Magn Reson Imaging 19:179–189
20. Senft C, Seifert V, Hermann E, Franz K, Gasser T (2008) Usefulness of intraoperative ultra low-field magnetic resonance imaging in glioma surgery. Neurosurgery 63:257–266
21. Nimsky C, Ganslandt O, Von Keller B, Romstock J, Fahlbusch R (2004) Intraoperative high-field-strength MR imaging: implementation and experience in 200 patients. Radiology 233:67–78
22. Nimsky C, Ganslandt O, Hastreiter P, Wang R, Benner T, Sorensen AG, Fahlbusch R (2005) Preoperative and intraoperative diffusion tensor imaging-based fiber tracking in glioma surgery. Neurosurgery 56:130–137
23. Nimsky C, Ganslandt O, Hastreiter P, Wang R, Benner T, Sorensen AG, Fahlbusch R (2007) Preoperative and intraoperative diffusion tensor imaging-based fiber tracking in glioma surgery. Neurosurgery 61:178–185
24. Nimsky C, Grummich P, Sorensen AG, Fahlbusch R, Ganslandt O (2005) Visualization of the pyramidal tract in glioma surgery by integrating diffusion tensor imaging in functional neuronavigation. Zentralbl Neurochir 66:133–141
25. Wirtz CR, Tronnier VM, Albert FK, Knauth M, Bonsanto MM, Staubert A, Pastyr O, Kunze S (1998) Modified headholder and operating table for intra-operative MRI in neurosurgery. Neurol Res 20:658–661
26. Wirtz CR, Bonsanto MM, Knauth M, Tronnier VM, Albert FK, Staubert A, Kunze S (1997) Intraoperative magnetic resonance imaging to update interactive navigation in neurosurgery: method and preliminary experience. Comput Aided Surg 2:172–179
27. Wirtz CR, Tronnier VM, Bonsanto MM, Knauth M, Staubert A, Albert FK, Kunze S (1997) Image-guided neurosurgery with intraoperative MRI: update of frameless stereotaxy and radicality control. Stereotact Funct Neurosurg 68:39–43
28. Knauth M, Aras N, Wirtz CR, Dorfler A, Engelhorn T, Sartor K (1999) Surgically induced intracranial contrast enhancement: potential source of diagnostic error in intraoperative MR imaging. AJNR Am J Neuroradiol 20:1547–1553
29. Wirtz CR, Knauth M, Stamov M, Bonsanto M, Metzner R, Kunze S, Tronnier VM (2002) Clinical impact of intraoperative magnetic resonance imaging on central nervous system neoplasia. Tech Neurosurg 7:326–331
30. Ahmadi R, Dictus C, Hartmann C, Zurn O, Edler L, Hartmann M, Combs S, Herold-Mende C, Wirtz CR, Unterberg A (2009) Long-term outcome and survival of surgically treated supratentorial low-grade glioma in adult patients. Acta Neurochir (Wien) 151 (11):1359–1365

Intraoperative Imaging in Neurosurgery: Where Will the Future Take Us?

Ferenc A. Jolesz

Abstract Intraoperative MRI (ioMRI) dates back to the 1990s and since then has been successfully applied in neurosurgery for three primary reasons with the last one becoming the most significant today: (1) brain shift-corrected navigation, (2) monitoring/controlling thermal ablations, and (3) identifying residual tumor for resection. IoMRI, which today is moving into other applications, including treatment of vasculature and the spine, requires advanced 3 T MRI platforms for faster and more flexible image acquisitions, higher image quality, and better spatial and temporal resolution; functional capabilities including fMRI and DTI; non-rigid registration algorithms to register pre- and intraoperative images; non-MRI imaging improvements to continuously monitor brain shift to identify when a new 3D MRI data set is needed intraoperatively; more integration of imaging and MRI-compatible navigational and robot-assisted systems; and greater computational capabilities to handle the processing of data. The Brigham and Women's Hospital's "AMIGO" suite is described as a setting for progress to continue in ioMRI by incorporating other modalities including molecular imaging. A call to action is made to have other researchers and clinicians in the field of image guided therapy to work together to integrate imaging with therapy delivery systems (such as laser, MRgFUS, endoscopic, and robotic surgery devices).

F.A. Jolesz
B. Leonard Holman Professor of Radiology, Division of MRI and Image Guided Therapy Program, Department of Radiology, Brigham and Women's Hospital, Harvard Medical School, 75 Francis Street, Boston, MA 02115, USA
e-mail: jolesz@bwh.harvard.edu

Keywords Image guided therapy · Imaging · Interventional · Intraoperative MRI (ioMRI) · Magnetic resonance · MR · Neurosurgery

Introduction

Since the early 1990s when we introduced intraoperative MRI (ioMRI) to the field of neurosurgery, it has greatly developed and the number of users and clinical applications have increased [1–10]. It is now important to look back and evaluate the progress of ioMRI to assess what has happened during almost two decades of activity and to identify to the best of our abilities where we are headed.

The original reasons to develop ioMRI were the following:

1. Brain shift-corrected navigation: The navigational systems used in operating rooms rely on preoperative images that do not reflect changes in brain anatomy due to deformations and shifts during surgery. This situation has caused inaccurate targeting and major limitations for neuronavigation. Today, by updating information on the brain using a 3D image database, navigation is made more accurate throughout the entire surgical procedure [11, 12].
2. Monitoring/controlling thermal ablations: The original idea of MRI-guided interstitial laser brain surgery leveraged the temperature sensitivity of MRI to allow for temperature monitoring during the procedure [13–20]. Today, radiofrequency (RF) and focused ultrasound thermal ablations can similarly be controlled through MRI [21–26].
3. Identifying residual tumor: MRI allows the clinician to verify completeness of tumor removal at the end of surgery and, if needed, to perform an additional tumor resection. The original vision for ioMRI focused on correcting for brain shift and monitoring temperature, while today most users apply to perform ioMRI for the third reason: tumor control [4, 27–29].

DOI 10.1007/978-3-211-99651-5_4, © Springer-Verlag/Wien 2011

Since its introduction, ioMRI, conceptually and in real practice, has grown and changed significantly.

Present Benefits and Capabilities

The original full access open MRI, like the SIGNA SP (General Electric Healthcare Technologies, Waukesha, WI), was replaced with open limited access low and midfield magnets and high (1.5 T) and ultra high field (3 T) closed bore MRI scanners [6, 9, 10, 30–32]. Although, the SIGNA SP represented the best configuration, it is at midfield and, therefore, not optimal for neurosurgery. Today most neurosurgeons want higher field strength and more advanced image acquisition technology that is only available in high field advanced systems to obtain higher image quality and better spatial and temporal resolution.

Advanced 3 T imaging platforms achieve faster and more flexible image acquisitions that improve localization, targeting, monitoring, and therapy control. Advance imaging methods functional MRI (fMRI) and diffusion tensor imaging (DTI) have been introduced into neurosurgery and integrated into intraoperative imaging [33–35].

As far as clinical applications are concerned, ioMRI has been successfully developed and implemented for multiple procedures, including:

- Biopsies and placement of electrodes
- Craniotomies for image-guided resection of benign and malignant intracranial tumors
- Intra-cranial cyst drainages and
- Thermal ablations for malignant and benign tumors.

Future ioMRI Applications

In the future, this application pool will expand to:

Bening tumors (skull base): MRI-enhanced neuroendoscopy can be faster and safer than conventional neuroendoscopy and minimize the possibility of complications. A strong need exists to develop MRI-compatible flexible endoscopes with position tracking coils. The combination of the two techniques may provide the best surgical guidance. The most promising application is endoscopic transphenoidal surgery for midline skull base and parasellar lesions and transventricular endoscopic removal for extraventricular tumors.

Neurovascular abnormalities and stroke: ioMRI provides real-time perfusion and diffusion imaging to intraoperatively diagnose acutely developed vascular occlusion and to monitor the condition of the brain during surgeries and/or endovascular procedures. Intraoperative imaging of vascular anatomy, including feeding arteries and the draining veins of an intracranial arteriovenous malformation (AVM), allows the neurosurgeon to intraoperatively assess vessels and surrounding areas and make decisions about the need to completely and safely resect or obliterate a vascular malformation.

Various diseases of the spine: Spinal surgeries with IMR will include: lumbar discectomies, anterior cervical discectomies with fusion, cervical vertebrectomies, foraminotomies, and laminectomies. Through ioMRI, the accuracy of localization and adequacy of decompression can be assessed. Future applications may also include: resection of spine and spinal cord, tumors, and spinal endoscopy. Temperature sensitive imaging for laser discectomy and vertebroplasty can be performed with ioMRI guidance to prevent the thermal damage of the nerve roots and spinal cord.

ioMRI Approaches

The "tumor control" method of ioMRI is a practical and well accepted use of the technology, though it is best applied, not as a single imaging session at the completion of surgery when the clinician cannot take full advantage of ioMRI, but throughout surgery to provide corrected, brain shift-compensated guidance (with serial imaging and navigation). The goal of more complete and effective tumor resection can only be accomplished if we have better techniques to detect the full extent of infiltrative brain tumors. ioMRI is part of this solution along with other multimodality-based molecular imaging (optical, nuclear, or other). Besides tumor margin detection, we need more detailed information about the functional and structural anatomy of the normal brain tissue that surrounds the tumor (for MRI such detail comes through multiparametric imaging: T1, T2, fMRI, DTI perfusion imaging).

Managing the Brain Shift Challenge

Navigational systems fully integrated with ioMRI are also part of improved image guidance [8, 11, 36–39]. For example, it is necessary to monitor brain shift with a non-MRI technique for continuous monitoring that helps the surgeon/neuroradiologist to decide when a new MRI 3D dataset should be obtained. Development of an integrated system to improve visualization, navigation, and monitoring is a necessary step in this direction.

Today we know it is possible to create an augmented reality visualization of the intraoperative configuration of the patient's brain merged with high resolution preoperative imaging data, including DTI and fMRI to better localize the tumor and critical healthy tissues. Brain shift-corrected imaging requires the use of non-rigid registration algorithms to compensate for displacements [40–42]. Massive computational needs must support these capabilities that entail online usage in reasonable time frames of less than 5 min. One of the main reasons for this computational load is that, to properly account for ongoing brain shifts, fMRI and DTI must be accurately co-registered and updated.

Methods of monitoring brain shift now include:

Laser Range Scanner (LRS): Devices, mostly used in robotics applications, that emit and receive a laser beam and by measuring difference of phase, time of flight or frequency shift depth is measured.

Stereo camera imaging: Imaging from a type of camera with two or more lenses that can capture three-dimensional images.

Transcranial US (ITUM): A type of device, at the prototype stage, that uses the shear mode of transcranial ultrasound transmission to intraoperatively monitor brain shift. MRI can then be obtained with the device spatially registered to the MRI reference coordinates [43].

Further Development

ioMRI allows for the introduction of new surgical approaches and/or techniques in vascular neurosurgery, spine surgery, and skull base surgery (using image guided and registered neuroendoscopy). Further moving ioMRI forward in neurosurgery is the already-underway integration of ioMRI with image guided robots that provide, through remote manipulation, an alternative solution to limited access. Already, for many types of neurosurgical procedures, companies have developed MRI-compatible robotic systems and manipulators [44–51]. Today most systems still lack the clinical validation that is necessary for the surgical robot to execute not only biopsies but also complex surgical manipulations.

ioMRI today has also moved beyond MRI-guided and controlled thermal ablations for interstitial laser therapy [13, 14, 16, 17, 19] to MRI-guided focused ultrasound surgery (MRgFUS) as well as the targeted ablative treatment of brain tumors via drug delivery through an open blood-brain-barrier (BBB) [23–25, 52–57]. FUS-induced neuromodulation is a complement to functional neurosurgical applications for coagulative lesions [57–59].

Greater progress and expansion for ioMRI requires the development of new, more advanced imaging methods, navigational techniques, surgical instruments and tools; the more efficient use of computing technologies; and the integration of diagnostic and therapy devices with navigational tools (computer-assisted surgery). A need exists for a multifocused, multidisciplinary effort involving researchers and clinicians to explore and refine ioMRI to make it as cost-effective and as widely accessible to a multidisciplinary pool of users.

AMIGO: Merging ioMRI and Other Modalities

At the Brigham and Women's Hospital, we are taking a lead in this effort through the development and execution of a multimodality approach to intraoperative imaging by integrating the components of a rich multimodal and translational clinical research environment to carry out open and minimally invasive surgeries and percutaneous interventions. Multimodality IGT provides comprehensive information derived from different physical and biological properties. Combined multimodalities provide anatomical, metabolic, and functional information – a previously stated goal for ioMRI. Images can be complemented with newly developed multiple molecular probes (nuclear, optical, mass spectrometer, etc.). The use of multiple molecular probes improves the sensitivity and specificity of cancer-relevant applications over single mode imaging. To achieve this we must expand our imaging platform for image guided neurosurgery to include all modalities, especially those applicable to molecular imaging (PETCT, MRI, optical imaging).

The validation of imaging tools and molecular imaging agents in a multimodal surgical setting is possible because, during surgeries, multiple tissue samples can be obtained for pathology that can validate imaging findings at the same location. Navigational and registration methods for multimodal registration can be used to compare multiple probes that are measuring exactly the same tissue region.

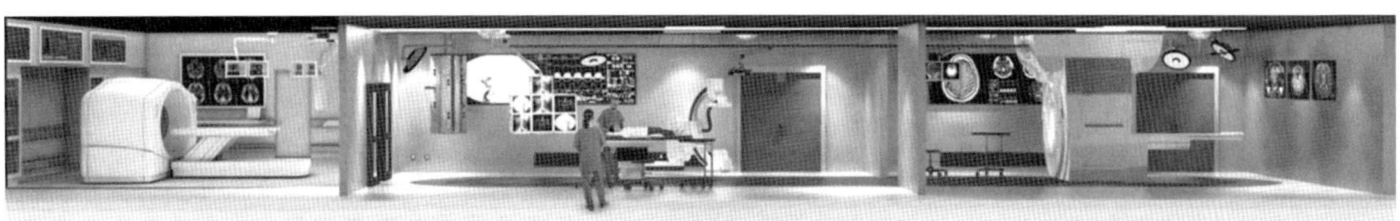

Fig. 1 Advanced Multimodality Image Guided OR (AMIGO). The middle room is an operating room with surgical microscope, angiography, ultarsound and optical imaging. The room on the left has a PETCT and on the right a 3T MRI which is seiling mounted and can move into the operating room to image the patient on the operating room table (IMRIS, Winnipeg, Canada)

The BWH's Advanced Multimodality Image Guided Operating (AMIGO) Suite (see Fig. 1), opening in 2010, is uniquely designed to support, alongside routine clinical procedures, the next phase of clinical and research activity in ioMRI that will incorporate multimodal imaging. The logistics of the suite are such that multidisciplinary teams will be in close cooperation with one another during procedures that might involve the use of an array of on-site (i.e., in the suite itself) modalities from 3D ultrasound, fluoroscopy, MRI, and PET/CT to carry out a variety of procedures.

The AMIGO and suites like it are at the forefront by providing settings for practice, refinement, improvement, validation, and innovation. Indeed, the future of intraoperative imaging in neurosurgery depends on such settings and teams and their increased application of advanced technologies and multimodality imaging. Integration of imaging with therapy delivery systems (laser, MRgFUS, endoscopic and robotic surgery devices) will characterize the next phase of this emerging field.

Conflict of interest statement Dr. Jolesz has received cosultant fees from General Electric, who pioneered this system.

References

1. Black PM, Alexander E 3rd, Martin C et al (1999) Craniotomy for tumor treatment in an intraoperative magnetic resonance imaging unit. Neurosurgery 45(3):423–431
2. Dimaio SP, Archip N, Hata N et al (2006) Image-guided neurosurgery at Brigham and Women's Hospital. IEEE Eng Med Biol Mag 25(5):67–73
3. Hall WA, Martin AJ, Liu H et al (1998) High-field strength interventional magnetic resonance imaging for pediatric neurosurgery. Pediatr Neurosurg 29(5):253–259
4. Jolesz FA, Talos IF, Schwartz RB et al (2002) Intraoperative magnetic resonance imaging and magnetic resonance imaging-guided therapy for brain tumors. Neuroimaging Clin N Am 12 (4):665–683
5. Lewin JS, Metzger AK (2001) Intraoperative MR systems. Low-field approaches. Neuroimaging Clin N Am 11(4):611–628
6. Schenck JF, Jolesz FA, Roemer PB, Cline HE, Lorensen WE, Kikinis R et al (1995) Superconducting open-configuration MR imaging system for image-guided therapy. Radiology 195 (3):805–814
7. Schwartz RB, Hsu L, Wong TZ et al (1999) Intraoperative MR imaging guidance for intracranial neurosurgery: experience with the first 200 cases. Radiology 211(2):477–488
8. Schulder M, Liang D, Carmel PW (2001) Cranial surgery navigation aided by a compact intraoperative magnetic resonance imager. J Neurosurg 94(6):936–945
9. Steinmeier R, Fahlbusch R, Ganslandt O et al (1998) Intraoperative magnetic resonance imaging with the magnetom open scanner: concepts, neurosurgical indications, and procedures: a preliminary report. Neurosurgery 43(4):739–747, discussion 747–748
10. Sutherland GR, Kaibara T, Louw D, Hoult DI, Tomanek B, Saunders J (1999) A mobile high-field magnetic resonance system for neurosurgery. J Neurosurg 91(5):804–813
11. Jolesz FA, Kikinis R, Talos IF (2001) Neuronavigation in interventional MR imaging. Frameless stereotaxy. Neuroimaging Clin N Am 11(4):685–689
12. Nabavi A, Black PM, Gering DT et al (2001) Serial intraoperative magnetic resonance imaging of brain shift. Neurosurgery 48 (4):787–797, discussion 797–798
13. Anzai Y, Lufkin R, DeSalles A, Hamilton DR, Farahani K, Black KL (1995) Preliminary experience with MR-guided thermal ablation of brain tumors. AJNR Am J Neuroradiol 16(1):39–48, discussion 49–52
14. Ascher PW, Justich E, Schröttner O (1991) Interstitial thermotherapy of central brain tumors with the Nd:YAG laser under real-time monitoring by MRI. J Clin Laser Med Surg 9(1):79–83
15. Bettag M, Ulrich F, Schober R et al (1991) Stereotactic laser therapy in cerebral gliomas. Acta Neurochir Suppl (Wien) 52:81–83
16. Fan M, Ascher PW, Schröttner O, Ebner F, Germann RH, Kleinert R (1992) Interstitial 1.06 Nd:YAG laser thermotherapy for brain tumors under real-time monitoring of MRI: experimental study and phase I clinical trial. J Clin Laser Med Surg 10(5):355–356
17. Kahn T, Bettag M, Ulrich F et al (1994) MRI-guided laser-induced interstitial thermotherapy of cerebral neoplasms. J Comput Assist Tomogr 18:519–532
18. Kettenbach J, Silverman SG, Hata N et al (1998) Monitoring and visualization techniques for MR-guided laser ablations in an open MR system. J Magn Reson Imaging 8(4):933–943
19. McDannold NJ, Jolesz FA (2000) Magnetic resonance image-guided thermal ablations. Top Magn Reson Imaging 11(3): 191–202
20. Stollberger R, Ascher PW, Huber D, Renhart W, Radner H, Ebner F (1998) Temperature monitoring of interstitial thermal tissue coagulation using MR phase images. J Magn Reson Imaging 8(1):188–196
21. Cline HE, Hynynen K, Watkins RD et al (1995) Focused US system for MR imaging-guided tumor ablation. Radiology 194 (3):731–737
22. Hynynen K, Vykhodtseva NI, Chung AH, Sorrentino V, Colucci V, Jolesz FA (1997) Thermal effects of focused ultrasound on the brain: determination with MR imaging. Radiology 204(1):247–253
23. Jolesz FA, Hynynen K (2002) Magnetic resonance image-guided focused ultrasound surgery. Cancer J 8(suppl 1):S100–S112
24. Jolesz FA, Hynynen K, McDannold N, Tempany C (2005) MR imaging-controlled focused ultrasound ablation: a noninvasive image-guided surgery. Magn Reson Imaging Clin N Am 13(3):545–60
25. Jolesz FA, McDannold N (2008) Current status and future potential of MRI-guided focused ultrasound surgery. J Magn Reson Imaging 27(2):391–399
26. McDannold N, Hynynen K, Wolf D, Wolf G, Jolesz F (1998) MRI evaluation of thermal ablation of tumors with focused ultrasound. J Magn Reson Imaging 8(1):91–100
27. Claus EB, Horlacher A, Hsu L (2005) Survival rates in patients with low-grade glioma after intraoperative magnetic resonance image guidance. Cancer 103(6):1227–1233
28. Mittal S, Black PM (2006) Intraoperative magnetic resonance imaging in neurosurgery: the Brigham concept. Acta Neurochir Suppl 98:77–86
29. Nimsky C, Fujita A, Ganslandt O, Von Keller B, Fahlbusch R (2004) Volumetric assessment of glioma removal by intraoperative high-field magnetic resonance imaging. Neurosurgery 55(2): 358–370, discussion 370–371
30. Bradley WG (2002) Achieving gross total resection of brain tumors: intraoperative MR imaging can make a big difference. AJNR Am J Neuroradiol 23(3):348–349
31. Nimsky C, Ganslandt O, Von Keller B, Romstöck J, Fahlbusch R (2004) Intraoperative high-field-strength MR imaging: implementation and experience in 200 patients. Radiology 233(1):67–78

32. Truwit CL, Hall WA (2006) Intraoperative magnetic resonance imaging-guided neurosurgery at 3-T. Neurosurgery 58(4 suppl 2): ONS-338–345, discussion ONS-345–346
33. Hall WA, Liu H, Truwit CL (2005) Functional magnetic resonance imaging-guided resection of low-grade gliomas. Surg Neurol 64(1):20–27, discussion
34. Golby AJ, McConnell KA (2004) Functional brain mapping options for minimally invasive surgery. In: Black PM, Proctor M (eds) Minimally invasive neurosurgery. Humana Press, Totawa, NJ, pp 87–106
35. Nimsky C, Ganslandt O, Kober H et al (1999) Integration of functional magnetic resonance imaging supported by magnetoencephalography in functional neuronavigation. Neurosurgery 44 (6):1249–1255, discussion 1255–1256
36. Gering DT, Nabavi A, Kikinis R et al (2001) An integrated visualization system for surgical planning and guidance using image fusion and an open MR. J Magn Reson Imaging 13(6):967–975
37. Nabavi A, Gering DT, Kacher DF et al (2003) Surgical navigation in the open MRI. Acta Neurochir Suppl 85:121–125
38. Nimsky C, Ganslandt O, Cerny S, Hastreiter P, Greiner G, Fahlbusch R (2000) Quantification of, visualization of, and compensation for brain shift using intraoperative magnetic resonance imaging. Neurosurgery 47(5):1070–1079, discussion 1079–1080
39. Nimsky C, Ganslandt O, Hastreiter P, Fahlbusch R (2001) Intraoperative compensation for brain shift. Surg Neurol 56(6):357–364, discussion 364–365
40. Clatz O, Delingette H, Talos IF et al (2005) Hybrid formulation of the model-based non-rigid registration problem to improve accuracy and robustness. Med Image Comput Comput Assist Interv 8(Pt 2):295–302
41. Ferrant M, Nabavi A, Macq B et al (2002) Serial registration of intraoperative MR images of the brain. Med Image Anal 6(4):337–359
42. Warfield SK, Haker SJ, Talos IF et al (2005) Capturing intraoperative deformations: research experience at Brigham and Women's Hospital. Med Image Anal 9(2):145–162
43. White PJ, Whalen S, Tang SC, Clement G, Jolesz F, Golby AJ (2009) An intraoperative brain shift monitor using shear mode transcranial ultrasound: preliminary results. J Ultrasound Med 28(2):191–203
44. Chinzei K, Miller K (2001) Towards MRI guided surgical manipulator. Med Sci Monit 7(1):153–163
45. Chinzei K, Warfield S, Hata N, Tempany C, Jolesz F, Kikinis R (2003) Planning, simulation and assistance with intraoperative MRI. Minim Invasive Ther Allied Technol 12(1):59–64
46. DiMaio SP, Pieper S, Chinzei K et al (2007) Robot-assisted needle placement in open MRI: system architecture, integration and validation. Comput Aided Surg 12(1):15–24
47. Elhawary H, Tse ZT, Hamed A, Rea M, Davies BL, Lamperth MU (2008) The case for MR-compatible robotics: a review of the state of the art. Int J Med Robot 4(2):105–113
48. Elhawary H, Zivanovic A, Davies B, Lampérth M (2006) A review of magnetic resonance imaging compatible manipulators in surgery. Proc Inst Mech Eng 220(3):413–424
49. Masamune K, Kobayashi E (1995) Development of an MRI-compatible needle insertion manipulator for stereotactic neurosurgery. J Image Guid Surg 1(4):242–248
50. Sutherland GR, Latour I, Greer AD (2008) Integrating an image-guided robot with intraoperative MRI: a review of the design and construction of neuroArm. IEEE Eng Med Biol Mag 27(3):59–65
51. Sutherland GR, Latour I, Greer AD, Fielding T, Feil G, Newhook P (2008) An image-guided magnetic resonance-compatible surgical robot. Neurosurgery 62(2):286–292, discussion 292–293
52. Hynynen K, McDannold N, Vykhodtseva N, Jolesz FA (2001) Noninvasive MR imaging-guided focal opening of the blood–brain barrier in rabbits. Radiology 220(3):640–646
53. Kinoshita M, McDannold N, Jolesz FA, Hynynen K (2006) Targeted delivery of antibodies through the blood–brain barrier by MRI-guided focused ultrasound. Biochem Biophys Res Commun 340(4):1085–1090
54. Kinoshita M, McDannold N, Jolesz FA, Hynynen K (2006) Noninvasive localized delivery of Herceptin to the mouse brain by MRI-guided focused ultrasound-induced blood–brain barrier disruption. Proc Natl Acad Sci U S A 103(31):11719–11723
55. Treat LH, McDannold N, Vykhodtseva N, Zhang Y, Tam K, Hynynen K (2007) Targeted delivery of doxorubicin to the rat brain at therapeutic levels using MRI-guided focused ultrasound. Int J Cancer 121(4):901–907
56. Vykhodtseva N, McDannold N, Hynynen K (2006) Induction of apoptosis in vivo in the rabbit brain with focused ultrasound and optison. Ultrasound Med Biol 32(12):1923–1929
57. Yoo SS, Lee JH, Zhang Y et al (2008) FUS-mediated reversible modulation of region-specific brain function. Proc MRgFUS 2008:10
58. Colucci V, Strichartz G, Jolesz F, Vykhodtseva N, Hynynen K (2009) Focused ultrasound effects on nerve action potential in vitro. Ultrasound Med Biol 35(10):1737–1747
59. Currier DP, Greathouse D, Swift T (1978) Sensory nerve conduction: effect of ultrasound. Arch Phys Med Rehabil 59(4): 181–185

Intraoperative MRI- Ultra Low Field Systems

Development and Design of Low Field Compact Intraoperative MRI for Standard Operating Room

Moshe Hadani

Abstract *Objectives*: To present the development of a compact low field intraoperative MR image guidance system and its application in brain surgery.

Methods: The PoleStar ioMRI system (Odin Medical Technologies, Israel and Medtronic, Inc. USA) was developed for use in a standard operating room. Its primary physical fixed parameters are magnetic field of 0.15 T and field of view of 20×16cm. The magnet is mounted on a transportable gantry and can be positioned under the surgical table when not in use for scanning. Additional functionality includes integrated navigation, and system operation by the surgeons.

Results: The PoleStar system integrates into existing operating rooms requiring only slight modification of the surgical environment. Standard instruments can be used. The system's imaging allows it to be used for the following indications: pituitary tumors, low grade gliomas (including awake surgery), high grade gliomas, intraventricular tumors, accurate navigation to small lesions such as cavernous angiomas or metastases, drainage of cysts and brain abscesses. The image quality, which is comparable to post operative diagnostic high field imaging, enables high quality resection control.

More than 6,000 brain surgeries were done with the system in 50 centers in the US and Europe.

Conclusion: The low field intraoperative MRI system is a valuable tool in the modern operating room.

Keywords Compact ioMRI · Image-guided surgery · ioMRI · Intraoperative magnetic resonance imaging · Low field MRI · Resection control · Surgical neuronavigation

M. Hadani
Department of Neurosurgery, Sheba Medical Center, Sackler School of Medicine, Tel Aviv University, Tel Hashomer 52621, Israel
e-mail: moshe.hadani@sheba.health.gov.il

Introduction

Intraoperative magnetic resonance imaging (ioMRI) was introduced in 1997 to complement standard neuronavigation with updated, high resolution MR images during surgery [1] The first system was a 0.5 T MRI scanner (GE Signa SP) which weighted 6,000 kg and was installed in a special room, outside of the operating rooms complex. Our site, among a few others, had the opportunity to operate the system. The surgical environment was different from the standard. Working outside of the operating room complex was problematic and the cost of the magnet and the building was high. At the same time a group of MRI physicists and engineers in Israel developed a small, low field MRI scanner of 0.12 T, which weighted only 500 kg. The challenge was to bring this scanner to function in a standard neurosurgery operating room.

The goals for the clinical design of system were:

- Provide optimal MR imaging for navigation and tumor resection control.
- Integrated navigation capabilities
- Integration into existing operating rooms, allowing the use of standard surgical tools and equipment.
- Minimize interference with routine surgical procedures.
- No requirement for structural changes to the building and low cost of purchase and installation.
- Provide full control by the surgeon including MRI scanning.

Materials and Methods

The following were the fixed physical parameters of the PoleStar scanner: Low field magnetic strength (0.15 T in the PoleStar N20, which followed the original PoleStar N-10, Odin Medical Technologies Israel and Medtronic inc USA) The scanner consists of two vertical, parallel, disk-shaped permanent magnets located 27 cm from each

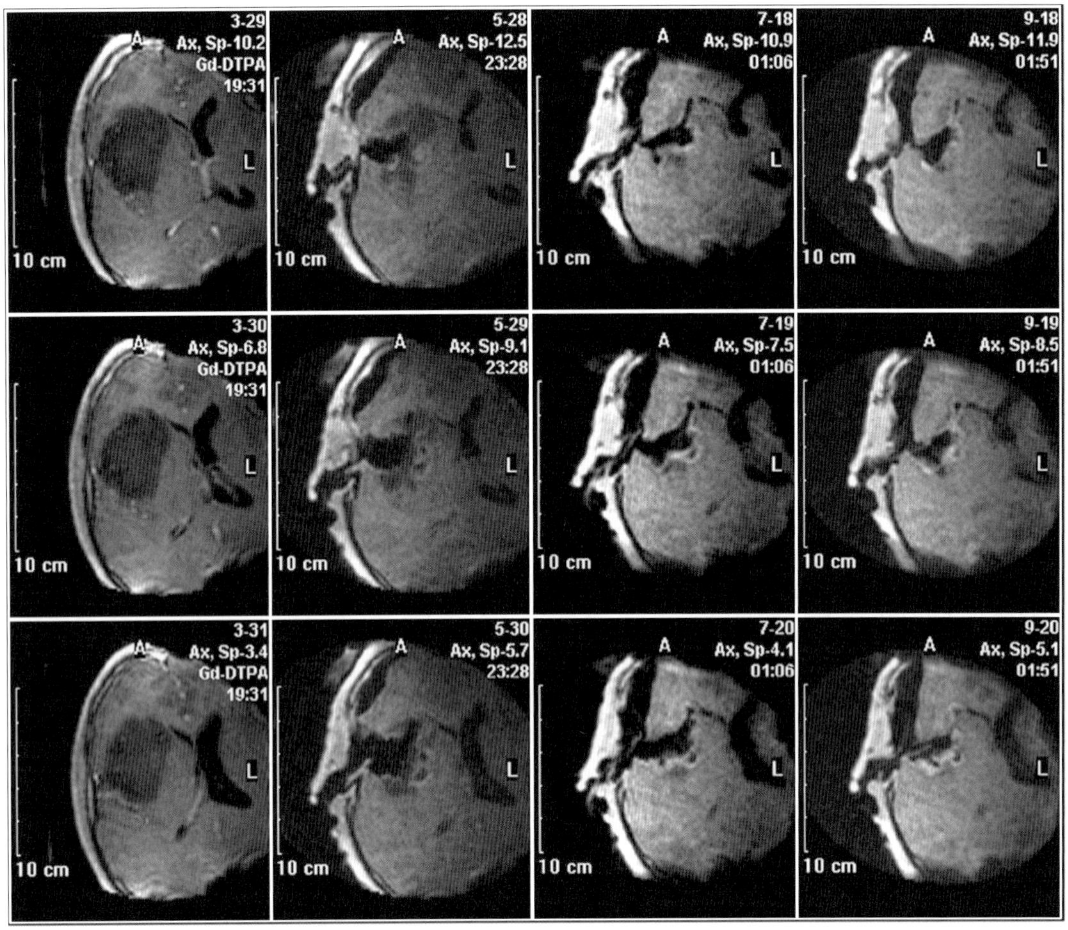

Fig. 1 The compare function shows consecutive T1 weighted axial sections of a patient with a grade II astrocytoma, illustrating occurring brain shift of 1.5 cm and residual tumor, that was located by intraoperative navigation and resected completely

other. This is the space for the positioning of the head. The field-of-view is 20 × 16 cm. The magnets are affixed to a U-shaped arm. The arm itself is mounted on a transportable gantry positioned below the operating table. For scanning the magnets are raised, by the system computer under tight manual control, so that the area to be imaged is well centered between the magnet poles. After scanning, the magnets are retracted under the OR table providing good access to the head during surgery.

A special MRI compatible head holder was designed to accommodate the limited space for the head between the magnet poles.

The following MRI sequences were developed: T1-weighted, T2-weighted, FLAIR and e-steady sequences. Image acquisition takes from 8 s to 13 min, depending on the selected MR sequence and slice thickness. Typically, 7-min T1-weighted images and 4 mm slice thickness are used as preoperative baseline imaging.

Image series from different scans can be displayed side by side, facilitating comparison between different stages of surgery as well as comparison of images acquired with different sequences, such as T1 and T2 contrasts (Fig. 1).

The scanner is integrated with a navigation station. Acquired images are immediately available for navigation. Patient registration is not required. Navigation on diagnostic images is also supported.

Results

Due to the low field and the compact size the scanner was installed in a standard operating room (Fig. 2). The only modification of the room was the installation of copper mesh in the walls to eliminate RF noise. Light, power and anesthesiology gas inlets are filtered to avoid interference with image acquisition.

When not in use, the scanner is placed in a special cabinet to allow the room to be used for any surgery. The low magnetic field of the system is largely confined to the area between the magnets and decays to 5 G 1.7 m from the

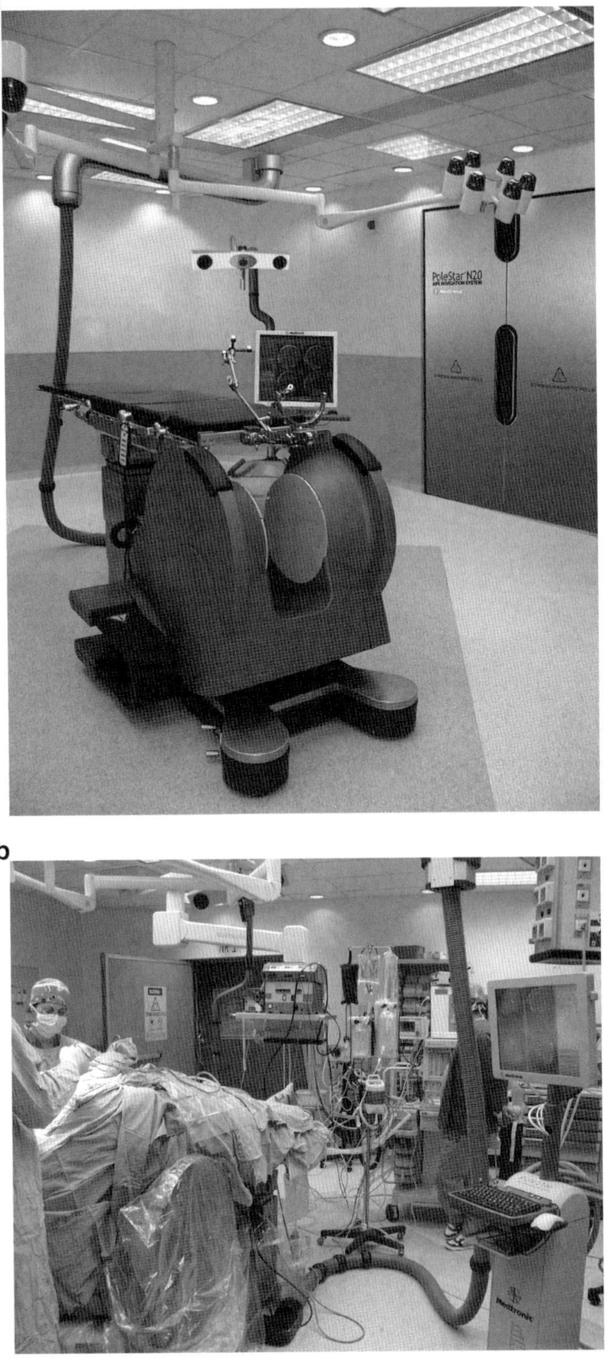

Fig. 2 (**a**) The PoleStar system in a standard operating room shielded for RF. On the right the "cabinet" for the magnet when not in use. The scanner is integrated with the Treon navigation system. (**b**) Operation room setup. Only anesthesia equipment is MRI compatible

magnet's isocenter. When the scanner is placed below the level of the OR table, the magnetic field strength in the operative field is below 50 G, enabling the use of standard surgical instruments.

All equipment and tools are the standard. This includes conventional operating tables, microscopes, chairs, ultrasonic aspirator, standard drill, bipolar stimulator, EEG recorder.

MRI scans are controlled by the surgeon or an assistant at the navigation workstation (Treon, Medtronic, Inc.)

Navigation is done on the last MRI set. No registration is needed, the magnet itself, rather than the patient's head, is automatically registered, and the accuracy is high [2].

More than 600 adult and pediatric cases were operated with the PoleStar ioMRI system in our center in Tel Aviv. Currently about 6,000 operations were done with the system worldwide.

Clinical applications included craniotomies for intraxial and extraaxial brain tumors, metastastic tumors, pituitary tumors, intraventricular lesions, cavernous angiomas, shunt placements, epilepsy surgery, awake surgeries, stereo tactic biopsies and cyst aspirations.

Discussion

Following the 10 years experience with ioMRI, there are currently 90 systems installed worldwide: about 40 high magnetic field systems (1.5 T and 3 T), 50 low field systems (0.15 T) and a few 0.3 T systems.

8,000–9,000 surgeries were performed with ioMRI.

The utility of ioMRI is mainly resection control, correction of brain shift, complication avoidance, and navigation to small lesions.

The design goals of the PoleStar compact system were met [3–5]. Its intraoperative images serve as the data for navigation and for resection control. The image quality of the low field system is inferior to that of the high field systems; however, it was found optimal for updating the navigation data and for the ability to navigate with high accuracy to small lesions. The PoleStar imaging enables high quality resection control, which is comparable to post-operative diagnostic high field imaging (Fig. 3).

All patients' positions are possible and manipulation of the operative table enables the surgeon to work in the most comfortable position.

For the anesthesiologist, [6] using the PoleStar ioMRI system allows preservation of working conditions that are similar to a regular operating room. The patient is accessible to the anesthesiologist at all times during the procedure, and conventional syringe pumps and warming devices can be used. It is also possible to perform electrophysiological monitoring in surgery for epilepsy, and to carry out surgery under intravenous sedation and intra-operative mapping in the awake state.

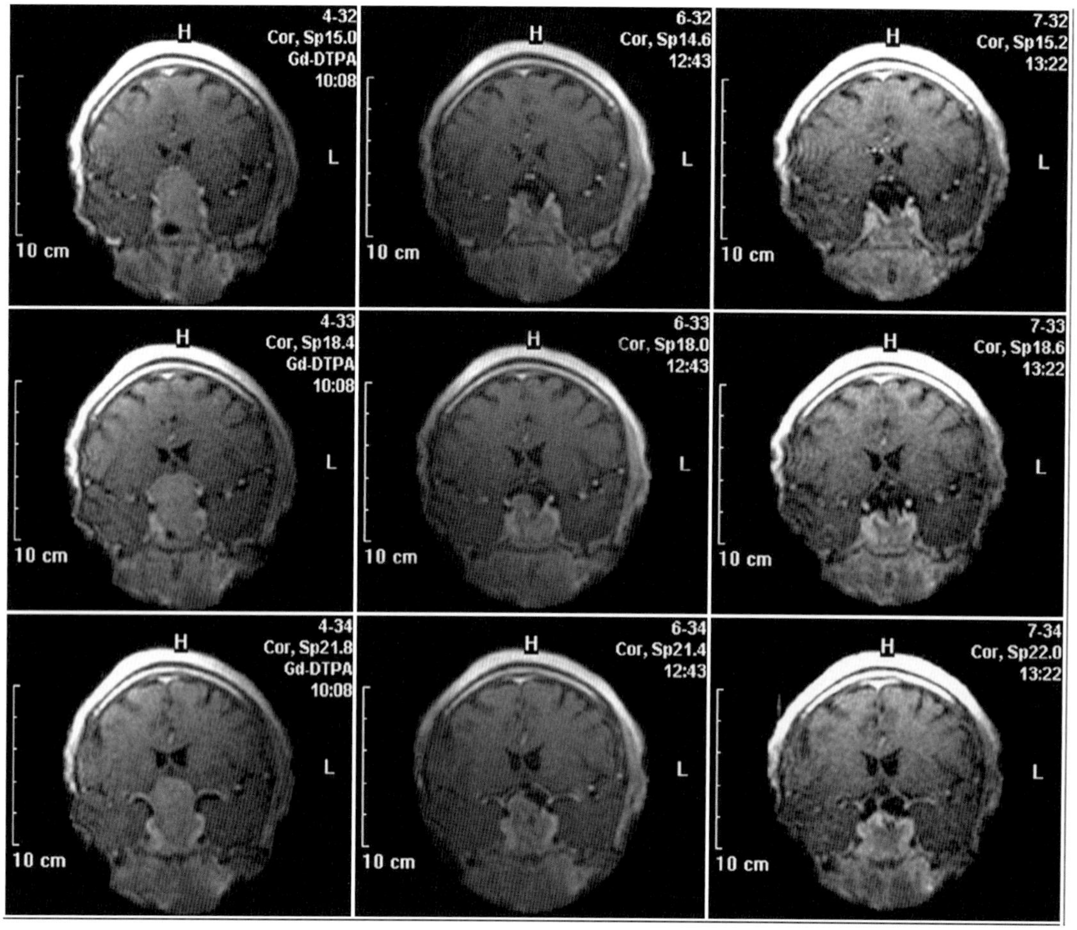

Fig. 3 Intraoperative extended resection of a pituitary macro adenoma. Compare mode

In exchange for the "lower quality" imaging the following advantages were achieved in the development of the PoleStar system:

Easy to use in a standard operating room with no need to change the normal flow of the operative procedure.

Safety, when using the system in a standard operating room environment.

Keeping the duration of the operation within the usual timeframe with only minor addition of time, and last but not least

The compact system is by far less expansive due to the lower cost of the components of the system and the low cost of installation in the operation room without the need for special building.

ioMRI should be part of the modalities used in brain surgery. It is useful in a subset of operations such as: pituitary tumor surgery, high and low grade gliomas, for resection control and complication avoidance, Navigation and resection of small lesions 1 cm or less such as cavernous angiomas or small metastatic tumors, drainage of cysts and abscesses, navigation during facedown procedures.

Conclusions

The development of a low field compact intraoperative MRI system was custom made to the clinical need.

This low field ioMRI system functions in a normal operating room modified only for radiofrequency interference. The operative environment is normal and standard instruments are used. Use of the system does not change the working habits in the OR.

The scanning and navigation capabilities of the system eliminate the inaccuracies that may result from brain shift. Image quality enables high quality resection control, which is comparable to post operative diagnostic high field imaging.

The main indications for the use of ioMRI are: pituitary tumors, low grade gliomas (awake), high grade gliomas, intraventricular tumors, accurate navigation to small lesions such as cavernous angiomas or metastases, drainage of cysts and brain abscesses.

Conflict of interest statement We declare that we have no conflict of interest.

References

1. Black PM, Moriarty T, Alexander E 3rd, Steig P, Woodard EJ, Gleason L, Martin CH, Kikinis R, Schwartz RB, Jolesz F (1997) Development and implementation of intraoperative magnetic resonance imaging and its neurosurgical applications. Neurosurgery 41(4):831–845
2. Salas S, Brimacombe M, Schulder M (2007) Stereotacti accuracy of a compact intraoperative MRI system. Stereotact Funct Neurosurg 85:69–74
3. Hadani M, Spiegelman R, Feldman Z, Berkenstadt H, Ram Z (2001) Novel, compact, intraoperative magnetic resonance imaging-guided system for conventional neurosurgical operating rooms. Neurosurgery 48(4):799–809
4. Hadani M, Schulder M, Bernays RL (2002) Compact 0.12-tesla intraoperative magnetic resonance image guidance system in the standard operating room. Tech Neurosurg 7(4)
5. Schulder M, Salas S, Brimacombe M, Fine P, Catrambone J, Maniker A, Carmel P (2006) Cranial surgery with an expanded compact intraoperative magnetic resonance imager. J Neurosurg 104:611–617
6. Berkenstadt H, Perel A, Ram Z, Feldman Z, Nahtomi-Shick O, Hadani M (2001) Anesthesia for magnetic resonance guided neurosurgery. Initial experience with a new open magnetic resonance imaging system. J Neurosurg Anesthesiol 13:158–162

Low Field Intraoperative MRI in Glioma Surgery

Volker Seifert, Thomas Gasser, and Christian Senft

Abstract The extent of resection marks one prognostic factor for patients with malignant gliomas. Among the methods used for the intraoperative control of the extent of resection, intraoperative magnetic resonance imaging (ioMRI) has become a very attractive method. It was introduced in the in the final decade of the last century. The first available system was a low magnetic field strength unit employing 0.5 Tesla (T). While currently high-field systems (1.5 T and above) are being developed, different low-field ioMRI systems (0.5 T and below) have been used for brain tumor resection in far more centers than high-field ioMRI, corresponding to a greater number of publications. Undoubtedly, high-field ioMRI systems offer superior image quality and faster acquisition times. Yet, low-field ioMRI has influenced intraoperative decision-making and improved brain tumor resection. With this article, we review the use of low-field ioMRI in glioma surgery.

Keywords Glioma surgery · Intraoperative MRI · Review

Surgical Treatment of Gliomas

Rickman Godlee performed the first successful resection of a glioma in 1884 [1]. Since then, numerous reports have stated beneficial effects of extensive tumor resections despite a nonetheless deleterious course of the disease. With the introduction of microneurosurgical techniques and refined imaging modalities, recent studies could show that a radiologically complete resection represents an independent prognostic factor for patients with malignant gliomas [2–6].

In contrast to e.g. abdominal oncological surgery, brain tumor resections cannot be performed with a safety margin. Due to the infiltrative nature of gliomas and the fact that their margins are frequently difficult to be visualized intraoperatively, postoperative imaging studies reveal unintentionally remaining tumor tissue quite frequently [3, 7]. To improve the extent of resection, and thus the prognosis for glioma patients, neurosurgeons have sought to develop different methods of intraoperative imaging to visualize tumor tissue. Compared to intraoperative ultrasound or intraoperative computed tomography, MRI offers superior image quality without radiation exposure to the patient and/or staff. Magnetic resonance imaging has become the gold standard for the diagnostic and follow-up imaging of gliomas. Intraoperative MRI seemed as the method of choice in the resection control of gliomas, and it was developed for mainly, but not exclusively, this reason [8–10].

Development of Low-Field ioMRI-Systems

Peter Black and Ferenc Jolesz from the Brigham and Women's Hospital in Boston pioneered intraoperative magnetic resonance imaging in the 1990s. In collaboration with General Electric Co. they developed the first ioMRI scanner to be used in a neurosurgical operating room. The *Signa SP* employed a magnetic field strength of 0.5 T and was nicknamed "double-donut" system due to the shape and appearance of the system – it consisted of two magnets with a vertical gap in which the patient's head was placed during surgery. It required major modifications of OR-infrastructure to meet the demands for low radiofrequency interference as well as adaptation regarding surgical tools, instruments, microscopes, etc., which all needed to be MR-compatible [11, 12]. While the provided images were consistently of

V. Seifert (✉) and C. Senft
Department of Neurosurgery, Johann Wolfgang Goethe-University, Schleusenweg 2-16, 60528 Frankfurt, Germany
e-mail: v.seifert@em.uni-frankfurt.de

T. Gasser
Department of Neurosurgery, Johann Wolfgang Goethe-University, Schleusenweg 2-16, 60528 Frankfurt, Germany
University of Essen, Essen, Germany

M.N. Pamir et al. (eds.), *Intraoperative Imaging*, Acta Neurochirurgica Supplementum, Vol. 109,
DOI 10.1007/978-3-211-99651-5_6, © Springer-Verlag/Wien 2011

good quality, one major concern with this system was the constraint working area of the surgeon, who stood in between the magnets (Fig. 1). Also, some restrictions applied regarding patient positioning.

Simultaneosly, Siemens Corp. developed a C-shaped resistive MRI scanner with a static magnetic field with strength of 0.2 T (*Magnetom Open*). In contrast to the *Signa SP* which marked the center of the operating theater, the *Magnetom Open* was set up at the one end of the operating room, separated from the surgical area by radiofrequency shielding, thus allowing for the use of standard instrumentarium during surgery. The patient had to be transferred to the magnet, which featured a 240° opening, allowing for safe placement of the anaesthetized patient's head into the scanner's field of view [13, 14]. However, image acquisition necessitated transferring the patient from the operating site to the scanner, which is time-consuming.

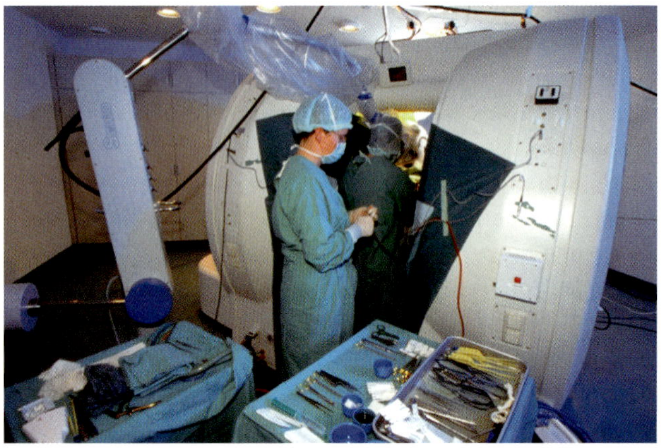

Fig. 1 Example of a brain tumor surgery perfomed with the Signa SP – the surgeon stands in between the magnets' gap using non-ferromagnetic instruments

While the *AIRIS II* MRI scanner (Hitachi Corp.), employing a magnetic field strength of 0.3 T, was developed primarily as a conventional diagnostic tool, it was also employed as an ioMRI scanner [15, 16]. It is an open MRI unit with two horizontally oriented magnets with a vertical opening of 17 in. Surgeries can be performed either in the adjacent operating room, or with the patient positioned on the scanner's table.

The *PoleStar* by Odin/Medtronic Inc. is one of the most frequently used low-field systems today with a static magnetic field strength of 0.12 (Model N-10) or 0.15 T (Model N-20), respectively [17, 18]. It was developed to overcome the necessity of using special, MRI-compatible instruments and surgical devices, demanded for by other ioMRI systems, yet avoiding cumbersome patient transfer to the scanner. The *PoleStar* was designed as a mobile MRI unit with two vertical magnets spaced 25 or 27 cm apart, respectively. During surgery, conventional instruments can be used while the magnet is parked underneath the operating table (Fig. 2). The scanner is moved upwards for intraoperative image acquisition [19, 20].

Image Quality in Low Field MRI

Although there is a span of different magnet designs, field strengths, and investigational concepts, there are many similarities in the information obtained in order to guide and

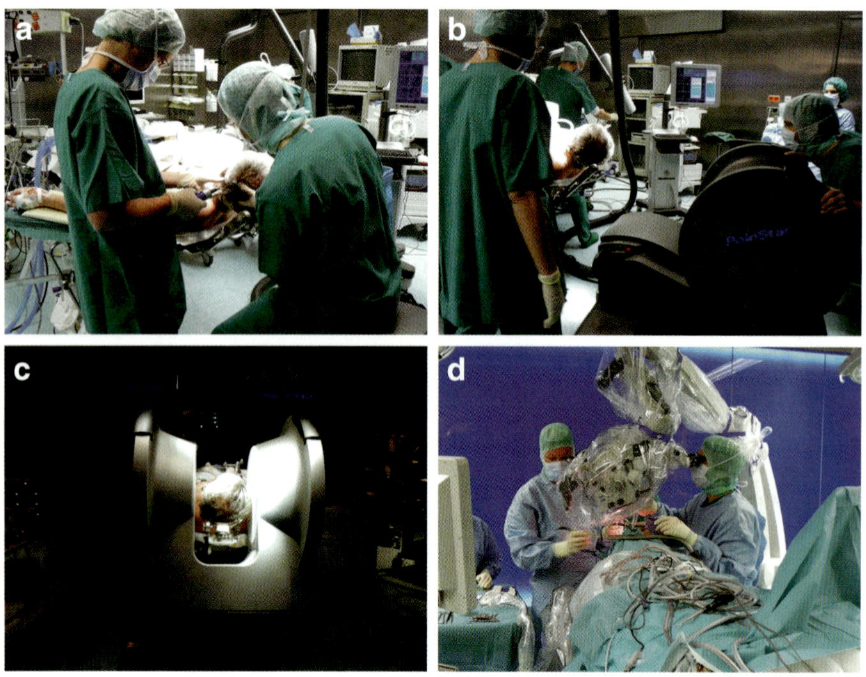

Fig. 2 Example of a brain tumor surgery performed with the PoleStar N-20. (**a**) Fixation of the head and application of the radiofrequency coil (**b**) Transfer of the magnet to its position underneath the operating table (**c**) The magnet is moved upwards for image acquisition (**d**) The magnet is lowered and tumor resection is performed with standard instruments in a microsurgical fashion

monitor neurosurgical procedures. All of the above mentioned systems have been successfully used to monitor craniotomy and extent of resection in patients with gliomas [15, 17, 19, 21–27].

However, each has its own set of advantages and disadvantages, and as ioMRI-technology still evolves, no single system has gained universal use. Image quality in MRI is directly linked to the field strength of the magnet and to the homogeneity and stability of the static and gradient magnetic fields. Undoubtedly, high field, i.e. 1.5 or even 3 T systems offer an excellent image quality that cannot be reached by low-field systems. They are, however, very expensive, and are yet limited to a small number of centers worldwide.

In ioMRI in general, there is a constant trade-off between signal-to-noise ratio, access to the patient, and usable field of view. The optimal design of a magnet with regard to homogeneity would be a complete sphere without opening, which is obviously impossible in both conventional "closed" and intraoperative "open" MRI systems [28]. To overcome this problem and to achieve an acceptable signal-to-noise ratio in low field open MRI systems, longer acquisition times are necessary. While weaker magnets are usually less expensive and can allow near real-time imaging, they suffer from poorer image resolution. High-field systems on the other hand are more expensive and permit only interruptive scanning.

From an image-quality point of view, cylindrical superconductive systems bear significant advantages relative to static magnetic field strength and homogeneity [29]. In the *Signa SP* scanner, the central segment of a cylindrical system was taken out, allowing for direct access to the patient in the scanner at the expense of decreased field strength at the imaging isocenter compared to 1.5 T. Nonetheless, image quality is still almost comparable to high field imaging, and sufficient for the delineation of both, contrast-enhancing and non contrast-enhancing lesions such as high- and low-grade gliomas [27].

In contrast to this system, e.g. the *PoleStar* ioMRI system offers more convenience for the surgeon with a larger working space, yet its field strength is even lower, and the magnet's field of view is considerably smaller, requiring accurate patient positioning and rendering a slightly lower signal-to-noise ratio. Still, the *PoleStar* provides good quality visualization of contrast-enhancing tumors and fair quality for non-enhancing lesions [20, 30]. To our personal experience, image quality in high-grade gliomas is comparable in both systems, but image quality in low-grade gliomas is to some extent better when using the *Signa SP* [19].

Contrast enhancing gliomas are displayed best on T1-weighted imaging with application of contrast agent, while usually higher doses of contrast agent are recommended for optimal lesion-to-white-matter-contrast [31]. Several groups have experienced difficulties with visualizing the tumor margins on regular T2-weighted imaging in non-enhancing tumors with different low field MRI units – (fluid attenuated) inversion recovery (FLAIR) sequences were found to be superior in these cases [12, 30, 32].

Indications for ioMRI

Implementing neuronavigation was a major step towards an improved visualization of the surgical field. It aids in tailoring craniotomies and localizing subcortical lesions. Yet, the usefulness of neuronavigation is limited once the tumor resection has begun. Surgically induced edema, csf loss, and tumor resection itself lead to anatomical alterations, the so-called "brain-shift" [33]. Consequently, neuronavigation, as it is based on preoperative imaging data, is not reliable in terms of determining residual tumor tissue intraoperatively.

Therefore, ioMRI should be superior to neuronavigation in tumor resection with the aid of frameless neuronavigation: it enables the surgeon to update anatomical data intraoperatively. The intraoperative update of the neuronavigation system helps to precisely localize and target remaining tumor tissue [24, 30]. Bergsneider et al. [34] indicated the superiority of ioMRI versus neuronavigation when they found that a higher percentage of tumor resection was possible with low-field strength ioMRI guidance versus neuronavigation alone.

Hence, in order to update neuro-anatomical information intraoperatively, intraoperative imaging techniques such as MRI or ultrasound are mandatory. In this respect, ultrasonographic imaging is not only more difficult to interpret but might also impose severe limitations in regards of reliability of findings, even for experienced surgeons [35–37]. Consequently, intraoperative imaging in glioma surgery is the domain of MRI, allowing even for the incorporation of preoperatively acquired high-resolution datasets. As outlined above, image quality issues might restrict the reliability of ioMRI in non-contrast enhancing gliomas. Yet, no such limitations apply to ioMRI-guidance in enhancing lesions amenable to surgical resection.

Influence of ioMRI on the Course of Surgery

While intraoperative magnetic resonance imaging has evolved as a new technology in neurosurgery from the 1990s, first reports dealing with ioMRI systems focused primarily on the feasibility of their use. Until today, more than 800 glioma patients have reportedly undergone surgical resection with the aid of any low field strength ioMRI. With the increasing experience of applying these methods in the neurosurgical routine and the knowledge of their safety, the

Table 1 Studies reporting the use of low-field intraoperative MRI in low-grade gliomas with a minimum of ten patients

Author	Year	System used	No. of patients	Increased resection due to intraoperative imaging
Black et al.	1999	Signa SP	29	n.r.
Seifert et al.	1999	Signa SP	13	n.r.
Wirtz et al.	2000	Magnetom Open	29	45%
Zimmermann et al.	2000	Signa SP	16	n.r.
Bohinski et al.	2001	AIRIS II	10	40%
Zimmermann et al.	2001	Signa SP	11	n.r.
Buchfelder et al.	2002	Magnetom Open	11	14%
Nimsky et al.	2002	Magnetom Open	47	38%
Nimsky et al.	2003	Magnetom Open	52	40%
Schulder et al.	2003	PoleStar N-10	12	n.r.
Claus et al.	2005	Signa SP	156	n.r.
Nimsky et al.	2005	Magnetom Open	61	29%
Senft et al.	2008	PoleStar N-20	21[a]	47%

Abbreviations: n.r. not reported
[a]Non-enhancing gliomas

Table 2 Studies reporting the use of low-field intraoperative MRI in high-grade gliomas with a minimum of ten patients

Author	Year	System used	No. of patients	Increased resection due to intraoperative imaging
Tronnier et al.	1997	Magnetom Open	10	n.r.
Black et al.	1999	Signa SP	19	n.r.
Knauth et al.	1999	Magnetom Open	41	41%
Seifert et al.	1999	Signa SP	12	n.r.
Wirtz et al.	2000	Magnetom Open	68	63%
Zimmermann et al.	2000	Signa SP	16	n.r.
Bohinski et al.	2001	AIRIS II	30	56%
Zimmermann et al.	2001	Signa SP	14	n.r.
Nimsky et al.	2002	Magnetom Open	48	10%
Trantakis et al.	2003	Signa SP	68	n.r.
Nimsky et al.	2003	Magnetom Open	54	13%
Schulder et al.	2003	PoleStar N-10	25	n.r.
Bergsneider et al.	2005	Magnetom Open	10	n.r.
Hirschberg et al.	2005	Signa SP	32	52%
Schneider et al.	2005	Signa SP	31	71%
Senft et al.	2008	PoleStar N-20	42[a]	28%

Abbreviations: n.r. not reported
[a]Contrast-enhancing gliomas

influence of ioMRI on the surgical routine and clinical benefit of the patients has become more important.

In both, high- and low-grade glioma cases, all investigators who reported on the influence of intraoperative low field MRI on the course of surgery stated that intraoperative scanning had revealed residual tumor tissue in a significant number of cases. The percentage of patients with an extended resection after depiction of residual tumor-tissue on intraoperative images is reported to range between 14 and 75% (Table 1) [14, 15, 24, 30, 38–40]. Correspondingly, in high-grade glioma cases the respective figures are 10–71% (Table 2) [14, 15, 22, 24, 30, 40–42]. As a consequence, the rates of complete resection have increased by usually greater than 20% [43]. Evidently, the use of low field ioMRI has had a major influence on the course of surgery in a large number of patients.

Influence of ioMRI on Patient Outcome

In studies addressing postoperative morbidity, complication rates lay between 5 and 18% directly postoperatively in all but one series [15, 21, 27, 30, 32, 42, 44, 45], where an early complication rate of 53% in a group of 13 patients was observed [34]. Permanent deficits occurred in constantly less than 10% of the patients, which is comparable to the complication rates in conventional glioma surgery. In our own series of patients, an extended resection after ioMRI scans had revealed residual tumor did not correlate with postoperative morbidity [30]. To prevent patient injury and neurological deterioration due to overly aggressive resection, the use of ioMRI can also be combined with intraoperative monitoring techniques, such as motor or sensory evoked potentials during surgery, even when applied in the fringe field [46]. As a result, there are no obstacles to conclude that, after careful patient selection, surgical resection of gliomas can be increased to a maximum extent with acceptable risks for the patients, given the proven benefit of maximum resection.

Yet, only few studies have aimed to evaluate the influence of intraoperative low field MRI on the clinical course of glioma patients so far. As mentioned earlier, most studies have focused on the feasibility, safety, and influence on the course of surgery in the application of ioMRI in glioma surgery. In a large series of low-grade glioma patients, Claus et al. [2] found a trend towards prolonged survival of patients who had undergone total vs. subtotal resection in an ioMRI-environment. Similar findings were reported by Trantakis et al. [47] in patients with high-grade gliomas. Using two different low field systems, Wirtz et al. [40] and Schneider et al. [42] independently reported statistically significant prolonged survival times for high-grade glioma patients who had undergone total vs. subtotal tumor resection with the aid of ioMRI. These results add to the growing evidence that extent of resection translates into prolonged survival in glioma patients [4]. However, all theses studies did not compare patients treated under ioMRI-guidance with a control group of patients. Hirschberg et al. [41] presented the only matched group-analysis in a series of glioblastoma patients undergoing intraoperative low-field ioMRI-guided vs. standard microsurgery and found a trend in favor of ioMRI, but no statistically significant differences in overall survival between the groups. Therefore, the true benefit of ioMRI has not yet been proven, in contrast to other means of intraoperative resection control, e.g. administration of fluorescent porphyrins [5, 6]. Such studies are utterly needed today.

Comparison with High Field Systems

Even though the superiority of high field ioMRI systems over low field ioMRI systems seems obvious in terms of image resolution and quality, only few reports have specifically addressed this issue. While Nimsky et al. [39] described a clearly better image quality and a smoother workflow with a high field system, the rates of extended resection were comparable between the low and high field system, and Bergsneider et al. [34] found no difference in the extent of resection when comparing a low field vs. a high field ioMRI. High field systems might offer faster acquisition times and might allow for a greater variety of imaging sequences, but, as outlined before, low field systems, too, can provide the surgeon with reliable information about the extent of resection. To our own experience, this is definitely true at least for contrast enhancing, high-grade tumors. In non-enhancing, low-grade tumors, high field systems surely present an improved spatial resolution.

The question whether high and low field ioMRI differ in terms of patient benefit or clinical outcome remains nonetheless unanswered. This is a crucial concern, however, especially when looking at the setup and installation costs of the different available ioMRI systems. One distinct advantage of low field ioMRI systems over high field ones certainly is the possibility to perform intraoperative electrophysiological monitoring of eloquent function employing sensory or motor evoked potential with the patient being in the fringe field of the magnet without disturbances [46].

The Future of ioMRI in Glioma Surgery

Advances in technology have increasingly improved the precision of intracranial surgery, and ioMRI is the latest development in this field. The potential impact on the management of patients with brain tumors is obvious. The use of low field MRI scanners in glioma surgery is safe, reliable and most useful in assessing the extent of resection of intrinsic, infiltrating brain tumors whose boundaries cannot be clearly distinguished with the surgeon's eyes. While several retrospective analyses have documented the benefit of implementing ioMRI into the neurosurgical routine in glioma surgery by means of increasing the extent of resection, prospective randomized studies are still lacking that might prove the benefit of ioMRI compared to the standard microneurosurgical resection of brain tumors. Further, use of ioMRI itself has not been proven to prolong survival in patients with glial tumors. Although beneficial effects are suggested by previous studies, there is no high-class evidence to promote the use of ioMRI today, and pursuant studies are needed.

One clear advantage over the administration of fluorescent porphyrins to visualize tumor tissue intraoperatively is the usability of ioMRI also in low-grade gliomas on the one hand, and the implementation of functional anatomical data on the other. In the future, not only pre-operative functional MRI datasets might be incorporated into neuronavigation, but also intraoperative diffusion weighted imaging to depict white matter tracts seems feasible in both, high field and low field ioMRI systems [48–50].

Conclusions

For obvious reasons, glioma patients will not be cured by neurosurgical intervention. Additional treatment modalities are and will remain mandatory to prolong survival and to maintain quality of life for these patients. However, maximum tumor resection without induction of disabling neurological deficits appears to be one of the strongest predictive factors. Therefore, the neurosurgeon's abilities and the advances of modern aides such as ioMRI will certainly translate into benefit for our patients. In this respect, upcoming studies will yet have to demonstrate the true value of ioMRI.

Conflict of interest statement T. Gasser serves as a clinical consultant to Medtronic, but the company provided no payment or any other benefits with respect to this work. V. Seifert and C. Senft declare to have no potentially conflicting interests.

References

1. Bennett AH, Godlee RJ (1974) A case of cerebral tumor – the surgical treatment. CA Cancer J Clin 24:171–181 (excerpt from Trans R Med Chir Soc Lond 168:243–275, 1885)
2. Claus EB, Horlacher A, Hsu L, Schwartz RB, Dello-Iacono D, Talos F, Jolesz FA, Black PM (2005) Survival rates in patients with

low-grade glioma after intraoperative magnetic resonance image guidance. Cancer 103:1227–1233
3. McGirt MJ, Chaichana KL, Gathinji M, Attenello FJ, Than K, Olivi A, Weingart JD, Brem H, Quinones-Hinojosa A (2009) Independent association of extent of resection with survival in patients with malignant brain astrocytoma. J Neurosurg 110:156–162
4. Sanai N, Berger MS (2008) Glioma extent of resection and its impact on patient outcome. Neurosurgery 62:753–764, discussion 264–756
5. Stummer W, Pichlmeier U, Meinel T, Wiestler OD, Zanella F, Reulen HJ (2006) Fluorescence-guided surgery with 5-aminolevulinic acid for resection of malignant glioma: a randomised controlled multicentre phase III trial. Lancet Oncol 7:392–401
6. Stummer W, Reulen HJ, Meinel T, Pichlmeier U, Schumacher W, Tonn JC, Rohde V, Oppel F, Turowski B, Woiciechowsky C, Franz K, Pietsch T (2008) Extent of resection and survival in glioblastoma multiforme: identification of and adjustment for bias. Neurosurgery 62:564–576, discussion 564–576
7. Albert FK, Forsting M, Sartor K, Adams HP, Kunze S (1994) Early postoperative magnetic resonance imaging after resection of malignant glioma: objective evaluation of residual tumor and its influence on regrowth and prognosis. Neurosurgery 34:45–60, discussion 60–61
8. Bernays RL, Kollias SS, Khan N, Brandner S, Meier S, Yonekawa Y (2002) Histological yield, complications, and technological considerations in 114 consecutive frameless stereotactic biopsy procedures aided by open intraoperative magnetic resonance imaging. J Neurosurg 97:354–362
9. Hall WA, Liu H, Martin AJ, Truwit CL (2000) Intraoperative magnetic resonance imaging. Top Magn Reson Imaging 11: 203–212
10. Senft C, Seifert V, Hermann E, Gasser T (2009) Surgical treatment of cerebral abscess with the use of a mobile ultralow-field MRI. Neurosurg Rev 32:77–85
11. Black PM, Moriarty T, Alexander E 3rd, Stieg P, Woodard EJ, Gleason PL, Martin CH, Kikinis R, Schwartz RB, Jolesz FA (1997) Development and implementation of intraoperative magnetic resonance imaging and its neurosurgical applications. Neurosurgery 41:831–842, discussion 842–845
12. Seifert V, Zimmermann M, Trantakis C, Vitzthum HE, Kuhnel K, Raabe A, Bootz F, Schneider JP, Schmidt F, Dietrich J (1999) Open MRI-guided neurosurgery. Acta Neurochir (Wien) 141: 455–464
13. Tronnier VM, Wirtz CR, Knauth M, Lenz G, Pastyr O, Bonsanto MM, Albert FK, Kuth R, Staubert A, Schlegel W, Sartor K, Kunze S (1997) Intraoperative diagnostic and interventional magnetic resonance imaging in neurosurgery. Neurosurgery 40:891–900, discussion 900–902
14. Wirtz CR, Bonsanto MM, Knauth M, Tronnier VM, Albert FK, Staubert A, Kunze S (1997) Intraoperative magnetic resonance imaging to update interactive navigation in neurosurgery: method and preliminary experience. Comput Aided Surg 2:172–179
15. Bohinski RJ, Kokkino AK, Warnick RE, Gaskill-Shipley MF, Kormos DW, Lukin RR, Tew JM Jr (2001) Glioma resection in a shared-resource magnetic resonance operating room after optimal image-guided frameless stereotactic resection. Neurosurgery 48:731–742, discussion 742–744
16. Muragaki Y, Iseki H, Maruyama T, Kawamata T, Yamane F, Nakamura R, Kubo O, Takakura K, Hori T (2006) Usefulness of intraoperative magnetic resonance imaging for glioma surgery. Acta Neurochir Suppl 98:67–75
17. Hadani M, Spiegelman R, Feldman Z, Berkenstadt H, Ram Z (2001) Novel, compact, intraoperative magnetic resonance imaging-guided system for conventional neurosurgical operating rooms. Neurosurgery 48:799–807, discussion 807–809
18. Schulder M, Salas S, Brimacombe M, Fine P, Catrambone J, Maniker AH, Carmel PW (2006) Cranial surgery with an expanded compact intraoperative magnetic resonance imager. Technical note. J Neurosurg 104:611–617
19. Ntoukas V, Krishnan R, Seifert V (2008) The new generation polestar n20 for conventional neurosurgical operating rooms: a preliminary report. Neurosurgery 62:82–89, discussion 89–90
20. Schulder M, Carmel PW (2003) Intraoperative magnetic resonance imaging: impact on brain tumor surgery. Cancer Control 10: 115–124
21. Black PM, Alexander E 3rd, Martin C, Moriarty T, Nabavi A, Wong TZ, Schwartz RB, Jolesz F (1999) Craniotomy for tumor treatment in an intraoperative magnetic resonance imaging unit. Neurosurgery 45:423–431, discussion 431–433
22. Knauth M, Wirtz CR, Tronnier VM, Aras N, Kunze S, Sartor K (1999) Intraoperative MR imaging increases the extent of tumor resection in patients with high-grade gliomas. AJNR Am J Neuroradiol 20:1642–1646
23. Metzger AK, Lewin JS (2001) Optimizing brain tumor resection. Low-field interventional MR imaging. Neuroimaging Clin N Am 11:651–657, ix
24. Nimsky C, Ganslandt O, Tomandl B, Buchfelder M, Fahlbusch R (2002) Low-field magnetic resonance imaging for intraoperative use in neurosurgery: a 5-year experience. Eur Radiol 12: 2690–2703
25. Ram Z, Hadani M (2003) Intraoperative imaging – MRI. Acta Neurochir Suppl 88:1–4
26. Schulder M, Sernas TJ, Carmel PW (2003) Cranial surgery and navigation with a compact intraoperative MRI system. Acta Neurochir Suppl 85:79–86
27. Zimmermann M, Seifert V, Trantakis C, Kuhnel K, Raabe A, Schneider JP, Dietrich J, Schmidt F (2000) Open MRI-guided microsurgery of intracranial tumours. Preliminary experience using a vertical open MRI-scanner. Acta Neurochir (Wien) 142: 177–186
28. Hinks RS, Bronskill MJ, Kucharczyk W, Bernstein M, Collick BD, Henkelman RM (1998) MR systems for image-guided therapy. J Magn Reson Imaging 8:19–25
29. Lewin JS (1999) Interventional MR imaging: concepts, systems, and applications in neuroradiology. AJNR Am J Neuroradiol 20:735–748
30. Senft C, Seifert V, Hermann E, Franz K, Gasser T (2008) Usefulness of intraoperative ultralow-field magnetic resonance imaging in glioma surgery. Neurosurgery 63:257–266, discussion 266–267
31. Knauth M, Wirtz CR, Aras N, Sartor K (2001) Low-field interventional MRI in neurosurgery: finding the right dose of contrast medium. Neuroradiology 43:254–258
32. Nimsky C, Ganslandt O, Buchfelder M, Fahlbusch R (2003) Glioma surgery evaluated by intraoperative low-field magnetic resonance imaging. Acta Neurochir Suppl 85:55–63
33. Roberts DW, Hartov A, Kennedy FE, Miga MI, Paulsen KD (1998) Intraoperative brain shift and deformation: a quantitative analysis of cortical displacement in 28 cases. Neurosurgery 43:749–758, discussion 758–760
34. Bergsneider M, Sehati N, Villablanca P, McArthur DL, Becker DP, Liau LM (2005) Mahaley Clinical Research Award: extent of glioma resection using low-field (0.2 T) versus high-field (1.5 T) intraoperative MRI and image-guided frameless neuronavigation. Clin Neurosurg 52:389–399
35. Erdogan N, Tucer B, Mavili E, Menku A, Kurtsoy A (2005) Ultrasound guidance in intracranial tumor resection: correlation with postoperative magnetic resonance findings. Acta Radiol 46:743–749
36. Rygh OM, Selbekk T, Torp SH, Lydersen S, Hernes TA, Unsgaard G (2008) Comparison of navigated 3D ultrasound findings with

histopathology in subsequent phases of glioblastoma resection. Acta Neurochir (Wien) 150:1031–1044

37. Tronnier VM, Bonsanto MM, Staubert A, Knauth M, Kunze S, Wirtz CR (2001) Comparison of intraoperative MR imaging and 3D-navigated ultrasonography in the detection and resection control of lesions. Neurosurg Focus 10:E3
38. Buchfelder M, Fahlbusch R, Ganslandt O, Stefan H, Nimsky C (2002) Use of intraoperative magnetic resonance imaging in tailored temporal lobe surgeries for epilepsy. Epilepsia 43:864–873
39. Nimsky C, Ganslandt O, Fahlbusch R (2005) Comparing 0.2 tesla with 1.5 tesla intraoperative magnetic resonance imaging analysis of setup, workflow, and efficiency. Acad Radiol 12:1065–1079
40. Wirtz CR, Knauth M, Staubert A, Bonsanto MM, Sartor K, Kunze S, Tronnier VM (2000) Clinical evaluation and follow-up results for intraoperative magnetic resonance imaging in neurosurgery. Neurosurgery 46:1112–1120, discussion 1120–1122
41. Hirschberg H, Samset E, Hol PK, Tillung T, Lote K (2005) Impact of intraoperative MRI on the surgical results for high-grade gliomas. Minim Invasive Neurosurg 48:77–84
42. Schneider JP, Trantakis C, Rubach M, Schulz T, Dietrich J, Winkler D, Renner C, Schober R, Geiger K, Brosteanu O, Zimmer C, Kahn T (2005) Intraoperative MRI to guide the resection of primary supratentorial glioblastoma multiforme – a quantitative radiological analysis. Neuroradiology 47:489–500
43. Oh DS, Black PM (2005) A low-field intraoperative MRI system for glioma surgery: is it worthwhile? Neurosurg Clin N Am 16:135–141
44. Bernstein M, Al-Anazi AR, Kucharczyk W, Manninen P, Bronskill M, Henkelman M (2000) Brain tumor surgery with the Toronto open magnetic resonance imaging system: preliminary results for 36 patients and analysis of advantages, disadvantages, and future prospects. Neurosurgery 46:900–907, discussion 907–909
45. Zimmermann M, Seifert V, Trantakis C, Raabe A (2001) Open MRI-guided microsurgery of intracranial tumours in or near eloquent brain areas. Acta Neurochir (Wien) 143:327–337
46. Szelenyi A, Gasser T, Seifert V (2008) Intraoperative neurophysiological monitoring in an open low-field magnetic resonance imaging system: clinical experience and technical considerations. Neurosurgery 63:268–275, discussion 275–276
47. Trantakis C, Winkler D, Lindner D, Strauss G, Nagel C, Schneider JP, Meixensberger J (2003) Clinical results in MR-guided therapy for malignant gliomas. Acta Neurochir Suppl 85:65–71
48. Nimsky C, Ganslandt O, Hastreiter P, Wang R, Benner T, Sorensen AG, Fahlbusch R (2007) Preoperative and intraoperative diffusion tensor imaging-based fiber tracking in glioma surgery. Neurosurgery 61:178–185, discussion 186
49. Ozawa N, Muragaki Y, Nakamura R, Lseki H (2008) Intraoperative diffusion-weighted imaging for visualization of the pyramidal tracts. Part II: clinical study of usefulness and efficacy. Minim Invasive Neurosurg 51:67–71
50. Schulder M, Azmi H, Biswal B (2003) Functional magnetic resonance imaging in a low-field intraoperative scanner. Stereotact Funct Neurosurg 80:125–131

Intraoperative MRI (ioMRI) in the Setting of Awake Craniotomies for Supratentorial Glioma Resection

Pierpaolo Peruzzi, Erika Puente, Sergio Bergese, and E. Antonio Chiocca

Abstract Both awake craniotomy under conscious sedation and use of intraoperative MRI can increase the efficiency and safety of glioma resections. In contrast to craniotomies under general anesthesia, neurosurgery under conscious sedation requires several changes to the routine operative setup when performed in the ioMRI environment. This work reports our experience with awake craniotomies under conscious sedation using ioMRI.

Seven patients underwent awake-craniotomies for resection of supratentorial gliomas using ioMRI at the Ohio State University Medical Center and James Cancer Hospital by a single surgeon.

ioMRI can be safely employed in patients who are undergoing craniotomies under conscious sedation. Particularly important is the evaluation by the anesthesiologist whether the patient is a good candidate to sustain a likely longer than average procedure in a setting where his active cooperation is not only required, but also the essential aspect of this procedure.

Keywords Conscious sedation · Craniotomy · Glioma · Intraoperative MRI

Abbreviation

ioMRI intraoperative Magnetic Resonance Imaging

P. Peruzzi and E.A. Chiocca (✉)
Department of Neurological Surgery, The Ohio State University College of Medicine and James Cancer Hospital, N-1017 Doan Hall, 410 West Tenth Avenue, Columbus, OH, 43210, USA
e-mail: EA.Chiocca@osumc.edu

E. Puente and S. Bergese
Department of Anesthesiology, The Ohio State University College of Medicine and James Cancer Hospital, Columbus, OH, USA

After its initial introduction in 1994 at Brigham and Women's Hospital in Boston, intraoperative MRI (ioMRI) is being increasingly accepted as an adjunct in the surgical treatment of cerebral gliomas [1–3]. One of the rationales for its implementation in neuro-oncologic surgery derives from increasing evidence that extent of tumor resection correlates positively with survival [4–7]. Consequently, the ability to determine in the operating room if and how much tumor has been left behind, allows the surgeon to decide whether to abstain from or continue with further resection.

Moreover, recent publications have discussed the ability of this technology to aid in neuronavigation and reduce the error associated with intraoperative brain shift [8–10].

Data are scarce on the use of ioMRI in the subpopulation of patients harboring lesions located in eloquent areas that undergo surgery under conscious sedation. In comparison to craniotomies under general anesthesia, some may view the management of the awake patient during the scanning procedure as challenging. For some ioMRI solutions, such as the PoleStar (Medtronic, Inc., Minneapolis, MN), the patients is inside a Faraday copper-wire tent during the scan and thus visibility of the patient under conscious sedation is curtailed. Even with high-strength ioMRIs, the patient's face is hidden from view and thus lack of its visibility could be an issue in ensuring that adequate ventilation and patient comfort are not being affected.

We thus analyzed retrospectively whether we could perform ioMRI in patients undergoing surgical resections of gliomas under conscious sedation (CS). Over a total of 40 patients who underwent craniotomy under CS for resection of supratentorial gliomas we identified 7 cases (17%) where ioMRI was performed. The time frame of the analysis was from January 2005 to June 2009 and all cases were performed at the Ohio State University Medical Center and James Cancer Hospital by a single surgeon (EAC).

Here we describe three such cases with the aim of providing practical insights on the use of ioMRI in the consciously sedated patient undergoing glioma resections in eloquent areas.

M.N. Pamir et al. (eds.), *Intraoperative Imaging*, Acta Neurochirurgica Supplementum, Vol. 109,
DOI 10.1007/978-3-211-99651-5_7, © Springer-Verlag/Wien 2011

Case Reports

Case 1

This 40-year old right-handed male, in otherwise good health, presented to the emergency room (ER) with the first time occurrence of a generalized tonic-clonic (GTC) seizure. Brain Magnetic Resonance Imaging (MRI) showed a non enhancing right frontal lesion in proximity to the primary motor area. His neurologic exam, upon resolution of the ictal period, was unremarkable. The imaging features suggested a low grade glioma, primarily confined within gyri in the premotor strip and it was thus decided to try and attempt a radical resection under CS.

After conscious sedation was obtained with diprivan and dexmedetomidine in the operating room, a baseline ioMRI scan was obtained (Fig. 1, Ia). Thereafter, a right frontal craniotomy was performed and once the brain was exposed, cortical stimulation was used to localize motor cortex. As expected from the preoperative MRI, the motor cortex was localized in the gyrus posterior to the one that contained the lesion. Tumor debulking proceeded uneventfully testing the patient in the performance of requested motor and speech tasks. When the operating surgeon estimated that gross total resection of the tumor had occurred, another ioMRI was obtained. Additional diprivan was administered to sedate the patient and then the copper-wired tent (Starshield, Medtronic, Inc.) was placed on top and around the patient. After scanning for a period of approximately 16 min (T2 axial and FLAIR axial, 7 and 9 min each), the ioMRI suggested a gross total resection (Fig. 1, Ib) and no further removal was pursued. Importantly, the scanning process was well tolerated by the patient and no technical difficulties were encountered.

Postoperatively the patient had a slight decrease in strength in his left upper extremity, in the order of 5-/5 (Medical Research Council, MRC scale). However, this did not impair his functional status. A postoperative MRI performed within 24 h after surgery confirmed gross total resection of the tumor (Fig. 1, Ic–Id). The patient was discharged to home in stable conditions on postoperative

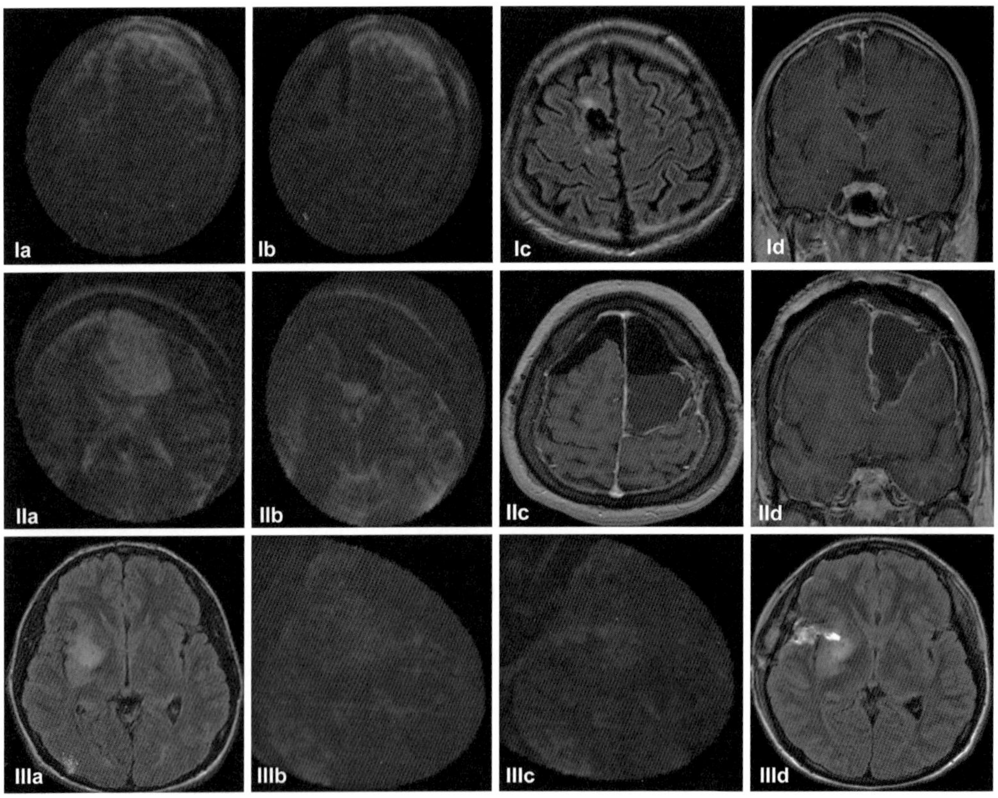

Fig. 1 *Upper row*: T2-weighted ioMR imaging obtained prior to tumor resection shows hyperintense signal in the right frontal lobe (Ia). Repeated scan after resection shows surgical cavity and removal of lesion (Ib), as confirmed by postoperative MRI, respectively axial FLAIR (Ic) and coronal T1-weighted with contrast (Id). *Middle row*: pre-resection ioMRI shows a large left frontal lesion hyperintense in T2-weighted sequences (IIa). Follow-up intraoperative scan shows residual tumor as a hyperintense area in the posteromedial part of the surgical cavity (IIb) which was thereafter addressed. Postoperative axial (IIc) and coronal (IId) T1-weighted images with constrast show gross total tumor resection. *Lower row*: Preoperative MRI is significant for a large left frontotemporal lesion (IIIa) with areas of contrast enhancement (IIIb). Postoperative imaging shows large surgical cavity without evidence of residual tumor (IIIc–IIId). In this case ioMRI was not obtained because of technical difficulties

day 4 with a diagnosis of WHO grade 2 oligodendroglioma, for which he subsequently received chemotherapy with temozolomide, and is currently neurologically stable 18 months after surgery without clinical or radiological evidence of tumor progression.

Case 2

This 44-year old right-handed female with a history of a left frontal WHO grade 2 oligoastrocytoma, partially resected 8 and 4 years prior to the current admission, was referred to our institution with increased frequency of seizure activity, manifesting as a right sided jacksonian progression, mainly involving her lower extremity. Her most recent brain MRI was consistent with tumor recurrence at the site of her left motor area and suggestive of likely malignant progression. Since it was felt that histological analysis would be necessary to guide further treatment and to improve seizure control, a re-resection of her recurrent lesion was attempted.

Once in the operating room, conscious sedation was induced using diprivan and dexmedetomidine and then a baseline ioMRI was obtained inside the copper-wire tent (Fig. 1, IIa). Cortical mapping for speech and motor cortex was performed with an Ojemann stimulator. During the surgical resection of the tumor, the patient was also periodically asked to move her right side and to talk with a speech pathologist present in the room. Once the lesion was judged to have been removed in a gross total fashion, a second ioMRI was obtained. This showed some residual tumor in the most medial part of the hemisphere, along the falx (Fig. 1, IIb). Further resection was then performed until the tumor was judged to have been resected in a gross total fashion.

In this second phase of the resection, the patient did not show intraoperative signs of neurological impairment. She was able to tolerate ioMRI well and no technical difficulties ensued. Postoperative MRI corroborated the preliminary findings of the gross total resection (Fig. 1, IIc–IId); Histologic evaluation upgraded her tumor to oligoastrocytoma with isolated areas of anaplastic progression.

Postoperatively, however, her neurological status was overall worsened as compared to her preoperative function, with new severe right sided weakness and impairment of fine motor skills most consistent with a supplementary motor area (SMA) syndrome. Eventually she needed 2 weeks of inpatient rehabilitation before being able to be discharged to home and to date, 6 months after surgery, she has recovered most of her motor functions and functional independence, seizure activity has been well controlled since surgery and she is still tumor free.

Case 3

This 18-year old left-handed male was referred to our clinics to be evaluated for a newly discovered FLAIR-hyperintense abnormality involving his right insular region (Fig. 1, IIIa), highly suspiscious for a low grade glioma. Apart from headaches he was neurologically asymptomatic. Surgical removal of the lesion was recommended both for diagnostic and prognostic purposes, and craniotomy under conscious sedation was planned in order to minimize surgical morbidity. Once in the operating room, after sedation was achieved, an initial ioMRI was obtained for baseline (Fig. 1, IIIb). The initial part of the craniotomy was uneventful, but when the patient was allowed to regain consciousness in order to proceed with the cortical mapping and tumor removal, he became progressively agitated and restless, to the point that induction of general anesthesia was necessary. It was decided, however, to continue with resection and the tumor was debulked until no clear neoplastic tissue was evident under the microscope. However, a frozen section of the cavity margin showed presence of scattered atypical cells dispersed within normal white matter. At this point an ioMRI was obtained, showing residual T2 hyperintensity in the more medial aspect of the tumor (Fig. 1, IIIc). Further resection was then attempted, but shortly thereafter perforating vessels feeding the basal ganglia were encountered and we desisted from further resection. Postoperatively, his neurological status remained intact. MR imaging showed a subtotal resection of the tumor mass, confirming the persistence of the medial and posterior portion of the lesion (Fig. 1, IIId). The patient was discharged to home 2 days after surgery with a final diagnosis of low grade astrocytoma.

Discussion

In the past few decades, improvements in the treatment of many neurological diseases have been tied to technological advances. Specifically, for the treatment of gliomas the introduction of intraoperative MRI, together with the use of stereotactic navigation, can be useful adjuncts to achieve the therapeutic goal of gross total resection. In fact, the extent of tumor removal appears to influence disease progression with numerous reports showing that the incidence of tumor recurrence and malignant transformation of low grade gliomas are significantly reduced [7, 8, 11, 12], while extended survival is achieved for higher grade lesions [5, 6]. In 40–70% of patients, the adjunct of ioMRI has been reported to lead to discovery of residual tumor [2, 13–15], with a greater than 20% increase in cases of total tumor resection [13, 16–18]. This advantage seems to be more prominent for low grade gliomas compared to high grade gliomas which often have signs of necrosis or grossly abnormal appearance [16, 18]. The predictive value of ioMRI for reliable detection of tumor residues has been validated even with the low-field strength units. Hirschl et al. have recently shown a 82% concordance between intraoperative and post-operative imaging; more importantly, they reported "false positive" results, i.e. residual tumor detected by intraoperative images while not identified in postoperative standard MR images, only in 1% of cases [10]. The question remains whether ioMRi should be applied to all craniotomies for glioma resection or if it should be dedicated only to selected cases. In our experience, we reserve ioMRI use for low grade tumors since its more normal appearance can escape intraoperative detection.

With lesions involving eloquent areas, ioMRI can also be performed with patients undergoing "awake" craniotomies. Little data is available in the literature reporting results of the combination of the two procedures. In their description of a series of 25 patients who underwent ioMRI for resection of low grade gliomas, Martin et al. included at least five patients (the exact number is not specified by the authors) who, in addition to intraoperative imaging were operated under conscious sedation because of the location of their lesions. In these five patients, despite the evidence of tumor remnant at ioMRI, total resection could not be achieved because of the onset of changes in neurological functions, and four experienced mild transient deficits in the immediate postoperative period, while the other one suffered a permanent left-sided paresis [7].

Another such case is reported by Tan and Leong, where a middle aged woman was diagnosed with a low grade glioma which was completely resected without major complications. The authors, though, stress the fact that the procedure was unduly lengthy because of the multiple intraoperative scans, leading to patient exhaustion during the procedure [19].

Awake craniotomies in the context of ioMRI were reported in 38 cases performed from 2005 to 2008 at the university of Kiel, Germany, where the authors mainly stressed the "emotional" aspect of the procedure, concluding that, despite being physically and psychologically demanding for the patients, it was overall well tolerated, leading them to adopt a standard approach by which all awake craniotomies for gliomas in their institution are performed with ioMRI implementation [20].

The role of the anesthesiologist is crucial both preoperatively, when it comes to determine if each single patient is a suitable candidate, medically and emotionally, for this stressful procedure, and, intraoperatively, with regards of maintaining an appropriate level of anesthesia and analgesia compatible with the need of the neurosurgeon to have the patient able to talk and to follow commands.

The main challenge for the anesthesiologist in awake craniotomy procedures is to provide adequate sedation and analgesia during the different stages of the procedure [21, 22]. The primary goal is to keep the patient awake and alert during brain mapping, allowing for full cooperation, while providing sufficient, safe and effective analgesia and guaranteeing comfort to the patient. It is paramount that the anesthesiologist evaluate patients who may benefit from this procedure thoroughly, since some patients may not be ideal candidates to undergo awake procedures. During this phase, the assessment of the patients' level of comfort and cooperation with the described procedure is made. Also, possible contraindications to the procedure, like esophageal reflux, obesity and large vascular tumors are ruled out. Patients should be counseled before the surgery and optimally have the opportunity to interact with other patients that have gone through this procedure. We have observed that sometimes the awake technique in patients of younger age, like the one reported in our Case 3, and generally those with higher sympathetic tone is not successful. In our case, several attempts where made to adjust the anesthetic regimen, such as, increasing the level of α-2 agonists (dexedetomidine) and decreasing GABA receptor agonist drugs (like propofol or midazolam) with the intention of obtaining a higher degree of cooperation. However, in this patient, the fine balance between an adequate level of sedation and good cooperation was lost, and that resulted in oversedation with resultant loss of a meaningful cooperation. In general, when such situations happen, after discussing with the surgeons, it usually becomes necessary to convert to conventional general anesthesia techniques to achieve proper anesthesia levels.

The most popular techniques that are utilized are based on a combination of general anesthesia and an awake technique, better known as "asleep awake asleep" technique (AAA). This technique places patients' under general anesthesia before and after brain mapping. Therefore, it consists of an initial phase of general anesthesia, followed by an intraoperative awakening phase and finally, back to general anesthesia [23, 24]. The recent introduction of dexmedetomidine, a highly selective α2-agonist, with dose-dependent sedative, anxyolitic, and analgesic effects has provided an alternative to sedation that decreases respiratory suppression and reduces opioid administration. Dexmedetomidine allows minimal sedation, resulting in an awake and cooperative state that enables patient's to feel the effect of sedation and at the same time respond to cognitive tests, necessary to assess specific functions that may be impaired during tumor resection. The addition of ioMRI to awake craniotomy increases the complexity of the whole procedure for several aspects. The space constriction and the noise which the patient is subjected to during the scanning phase may not be well tolerated and may require anesthesia adjustments, increasing the Awake-Asleep phases needed throughout the case. Moreover, during the time the patient is inside of the Faraday cage, within the bore of the scanner, he will not be under the direct supervision or visibility of the anesthesiologist for the duration of the scan. During this period, it is essential to provide continuous ventilatory support, provide special attention to IV lines, drugs or contrast media infusions and inhalation anesthetics, and constantly supervise monitoring devices, in compliance with the American Society of Anesthesiologists (ASA) guidelines.

Due to the difficulties in monitoring and limited access to the patient, while in the cage, complications should be expected such as, inadequate or excessive sedation, pain, nausea or vomiting; airway management difficulties or obstruction, decrease in oxygen saturation, below 90%, hypoventilation, below 8 bpm, hemodynamic instability and new neurological symptoms and signs [13].

No statistically relevant data can be inferred from our experience of using ioMRI in the setting of awake craniotomies. However, we believe that our case series is representative of some of the most common situations encountered in the operating room and give us the opportunity to discuss our approach to this complex operative setting. Case 1 describes a situation where the ioMRI is mainly used as a confirmatory test of gross total resection. In our experience, the decision to use ioMRI is usually made "a priori", particularly in an awake case, since we believe that the approach of "scanning everybody whenever possible", like other authors suggest [20, 25], is not necessary. Instead, the decision of performing ioMRI should be dictated by different variables, like tumor location, radiological aspect, size, and surgical accessibility to the tumor. Case 2 portrays a situation where ioMRI proved valuable in determining surgeon's decision to carry on with tumor resection, eventually helping to achieve a gross total resection. This is the situation where a fine balance between extent of resection and preservation of neurological function has to be maintained. Our patient did experience some postoperative deficits despite a substantially uneventful procedure, as it has been described multiple times in the setting of awake craniotomies and most commonly secondary to postoperative brain swelling or postoperative regional ischemia [26] but these resolved on postoperative followup.

Lastly, our case 3 reminds how a balance between proper sedation and ability to raise consciousness needs to be achieved or else patients will suffer undue agitation, particularly as they awaken, leading to inability to implement the preoperative plan of action.

Conclusion

ioMRI can be safely employed in patients who are undergoing craniotomies under conscious sedation. Particularly important, in this setting, is the evaluation by the anesthesiologist whether the patient is a good candidate to sustain a likely longer than average procedure in a setting where his active cooperation is not only required, but also the essential aspect of this procedure.

Conflict of interest statement We declare that we have no conflict of interest.

References

1. Black PM, Moriarty T, Alexander ER, Stieg P, Woodard EJ, Gleason PL, Martin CH, Kikinis R, Schwartz RB, Jolesz FA (1997) Development and implementation of intraoperative magnetic resonance imaging and its neurosurgical applications. Neurosurgery 41:831–842, discussion 842–845
2. Maesawa S, Fujii M, Nakahara N, Watanabe T, Saito K, Kajita Y, Nagatani T, Wakabayashi T, Yoshida J (2009) Clinical indications for high-field 1.5 T intraoperative magnetic resonance imaging and neuro-navigation for neurosurgical procedures. Review of initial 100 cases. Neurol Med Chir (Tokyo) 49:340–349, discussion 349–350
3. Schwartz RB, Hsu L, Wong TZ, Kacher DF, Zamani AA, Black PM, Alexander ER, Stieg PE, Moriarty TM, Martin CA, Kikinis R, Jolesz FA (1999) Intraoperative MR imaging guidance for intracranial neurosurgery: experience with the first 200 cases. Radiology 211:477–488
4. Albert FK, Forsting M, Sartor K, Adams HP, Kunze S (1994) Early postoperative magnetic resonance imaging after resection of malignant glioma: objective evaluation of residual tumor and its influence on regrowth and prognosis. Neurosurgery 34:45–60, discussion 60–61
5. Hess KR (1999) Extent of resection as a prognostic variable in the treatment of gliomas. J Neurooncol 42:227–231
6. Lacroix M, Abi-Said D, Fourney DR, Gokaslan ZL, Shi W, DeMonte F, Lang FF, McCutcheon IE, Hassenbusch SJ, Holland E, Hess K, Michael C, Miller D, Sawaya R (2001) A multivariate analysis of 416 patients with glioblastoma multiforme: prognosis, extent of resection, and survival. J Neurosurg 95:190–198
7. Martin C, Alexander ER, Wong T, Schwartz R, Jolesz F, Black PM (1998) Surgical treatment of low-grade gliomas in the intraoperative magnetic resonance imager. Neurosurg Focus 4:e8
8. Hall WA, Kowalik K, Liu H, Truwit CL, Kucharezyk J (2003) Costs and benefits of intraoperative MR-guided brain tumor resection. Acta Neurochir Suppl 85:137–142
9. Hall WA, Liu H, Maxwell RE, Truwit CL (2003) Influence of 1.5-Tesla intraoperative MR imaging on surgical decision making. Acta Neurochir Suppl 85:29–37
10. Hirschl RA, Wilson J, Miller B, Bergese S, Chiocca EA (2009) The predictive value of low-field strength magnetic resonance imaging for intraoperative residual tumor detection. Clinical article. J Neurosurg 111:252–257
11. Albert FK, Forsting M (2003) Resection and prognosis. J Neurosurg 98:225–226, author reply 226

12. Berger MS, Deliganis AV, Dobbins J, Keles GE (1994) The effect of extent of resection on recurrence in patients with low grade cerebral hemisphere gliomas. Cancer 74:1784–1791
13. Senft C, Seifert V, Hermann E, Franz K, Gasser T (2008) Usefulness of intraoperative ultra low-field magnetic resonance imaging in glioma surgery. Neurosurgery 63:257–266, discussion 266–267
14. Staubert A, Pastyr O, Echner G, Oppelt A, Vetter T, Schlegel W, Bonsanto MM, Tronnier VM, Kunze S, Wirtz CR (2000) An integrated head-holder/coil for intraoperative MRI in open neurosurgery. J Magn Reson Imaging 11:564–567
15. Wirtz CR, Tronnier VM, Bonsanto MM, Knauth M, Staubert A, Albert FK, Kunze S (1997) Image-guided neurosurgery with intraoperative MRI: update of frameless stereotaxy and radicality control. Stereotact Funct Neurosurg 68:39–43
16. Nimsky C, Ganslandt O, Tomandl B, Buchfelder M, Fahlbusch R (2002) Low-field magnetic resonance imaging for intraoperative use in neurosurgery: a 5-year experience. Eur Radiol 12:2690–2703
17. Oh DS, Black PM (2005) A low-field intraoperative MRI system for glioma surgery: is it worthwhile? Neurosurg Clin N Am 16:135–141
18. Schulder M, Carmel PW (2003) Intraoperative magnetic resonance imaging: impact on brain tumor surgery. Cancer Control 10:115–124
19. Tan TK, Leong KW (2009) Awake craniotomy in an intraoperative MRI environment. Anaesthesia 64:575–576
20. Nabavi A, Goebel S, Doerner L, Warneke N, Ulmer S, Mehdorn M (2009) Awake craniotomy and intraoperative magnetic resonance imaging: patient selection, preparation, and technique. Top Magn Reson Imaging 19:191–196
21. Bergese SD, Puente EG (2009) Anesthesia in the intraoperative MRI environment. Neurosurg Clin N Am 20:155–162
22. Zorzi F, Saltarini M, Bonasin P (2008) Anesthetic management in awake craniotomy. Signa vitae 3:28–32
23. Conte V, Baratta P, Tomaselli P, Songa V, Magni L, Stocchetti N (2008) Awake neurosurgery: an update. Minerva Anestesiol 74:289–292
24. Piccioni F, Fanzio M (2008) Management of anesthesia in awake craniotomy. Minerva Anestesiol 74:393–408
25. Whittle IR, Borthwick S, Haq N (2003) Brain dysfunction following 'awake' craniotomy, brain mapping and resection of glioma. Br J Neurosurg 17:130–137
26. Duffau H, Lopes M, Denvil D, Capelle L (2001) Delayed onset of the supplementary motor area syndrome after surgical resection of the mesial frontal lobe: a time course study using intraoperative mapping in an awake patient. Stereotact Funct Neurosurg 76:74–82

Glioma Extent of Resection and Ultra-Low-Field ioMRI: Interim Analysis of a Prospective Randomized Trial

Christian Senft, Andrea Bink, Michael Heckelmann, Thomas Gasser, and Volker Seifert

Abstract Aiming at providing high-class evidence regarding the use of intraoperative MRI (ioMRI), we are conducting a prospective randomized controlled trial. Adult patients with contrast enhancing lesions suspicious of malignant gliomas scheduled to undergo radiologically complete tumor resection are eligible to enter this trial. After giving their informed consent, patients are randomized to undergo either ioMRI-guided or conventional microneurosurgical tumor resection. To assess the extent of resection, pre- and early postoperative high-field MR images are obtained to perform volumetric analyses. Primary endpoint of the study is the rate of radiologically complete tumor resections. After the inclusion of 35 patients, we performed an interim analysis. In six patients, histopathological examination revealed metastases, so they were excluded from further analyses. Thus, data from 29 patients with gliomas could be analyzed. There were no significant differences in patient age ($P = 0.28$) or preoperative tumor sizes ($P = 0.40$) between the two treatment groups. We observed a trend towards a higher rate of complete tumor resections in the ioMRI-group compared to the control group ($P = 0.07$). Postoperative tumor volumes were significantly lower in the ioMRI-group than in the control group ($P < 0.05$). The use of ioMRI appears to be associated with a higher rate of radiographically complete as well as near total tumor resections compared to conventional microneurosurgery.

Keywords Extent of resection · Glioma surgery · Intraoperative MRI · PoleStar

C. Senft (✉), M. Heckelmann, and V. Seifert
Department of Neurosurgery, Johann-Wolfgang-Goethe-University, Schleusenweg 2-16, 60528, Frankfurt, Germany
e-mail: c.senft@med.uni-frankfurt.de

A. Bink
Department of Neuroradiology, Johann-Wolfgang-Goethe-University, Frankfurt, Germany

T. Gasser
Department of Neurosurgery, Johann-Wolfgang-Goethe-University, Schleusenweg 2-16, 60528, Frankfurt, Germany
Department of Neurosurgery, University of Essen, Essen, Germany

Introduction

Intraoperative magnetic resonance imaging (ioMRI) has been used as a surgical adjunct in the resection of brain tumors for more than a decade [1]. Many groups reported that ioMRI-guidance is beneficial in detecting unintentionally remaining tumor tissue intraoperatively leading to extended tumor resections, irrespective of the field strength of the magnet [2–7]. Some studies have even demonstrated benefits in terms of survival when looking at the extent of resection as a prognostic factor [8, 9].

But these reports mainly represent retrospective cohort analyses, and only Hirschberg et al. [10] performed a matched-group analysis in an attempt to show superiority of ioMRI-guidance compared to conventional microneurosurgery. Using a low field strength system (*Signa SP*, 0.5 T) this study could not show differences between the ioMRI and the control group. An explanation for this result is the fact that the extent of tumor resections was comparable in both groups. This was unsurprisingly so, as one would expect the extent of resection to be the prognostic factor, and ioMRI might just be able to influence the extent of resection. Therefore, prospective randomized trials are mandatory to determine beneficial effects of ioMRI-guided brain tumor surgery.

Here, on the occasion of the second Meeting of the Intraoperative Imaging Society, we present the results of an interim analysis of such a trial. To our knowledge, no other such study has been conducted so far.

Material and Methods

Patients

Adult patients with contrast enhancing lesions on T1-weighted MRI suspicious of malignant gliomas who are scheduled to undergo radiologically complete tumor resections are

DOI 10.1007/978-3-211-99651-5_8,

eligible to enter this trial. Also, patients with known gliomas and contrast enhancing lesions suspicious of tumor recurrence may be included. Patients in which the tumor is located close to eloquent structures, e.g. motor cortex, corticospinal tract, basal ganglia, Broca's or Wernicke's area, in a way that the surgical goal would be a near total or partial resection to spare these structures are not included. The study is conducted at the Johann Wolfgang Goethe-University, Frankfurt am Main/Germany, in adherence to the guidelines of the International Conference on Harmonisation – Good Clinical Practice. This study was approved by the local ethics committee.

Treatment

After having given written informed consent, patients are randomized to undergo either ioMRI-guided or conventional microneurosurgical resection. Intraoperative MRI-guided neurosurgery implies the use of a mobile intraoperative ultra-low field ioMRI system (*PoleStar-N 20*, Odin Medical Technologies, Yokneam, Israel/Medtronic, Louisville, CO, USA). The system can be used for intraoperative image acquisition for neuronavigation with its integrated software (*StealthStation*, Medtronic, Louisville, CO, USA) as well as intraoperative resection control as described previously [7, 11]. All intraoperative imaging is conducted and evaluated by neurosurgeons. Conventional microneurosurgical resection implies the use of all standard neurosurgical instruments and techniques, e.g. the use of an ultrasonic aspirator as well as a neuronavigation system. Two neuronavigation systems are available at our department (*StealthStation* and *VectorVision*, BrainLAB, Heimstetten, Germany). Tools that are capable to detect or visualize tumor tissue intraoperatively, e.g. intraoperative ultrasound or fluorescence-guided surgery as described by Stummer et al. [12] are not allowed to be used in either group. Following surgery, the resected tissue is sent for independent histopathological analysis. Postsurgical treatment is conducted according to standard protocols and clinical guidelines, depending on tumor histology, previous treatment and patient preferences. All patients are regularly followed up with clinical and MRI examinations every 3 months.

Study Endpoints

The primary endpoint of this study is the number of patients without contrast enhancing tumor as determined by high field MRI. Secondary endpoints are the volume of residual tumor on postoperative MRI, duration of surgery and patient positioning, overall survival, and neurological deficits. All patients undergo high field MRI within 7 days prior to surgery as well as within 72 h after surgery. One experienced neuroradiologist (A.B.) who is blinded for the surgical treatment of the patients performs the analysis of high field MRI. Volumetric analyses are performed for both, pre- and postoperative imaging studies. As done previously [12], residual tumor is defined as contrast-enhancement with a volume >0.175 cm^3 on postoperative MRI.

Statistics

Statistical analyses were performed using commercially available software (BiAS for Windows 9.01, epsilon Verlag, Frankfurt/Germany). Nominal dichotomized data were compared with Fisher's exact test (number of complete resections, patient sex). After testing for Gaussian distribution using Kolmogorov-Smirnov's test, Student's T-tests were applied to compare patients' age and the duration of surgeries. If a Gaussian distribution could not be confirmed, Wilcoxon-Mann-Whitney-U-tests were used to test for differences in pre- and postoperative tumor volumes as well as the duration of patient positioning. P values lower than 0.05 were considered statistically significant.

Results

Patient Demographics

Between October 2007 and March 2009, a total of 35 Patients entered the study. 18 patients were randomized to undergo ioMRI-guided surgery (ioMRI-group), 17 were randomized to undergo conventional microsurgical tumor resection (control group). Histopathology revealed metastasis in six patients (three in each group) who were excluded from further analysis. With 17 male and 12 female patients overall, there was no sex imbalance between the groups (ioMRI-group: nine males, six females; control group: seven males, six females; $P = 1.00$). Mean age was 56.2 years (range: 35–84 years). There were no age differences between the ioMRI-group and the control group (mean: 53.9 vs. 58.6 years, respectively; $P = 0.28$). All patients were in good clinical condition with a median preoperative KPS score of 90 (range: 60–100). There were no differences between the ioMRI- and the control group (median KPS score 90 in both, $P = 0.40$). Preoperative tumor volumes were not statistically different between the groups ($P = 0.40$, Fig. 1).

Impact of a Low-Field Intraoperative MRI on the Surgical Results for High-Grade Gliomas

Talat Kırış and Osman Arıca

Abstract In this study the authors retrospectively evaluated the results of the operated intracranial high grade gliomas using low field intraoperative MRI system Polestar N 20+ Stealth Station (Medtronic, Co, USA) at German Hospital, Istanbul. Between November 2006 and October 2008, 11 patients underwent microsurgical tumor resection with the use of intraoperative MRI for WHO Grade III and IV gliomas. There were six males and five females, mean age was 53 (range 30–73), and mean follow-up duration was 19 months (range 4–31). Ten total, one subtotal resection was achieved, whereas intraoperative MRI assesment demonstrated five residual tumors. Histopathological examination revealed that eight tumors were Glioblastomas and three were anaplastic oligodendroglioma, anaplastic oligoastrocytoma and anaplastic ependymoma respectively. No complications directly related to the intaoperative scanning were observed and there was no mortality, but one patient with an insular tumor developed hemiparesis after the operation. Mean hospital stay was 4.8 day. Ten patients received additional radiotherapy and chemotherapy, one patient refused further therapy. Mean survival was 18.8 months for the entire group and 15.6 months for glioblastoma patients. In this small series of patients with high grade gliomas we found that the use of intraoperative MRI helps complete tumor removal and hence improves survival.

Keywords High grade glioma · Intracranial tumors · Intraoperative MRI · Microsurgery

T. Kırış (✉)
Department of Neurosurgery, Istanbul School of Medicine, Istanbul University, 34093, Capa, Istanbul, Turkey
Department of Neurosurgery, German Hospital, Istanbul, Turkey
e-mail: talatkrs@gmail.com

O. Arıca
Department of Neurosurgery, German Hospital, Istanbul, Turkey

Introduction

The prognosis of patients with high grade gliomas remains poor despite advances in aggressive therapy with surgical resection, radiotherapy and chemotherapy [1]. The goals of surgery in high grade gliomas are obtaining histopathological diagnosis, alleviating symptoms related increased intracranial pressure and compression of neural tissues, increasing survival and decreasing the need for corticosteroids. Growing evidence suggest that the extent of microsurgical resection is associated with longer life expectancy in high grade gliomas [2]. The availability of the intraoperative MRI has changed the principles of surgery for gliomas [3]. An intraoperative MRI scanner can acquire presurgical neuroradiological examinations for planning, intraoperative images for realtime neuronavigation and for comparing the extent of tumor resection with preoperative tumor volume [3–5]. Studies have shown improvement in the extent of tumor resection with the use of intraoperative MRI, but improved survival has not yet been proven [6–8]. In this study we report our results in neurosurgical resection of high grade gliomas in adults, with the help of a low field MRI scanner.

Patients and Methods

Within a period of 18 months between November 2007 and June 2009, 13 craniotomies (for 11 patients) were performed for removal of WHO grade III and IV Gliomas using the low field intraoperative MRI scanner Polestar N-20, at the German Hospital, Istanbul. The group included 6 male and 5 female patients with a mean age 53 (age range 30–73). One patient, operated earlier for a Grade II insular astrocytoma, had been operated two more times after the tumor was recurred as Glioblastoma (the third operation was performed for a distant seeding metastasis).

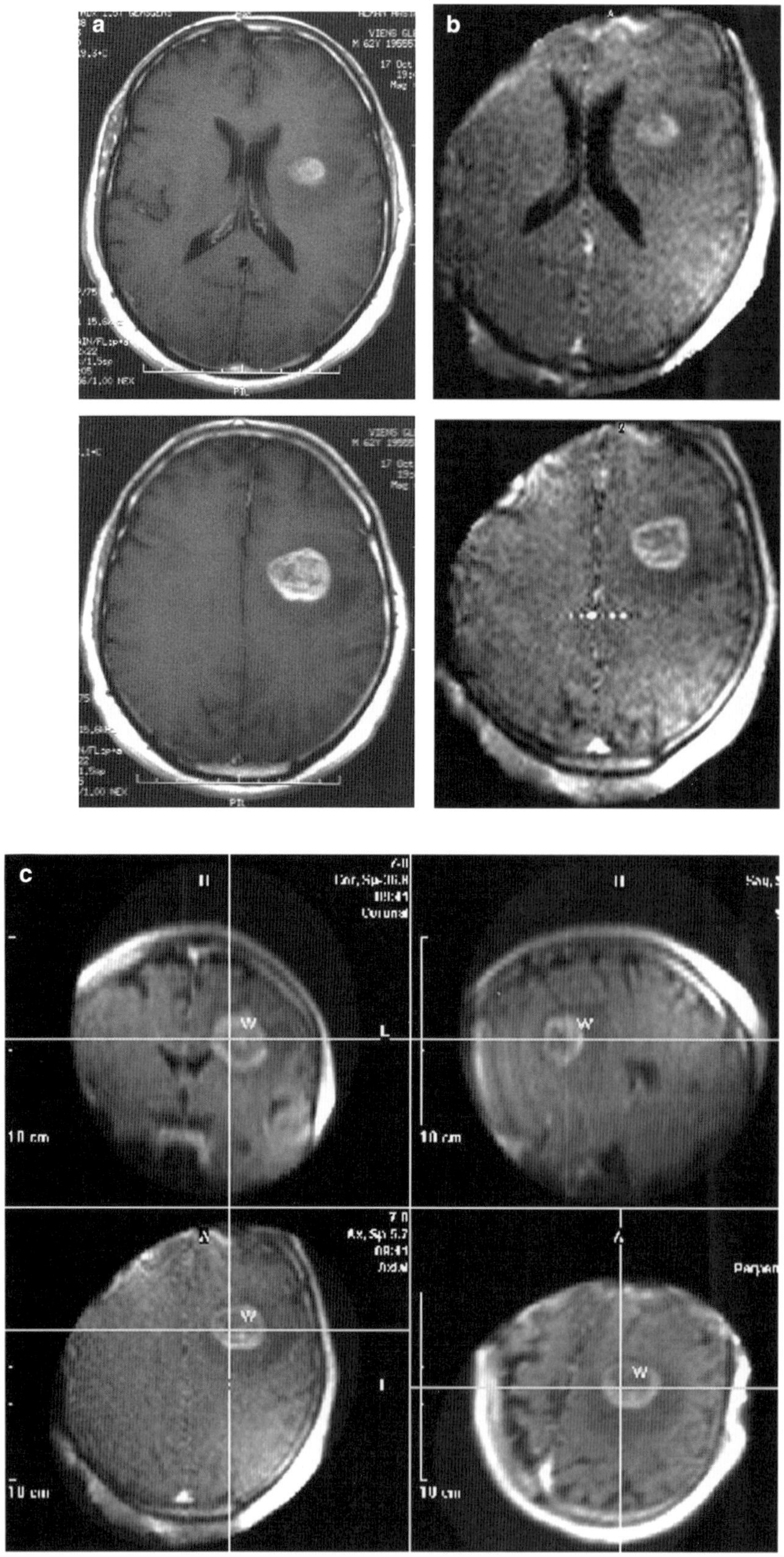

Fig. 1 (continued)

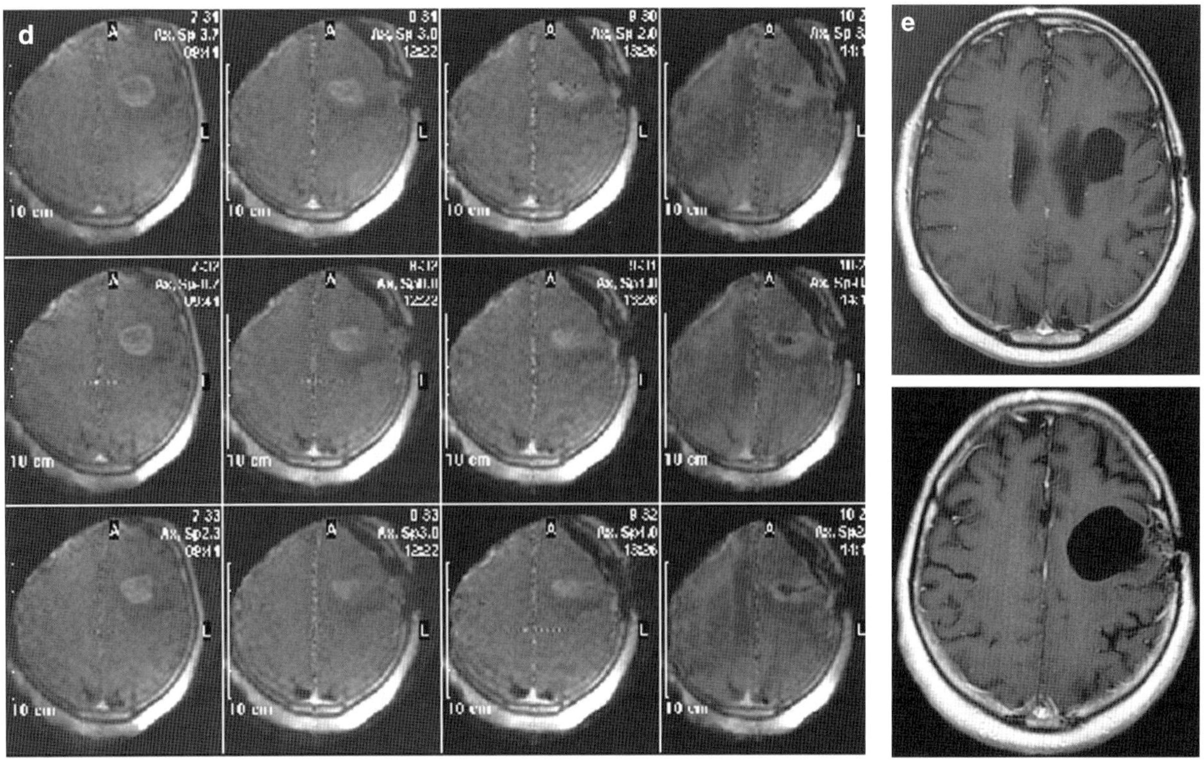

Fig. 1 (**a**) Preoperative T1 weighted postcontrast diagnostic images acquired with 1.5 T MRI scanner demonstrated a left deep seated frontal tumor. (**b**) T1 weighted postcontrast images acquired with Polestar before surgery. (**c**) Neuronavigation using the images acquired with Polestar before the beginning of surgery. (**d**) Intraoperative control MRI images for comparing the extend of resection. (**e**) Control MRI images 12 months after the operation

For the surgical procedure, the patient was positioned at the table with the non-magnetic headholder, designed for this system. The scanner was placed under the operating table. Patient reference frame and coil were attached to the headholder and the patient's head, respectively. The arms of the scanner were raised at a proper position. After the Starshield isolated the patient from the rest of the room, postcontrast (double dose) T1 weighted images were obtained. This image set was used for planning the craniotomy. Tumors were removed using standard microsurgical principles. Another intraoperative postcontrast T1 scanning was obtained for evaluating the tumor removal. Whenever rest tumor was detected, these images would be further used for real time neuronavigation. MRI scanning was repeated until complete resection was achieved (Fig. 1).

All patients except one (who refused any further therapy after microsurgery) received additional radiotherapy (a total dose of 60 G). One patient recruited to a study at the Radiation Oncology Department of Istanbul University, received a total dose of 66 G. Patients received radiotherapy, had also received adjuvant chemotherapy; namely temozolamide.

Results

In ten patients, total tumor resection was achieved. In one of the patients, brain stem infiltration prevented a total resection. Histopathological examination revealed that eight of the tumors operated were glioblastomas, one anaplastic oligodendroglioma, one anaplastic oligoastrocytoma and one anaplastic ependymoma. There was no mortality in this series. The patient operated previously for low grade astrocytoma, developed hemiparesis after the second operation.

Patients were positioned according to the surgical procedure, either the prone, supine or lateral. The average time for patient positioning and image acquisition in this series was 72 min (range 45–120 min). The average duration of surgery from incision to the last suture was 172 min. Intraoperative MRI demonstrated residual tumor in 5 of the 11 cases. Imaging sessions averaged 2.4 per surgery. Mean hospital stay was 4.8 days.

Mean follow-up was 19 months (4–31months). Mean survival for the entire series was 18.8 months, mean survival for glioblastoma patients was 15.6 months. On the last follow-up, four patients were disease free (2 Grade IV and 2 Grade III), one patient with subtotal resection did not show any progression, three patients demonstrated recurrences and three patients had died. One patient died of pneumonia 4 months after the operation, one patient who refused any further therapy died from recurrent tumor 7 months after the operation. One patient died 28, 12 and 3 months after the first, second and third operation, respectively. The second operation was performed for recurrence and the third for a seeding metastasis. No complications related to the use of intraoperative MRI had been observed. Table 1 summarizes the clinical features of the patients.

Table 1 Clinical features of the patients

Sex	
Female	5
Male	6
Age	
Mean	53
Range	30–73
Location	
Teomporal	2
Insular	1
Frontal	2
Parietal	2
Occipital	2
Thalamic	1
Serebellum-Brainstem	1
Incision	
Pterional	3
Horseshoe	1
Lineer	7
Time for patient positioning and image acquisition	
Mean	45–120 min
Range	72 min
Imaging sessions	
Mean	2.4
Range	2–4
Hospital stay	
Mean	4.8 days
Histopathology	
Glioblastoma	8
Anaplastic Oligodendroglioma	1
Anaplastic Oligoastrocytoma	1
Anaplastic Epandymoma	1
Ki-67 index	
Mean	31.15%
Range	9–80%
Follow-up	
Mean	19
Range	4–31
Survival	
Mean for Total Series	18.8 months
Mean for Glioblastoma Patients	15.6 months

Discussion

For high grade gliomas, establishment of universally relevant prognostic criteria and treatment options remains a great challenge. Tumor histopathology, patients' age and functional status are the only reliable prognostic factors. Although Class I evidence is deficient in determining the efficacy of surgery in improving survival and delaying tumor progression among patients with high grade gliomas, there is growing evidence that more extensive surgical resection may be associated with more favorable life expectancy [2]. Therefore some form of imaging modality like MRI, CT or ultrasound, which increase the percentage of gross total tumor resection should be of value.

During the past ten years, different intraoperative MRI systems have been introduced into the neurosurgical operating rooms, to allow realtime imaging during surgery [3, 5]. Intraoperative MRI systems with low- (0.15–0.5 T), high- (1.5 T) and ultrahigh- (3 T) field strength are available [3, 9–11]. High- and ultrahigh-field strength systems carry potential of better imaging quality and opportunity of advanced imaging features, such as diffusion, spectroscopy and anjiography. However the size and cost of high- and ultra-high-field strength magnets are pronounced disadvantages. Polestar N-20 is a compact and mobile system with field strength of 0.15 T. The magnet is formed by two vertical, parallel disk shaped arms and the permanent magnet docks under a standard OR table. Because of its low magnetic field strength, standard operating room and MRI-incompatible surgical instruments can be used. It provides more patient access since scanning and navigation are directly under the control of the neurosurgeon and thus eliminates the need of simultaneous presence of a neuroradiologist or an MRI technician.

Schulder et al. reported their experience in cranial surgery with the Polestar N-20 system [12]. Their report included 13 glioma cases. In their series, imaging sessions averaged 2.3 per surgery, which is almost identical with our experience 2.4 average imaging per surgery. As they stated, we also found that the T1 weighted images (7 min/4 mm) are the most accurate for evaluating the extent of tumor resection as well as for navigation. The extra time required for use of the system, averaged 1.1 h in their series.

Senft et al. reported their experience in glioma surgery (including low and high grade tumors) using the same system [8]. Patient positioning in their experience, took 33 min in average and additional time was used for image acquisition. In our experience, patient positioning + image acquisition lasted 72 min, which coincides with both reported series [11, 12]. Intraoperative scans after tumor resection revealed residual tumor in 47.6% of the patients with contrast enhanced tumors, in the series of Senft et al. In the present series residual tumor was demonstrated in 45.4% (all high grade contrast enhanced tumors) and intentional gross total resection was achieved in 90.9% of patients.

Hirschberg et al. evaluated the impact of intraoperative MRI on median survival for a series of patients harboring high grade gliomas [13]. They compared this group to a matched cohort of patients operated in a conventional manner. The intraoperative MRI scanner they used, was the Signa Sp/I (General Electric Medical Systems, WI, USA), an open vertical MRI scanner with 0.5 T field strength. The mean overall survival time in the study group was 14.5 months, compared 12.1 months for the matched control group. With a similar system Schneider et al. evaluated the influence of intraoperative MRI on the extent of resection and the median survival in patients with glioblastome multiforme [7]. The mean survival was 9.3 months, but when the patients were analyzed separately for gross-total and subtotal resections, the mean survival was 17.9 and 7.9 months, respectively. In our series, mean survival was 18.8 months for the whole group and 15.6 months for glioblastome multiforme patients.

The results of this small group of patients with high grade gliomas operated with the help of Polestar N-20, demonstrated that a low field strength MRI scanner is a useful surgical tool for evaluating the extent of tumor resection and for real time neuronavigation.

Conflict of interest statement We declare that we have no conflict of interest.

References

1. Oertel J, von Buttlar E, Schroeder HW, Gaab MR (2005) Prognosis of gliomas in the 1970s and today. Neurosurg Focus 18(4):E12
2. Sanai N, Berger M (2008) Glioma extent of resection and its impact on patients outcome. Neurosurgery 62(4):753–766
3. Albayrak B, Samdani AF, Black PM (2004) Intraoperative magnetic resonance imaging in neurosurgery. Acta Neurochir 146:543–557
4. Iseki H, Nakamura R, Muragaki Y, Suzuki T, Chernov M, Hori T, Takakura K (2008) Advanced computer aided intraoperative technologies for information-guided surgical management of gliomas: Tokyo Women's Medical University experience. Minim Invasive Neurosurg 51(5):285–291
5. Oh DS, Black PM (2005) A low-field intraoperative MRI system for glioma surgery: is it worthwhile? Neurosurg Clin N Am 16 (1):135 141, Review
6. Knauth M, Wirtz CR, Tronnier VM, Aras N, Kunze S, Sartor K (1999) Intraoperative MR imaging increases the extent of tumor resection in patients with high-grade gliomas. AJNR Am J Neuroradiol 20(9):1642–1646
7. Schneider JP, Trantakis C, Rubach M, Schulz T, Dietrich J, Winkler D, Renner C, Schober R, Geiger K, Brosteanu O, Zimmer C, Kahn T (2005) Intraoperative MRI to guide the resection of primary supratentorial glioblastoma multiforme – a quantitative radiological analysis. Neuroradiology 47(7):489–500
8. Senft C, Seifert V, Hermann E, Franz K, Gasser T (2008) Usefullness of introperative ultra-low field magnetic resonance imaging in glioma surgery. Neurosurgery 63(4 suppl 2):257–266
9. Nimsky C, Ganslandt O, Fahlbusch R (2005) Comparing 0.2 tesla with 1.5 tesla intraoperative magnetic resonance imaging analysis of setup, workflow and efficiency. Acad Radiol 12(9): 1065–1079
10. Pamir MN, Ozduman K, Dinçer A, Yildiz E, Peker S, Ozek MM (2010) First intraoperative, shared resource, ultra-high field 3-T magnetic resonance imaging system and its application in low grade glioma resection. J Neurosurg 112(1):57–69
11. Sutherland GR, Kaibara T, Louw D, Hoult DI, Tomanek B, Saunders J (1999) A mobile high-field magnetic resonance system for neurosurgery. J Neurosurg 91(5):804–813
12. Schulder M, Salas S, Brimacombe M, Fine P, Catrambone J, Maniker AH, Carmel PW (2006) Cranial surgery with an expanded compact intraoperative magnetic resonance imager. Technical note. J Neurosurg 104(4):611–617
13. Hirschberg H, Samset E, Hol PK, Tillung T, Lote K (2005) Impact of intraoperative MRI on the surgical results for high-grade gliomas. Minim Invasive Neurosurg 48(2):77–84

Intraoperative MRI and Functional Mapping

Thomas Gasser, Andrea Szelenyi, Christian Senft, Yoshihiro Muragaki, I. Erol Sandalcioglu, Ulrich Sure, Christopher Nimsky, and Volker Seifert

Abstract The integration of functional and anatomical data into neuronavigation is an established standard of care in many neurosurgical departments. Yet, this method has limitations as in most cases the data are acquired prior to surgery. Due to brain-shift the accurate presentation of functional as well as anatomical structures declines in the course of surgery.

In consequence, the acquisition of information during surgery about the brain's current functional state is of specific interest. The advancement of imaging technologies (e.g. fMRI, MEG, Intraoperative Optical Intrinsic Signal Imaging – IOIS) and neurophysiological techniques and the advent of intraoperative MRI all had a major impact on neurosurgery.

The combination of modalities such as neurophysiology and intraoperative MRI (ioMRI), as well as the acquisition of functional MRI during surgery (ifMRI) are in the focus of this work. Especially the technical aspects and safety issues are elucidated.

Keywords Brain mapping · Functional MRI · Intraoperative MRI · Neurophysiology

T. Gasser (✉)
Department of Neurosurgery, University of Duisburg-Essen, Hufelandstr. 55, 45147 Essen, Germany
Department of Neurosurgery, Goethe University, Schleusenweg 2-16, 60528 Frankfurt, Main, Germany
e-mail: thomas.gasser@uk-essen.de

A. Szelenyi, C. Senft, and V. Seifert
Department of Neurosurgery, Goethe University, Schleusenweg 2-16, 60528 Frankfurt, Main, Germany

Y. Muragaki
Department of Neurosurgery, Tokyo Women's Medical University, Tokyo, Japan

I.E. Sandalcioglu, and U. Sure
Department of Neurosurgery, University of Duisburg-Essen, Hufelandstr. 55, 45147 Essen, Germany

C. Nimsky
Department of Neurosurgery, University of Marburg, Marburg, Germany

Introduction

The success of resective surgery of brain lesions in close vicinity to eloquent cortex is closely linked to the preservation or improvement of the initial neurofunctional status. For that purpose, intraoperative electrophysiological monitoring (IOM) delivers information about the neurophysiological integrity of specific functional networks and pathways [1, 2]. Besides well-established and routinely employed methods such as sensory and motor evoked potentials (SEPs and MEPs), which test primarily the functional integrity of the corticospinal tract, cortical mapping allows for testing of even more complex functional networks (e.g. speech, reading, cognition).

Additionally, functional imaging technologies such as functional MRI and magnetic source imaging (MEG) play an increasing role in the preoperative planning of the approach and the resection borders [3–7]. Postoperatively, functional restitution and cortical reorganization may be documented by fMRI, presenting further insight into issues such as neuronal plasticity, which in turn is of growing interest to neurosurgeons as well.

To date neuronavigation is the technical core structure for the integration of image based functional information into the operative site. The usefulness of what may be called "functional neuronavigation" is well documented [1, 8–12] however, "functional neuronavigation" has technical limitations, primarily related to the fact, that the functional data is acquired preoperatively. Loss of cerebrospinal fluid and tumour resection may result in a significant intraoperative deformation of the brain resulting in an inaccuracy of the neuronavigation, which in turn can be compensated for by intraoperative imaging and regular updates of the navigational data sets [9–11].

The study group has developed two approaches to address this specific issue in order to increase accuracy of intraoperative functional mapping. The technological pathways being followed are:

Method 1: To perform functional MRI intraoperatively (intraoperative fMRI or ifMRI) employing a passive fMRI paradigm to visualize the sensorimotor cortex intraoperatively.

This method has been implemented in a 1.5 T, as well as in a 0.3 T environment [13].

Method 2: To routinely update intraoperative anatomical neuronavigation and to combine these data with conventional IOM. This method has been applied in a 0.15 T setup [12].

Materials and Methods

Method 1: Intraoperative Functional MRI

In the presented study, four patients (mean age: 39 years) with centrally located lesions (one glioblastoma WHO IV, one astrocytmoma WHO II, one bronchial carcinoma metastasis, one cavernoma) were evaluated under total intravenous anaesthesia (TIVA) with propofol 2% (2,6-diisopropylphenol; average dosage: 5.8 $mgkg^{-1}h^{-1}$) and fentanyl (1-phenethyl-4-(phenylpropionylamino)piperidine; average dosage: 0.23 $\mu gkg^{-1}h^{-1}$) at different stages of surgery. In order to acquire functional MRI, several technical prerequisites have to be met. Firstly, the installation of an intraoperative MR unit (ioMRI) is required. The neurosurgical operating suite in the Department of Neurosurgery, University Erlangen-Nuremberg, is equipped with such a 1.5-T scanner (Magnetom Sonata Maestro Class, Siemens Medical Solutions, Erlangen, Germany). Secondly, a passive functional MR-paradigm, eliciting an activation of the sensorimotor cortex under general anaesthesia has to be employed.

The study group has described this method's setup, safety and scope of application in detail previously [8, 13, 14]. In short, we applied a passive paradigm based on electrical stimulation of the median and tibial nerves [14]. For electrical stimulation an electromagnetically shielded coaxial lead (length: 8 m; resistance: 50 Ω) was designed. Shielding was achieved by connecting the conductor's shielding-mesh to the MRI-cage. Modified bipolar surface electrodes (Nicolet, Madison, WI, USA; Part Number: 019-401500) were utilized for both stimulated locations, applying 3-Hz square wave electrical pulses of 100 ms duration with an intensity of 3 mA above motor threshold. The impulse generator (Nicolet-Viking IV P, Madison, WI, USA) was located outside the operating suite and the conductor was threaded through a waveguide array into the operating theatre. After anaesthesiological induction and patient positioning, the stimulation electrodes were attached and the motor threshold was defined. After an initial anatomical and functional MR scan, surgery commenced and two further data sets were acquired during and at the end of the surgical procedure. The block-design stimulation paradigm alternated four rest and four activation periods of 33 s each. For functional imaging, slices parallel to the anterior–posterior commissural plane were acquired as T2*-weighted Echo Planar Imaging (EPI) sequences (TE 60 ms, TR 3,300 ms, flip-angle 90°, slice thickness 3 mm, FOV 220 mm, matrix 64×64) with data acquisition covering the whole cerebrum.

Employing Statistical Parametric Mapping (SPM, Wellcome Department of Imaging Neuroscience, London, Version 99), the functional time series were analyzed statistically. The data were motion corrected by rigid body spatial translation. After data smoothing, a design matrix according to the variables of the above mentioned boxcar stimulus function was created. The predictor vectors were convolved with a hemodynamic response function. The data were assessed statistically specifying P as 0.05 ($n=1$) for corrected and 0.001 ($n=3$) for uncorrected comparisons. For anatomical correlation the functional data with the realigned echo planar images were co-registered with a 3-D T1-weighted high-resolution data set.

A comparable procedure to the one described above has been applied by the study group in a different setting, namely in a 0.3 T ioMRI environment (Hitachi AIRIS II, Hitachi Medical Cooperation, Kashiwa, Japan) which is installed in the operating suite of the Department of Neurosurgery at Tokyo Women's Medical University, Tokyo, Japan. Minor modifications to the scanner software (Version 5.0 M) and an adaptation of the scanning parameters (echo planar sequence GE-EPI, TR 1,200 ms and TE 41.8 ms, flip angle 80°) were necessary to implement ifMRI.

Method 2: Combination of ioMRI and IOM

The combination of intraoperative MRI (ioMRI), neuronavigation, intraoperative neurophysiological localization (e.g. cortical mapping, phase reversal) and continuous functional monitoring promises to the neurosurgeon up-to-date functional and anatomical information. However, the interaction between the magnetic field (either static or alternating) and the electrodes, which are inserted in the scalp, may induce heat or an electric current. The maximum interaction within this specific ioMRI environment (PoleStar 0.15-T, Medtronic Surgical Navigation Technologies, Louisville, CO, USA) and the maximum electric current being delivered by the IOM system (ISIS intraoperative monitoring system, Inomed Co., Teningen, Germany) were first of all estimated in a precursor study evaluating effects such as induction of heat or directional forces in a phantom. Additionally, the effects on image quality were evaluated. The MRI data sets included the following axial sequences: T1-weighted

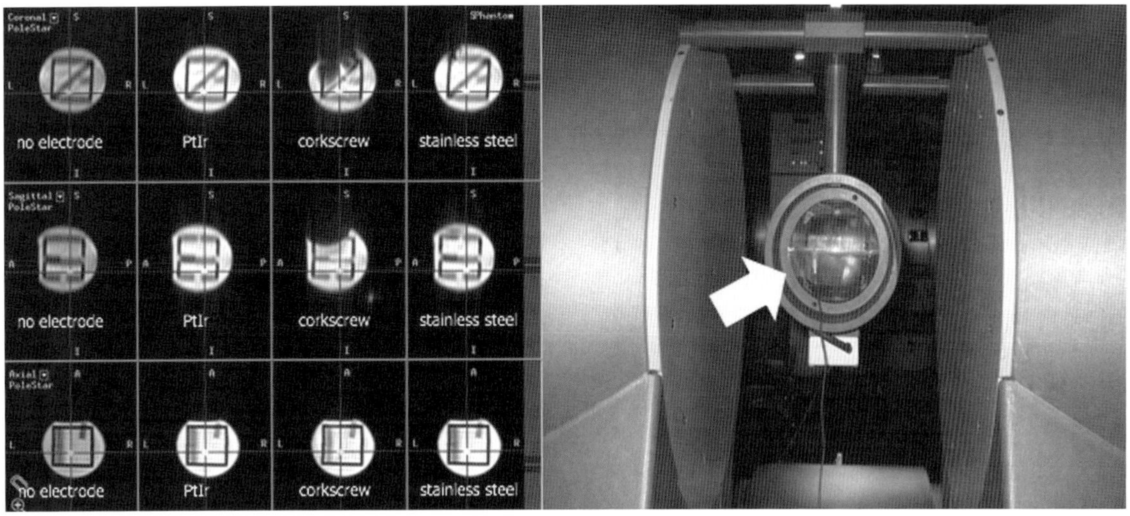

Fig. 1 Phantom prepared for standardized evaluation of artifacts originating from different electrodes. Left frame: comparison of the image artefacts, with the corkscrew electrodes producing a considerable signal wipe out (from left to right: no electrode; platinum iridium (PtIr) electrode; corkscrew electrode; steel electrodes. Right frame: actual setup with phantom placed in between the MR unit's aperture (Polestar N20) with electrode attached to the phantom's calibration sphere (*white arrow*)

(TR 40.00 ms, TE 3.00 ms, with and without gadolinium-DTPA) and T2-weighted (TR 3,000.00 ms TE 112 ms). After establishing safety criteria, the clinical feasibility was evaluated in a subsequent study.

Phantom Study

Standard CE-certified electrodes (stainless steel subdermal electroencephalography [EEG] needle electrodes, corkscrew design electrodes, and platinum/iridium [Pt/Ir]-subdermal EEG needle electrodes; Viasys Healthcare, Madison, WI; 0.4-mm diameter and 1.5-m lead length) were evaluated, by attaching the electrodes to a copper sulfate-filled phantom (PoleStar N20 specific equipment, Medtronic Surgical Navigation Technologies, Louisville, CO, USA) (Fig. 1). While imaging was performed with the PoleStar N20 (Medtronic Surgical Navigation Technologies, Louisville, COS, USA; scanning parameters, see above), induction of movement and heat was observed and measured. Image quality was analyzed for artifacts by comparing images with and without electrodes.

Clinical Study

In 29 patients (median age: 40 years) with supratentorial lesions (11 glioblastoma WHO IV, 15 astrocytoma WHO II-III, 1 cavernoma, 1 tuberculoma, oligodendroglioma) a neurosurgical procedure was performed with IOM and ioMRI. In 15 patients we additionally mapped the cortex with direct cortical stimulation (DCS). For IOM Pt/Ir electrodes were utilized (Fig. 2). ioMRI was performed at the start of surgery and at the presumed end of resection employing the following axial sequences: T1-weighted (TR 40.00 ms, TE 3.00 ms, with and without gadolinium-DTPA), T2-weighted (TR 3,000.00 ms, TE 112 ms).

During the scanning procedure the ION System was switched off and the head box was detached from the amplifier.

Results

Results of Method 1: Intraoperative Functional MRI

In all patients examined with the 1.5 T ioMRI, the somatosensory cortex could be identified by intraoperative fMRI. The signal characteristics varied in the course of surgery with changing BOLD signal intensities and co-activations of the assumed secondary sensory cortex (S2). Remarkably, an inversal of the BOLD response in nearly half of the measurements was observed. Analyzing the functional data sets by introducing a contrast of 1 suggested an increase of the deoxyhemoglobin concentration in the elicited somatosensory cortex. Microscope-based neuronavigation allowed the intraoperative correlation of anatomical and functional data with the exposed structures in the surgical field.

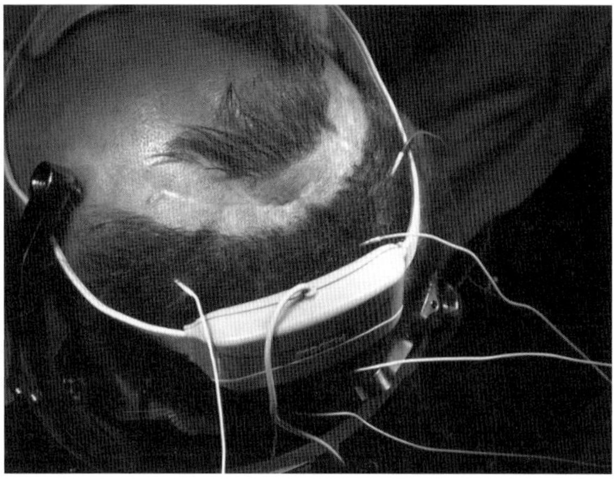

Fig. 2 Placement of the Platinum Iridium (PtIr) electrodes for IOM according to the international 10–20 EEG system in a patient with a recurrent astrocytoma. Note the location of electrodes within the HF-head coil (Medtronic Surgical Navigation, Louisville, CO, USA). To avoid heating and dislocation of the electrodes induced by the static and alternating magnetic field, all cables were braided, and looping of the electrode cables was avoided. The preamplifier was placed at a distance of 1 m from the patient's head at the sidebar of the operating table placed (not visible)

The average registration accuracy was 1.45 mm (standard error: 0.67 mm). Significant susceptibility artifacts were avoided by filling the resection cavity with saline. Applying SPM's statistical routines, the fitted response function (adjusted data versus time/scans) documented in all cases a high correlation between the temporal course of the paradigm and the cortical activation.

In a preliminary evaluation we could demonstrate that similar results were obtained in patients in whom intraoperative fMRI was performed employing a 0.3 T scanner.

Results of Method 2: Combination of ioMRI and IOM

Phantom Study

Primarily steel electrodes caused electrode-related artifacts. The most common artifacts were signal deletions and local field distortions. More importantly, this study demonstrated the inertness of Pt/Ir electrodes to MRI (Fig. 1); consequently, they were used for the patient study. Temperature changes were not observed in any of the utilized electrodes.

Clinical Study

In all collected ioMRI data sets, irrespective of the sequence, no image artifacts or changes in SNR (signal-to-noise-ratio) originating from the electrodes could be detected. There were no adverse effects related to the setup and the quality of the monitoring was not affected either.

Discussion

The integration of preoperatively acquired functional imaging and intraoperative neurophysiology employing neuronavigation has been implemented in several centres. However, only a few reports exist about intraoperative updates of functional information in combination with ioMRI [12]. Two different technical setups, which provide such a functional update, are in focus of the presented data.

Established methods of functional mapping and monitoring, such as direct cortical stimulation, phase reversal or evoked potentials, have still to be regarded as the gold standard of brain mapping. The combination with ioMRI could however facilitate the interpretation of neurophysiological information. Thus efforts were made to combine the technical components as described under method 2. The advantage of this method is, that it offers the high temporal resolution and the constant flow of information originating from IOM and electrophysiological mapping. In our setup, we have proven safety only for a 0.15 T environment, with its obviously reduced spatial resolution and the smaller field-of-view when compared to a 1.5 T MR unit. With careful selection of the electrode types, EEG and evoked potential recording, even in high-field MRI systems up to 7-T, has been described as safe [15].

The primary assets of ioMRI are the compensation of brain-shift and intraoperative resection control. Extended capabilities of ioMRI, namely functional MRI (fMRI) and diffusion tensor imaging (DTI), offer additional information to the neurosurgeon. To date, functional navigation relies on preoperatively acquired data. However, as described under method 1 the intraoperative acquisition and update of functional MRI is safe and feasible. In comparison to method 2, which propagates the combination of 0.15 T ioMRI and IOM, the functional information is updated only at a few times during surgery. This may be a disadvantage, yet the high anatomical resolution and the combination of up-to-date intraoperative fMRI and diffusion tensor imaging (DTI) provide a technical solution. By co-registration of ifRMI and DTI, the entire intracranial corticospinal tract can be visualized [16]. The application of ifMRI activation areas as seed points for fiber tracking algorithms in DTI data in order to delineate major white matter tracts intraoperatively can provide more exact data, reducing the risk for postoperative neurological deficits. Especially in surgery of larger, centrally located lesions with an increased shift of the adjacent gyri, the update of functional information may help to trace the sensorimotor cortex.

Conclusion

Neurophysiological monitoring with evoked potentials and DCS can be performed safely and with good quality within a low-field open MRI system. Alternatively, intraoperative fMRI, employing a 1.5 T MR unit and an appropriate paradigm, represents an equally safe and technically feasible method for near-real-time identification of eloquent brain areas despite brain shift during neurosurgical procedures.

Disclosure Thomas Gasser, M.D., Ph.D., serves as clinical consultant to Medtronic, but there has been no direct financial support of this study by the company.

References

1. Berger MS, Rostomily RC (1997) Low grade gliomas: functional mapping resection strategies, extent of resection, and outcome. J Neurooncol 34:85–101
2. Neuloh G, Pechstein U, Cedzich C, Schramm J (2004) Motor evoked potential monitoring with supratentorial surgery. Neurosurgery 54:1061–1072
3. Achten E, Jackson GD, Cameron JA, Abbott DF, Stella DL, Fabinyi GC (1999) Presurgical evaluation of the motor hand area with functional MR imaging in patients with tumors and dysplastic lesions. Radiology 210:529–538
4. Hill DL, Smith AD, Simmons A, Maurer CR Jr, Cox TC, Elwes R, Brammer M, Hawkes DJ, Polkey CE (2000) Sources of error in comparing functional magnetic resonance imaging and invasive electrophysiological recordings. J Neurosurg 93:214–223
5. Kober H, Nimsky C, Moller M, Hastreiter P, Fahlbusch R, Ganslandt O (2001) Correlation of sensorimotor activation with functional magnetic resonance imaging and magnetoencephalography in presurgical functional imaging: a spatial analysis. Neuroimage 14:1214–1228
6. Roux FE, Ibarrola D, Tremoulet M, Lazorthes Y, Henry P, Sol JC, Berry I (2001) Methodological and technical issues for integrating functional magnetic resonance imaging data in a neuronavigational system. Neurosurgery 49:1145–1157
7. Towle VL, Khorasani L, Uftring S, Pelizzari C, Erickson RK, Spire JP, Hoffmann K, Chu D, Scherg M (2003) Noninvasive identification of human central sulcus: a comparison of gyral morphology, functional MRI, dipole localization, and direct cortical mapping. Neuroimage 19:684–697
8. Gasser T, Sandalcioglu IE, Schoch B, Gizewski ER, Forsting M, Stolke D, Wiedemayer H (2005) Functional MRI in anaesthetized patients. A relevant step towards real-time intraoperative functional neuroimaging. Neurosurgery 57:94–99
9. Nabavi A, Black PM, Gering DT, Westin CF, Mehta V, Pergolizzi RS Jr, Ferrant M, Warfield SK, Hata N, Schwartz RB, Wells WM 3rd, Kikinis R, Jolesz FA (2001) Serial intraoperative magnetic resonance imaging of brain shift. Neurosurgery 48: 787–798
10. Nimsky C, Ganslandt O, Cerny S, Hastreiter P, Greiner G, Fahlbusch R (2000) Quantification of, visualization of, and compensation for brain shift using intraoperative magnetic resonance imaging. Neurosurgery 47:1070–1080
11. Nimsky C, Ganslandt O, Hastreiter P, Fahlbusch R (2001) Intraoperative compensation for brain shift. Surg Neurol 56: 357–365
12. Szelenyi A, Gasser T, Seifert V (2008) Intraoperative neurophysiological monitoring in an open low-field magnetic resonance imaging system: clinical experience and technical considerations. Neurosurgery 63:268–275
13. Gasser T, Ganslandt O, Sandalcioglu IE, Stolke D, Fahlbusch R, Nimksky C (2005) Intraoperative functional MRI: implementation and preliminary experience. Neuroimage 26:685–693
14. Gasser T, Sandalcioglu IE, Wiedemayer H, Hans V, Gizewski ER, Forsting M, Stolke D (2004) A novel passive functional MRI-paradigm for preoperative identification of the somatosensory cortex. Neurosurg Rev 27:106–112
15. Vasios CE, Angelone LM, Purdon PL, Ahveninen J, Belliveau JW, Bonmassar G (2006) EEG/(f)MRI measurements at 7 Tesla using a new EEG cap ("InkCap"). Neuroimage 33:1082–1092
16. Nimsky C, Ganslandt O, Hastreiter P, Wang R, Benner T, Sorensen AG, Fahlbusch R (2005) Intraoperative diffusion-tensor MR imaging: shifting of white matter tracts during neurosurgical procedures – initial experience. Radiology 234:218–225

Information-Guided Surgical Management of Gliomas Using Low-Field-Strength Intraoperative MRI

Yoshihiro Muragaki, Hiroshi Iseki, Takashi Maruyama, Masahiko Tanaka, Chie Shinohara, Takashi Suzuki, Kitaro Yoshimitsu, Soko Ikuta, Motohiro Hayashi, Mikhail Chernov, Tomokatsu Hori, Yoshikazu Okada, and Kintomo Takakura

Abstract

Background: Contemporary technological developments revolutionized management of brain tumors. The experience with information-guided surgery of gliomas, based on the integration of the various intraoperative anatomical, functional, and histological data, is reported.

Methods: From 2000 to 2009, 574 surgeries for intracranial gliomas were performed in our clinic with the use of intraoperative MRI (ioMRI) with magnetic field strength of 0.3 T, updated neuronavigation, neurochemical navigation with 5-aminolevulinic acid, serial intraoperative histopathological investigations of the resected tissue, and comprehensive neurophysiological monitoring. Nearly half of patients (263 cases; 45.8%) were followed more than 2 years after surgery.

Findings: Maximal possible tumor resection, defined as radiologically complete tumor removal or subtotal removal leaving the residual neoplasm within the vital functionally-important brain areas, was attained in 569 cases (99.1%). The median resection rate constituted 95%, 95%, and 98%, for WHO grade II, III, and IV gliomas, respectively. Actuarial 5-year survival was significantly worse in WHO grade IV gliomas (19%), but did not differ significantly between WHO grade III and II tumors (69% vs. 87%).

Conclusions: Information-guided management of gliomas using low-field-strength ioMRI provides a good opportunity for maximal possible tumor resection, and may result in survival advantage, particularly in patients with WHO grade III neoplasms.

Keyword Brain tumor resection · Glioma · Intraoperative MRI · Surgery · Updated intraoperative neuronavigation

Y. Muragaki (✉), T. Maruyama, and M. Hayashi
Faculty of Advanced Techno-Surgery, Institute of Advanced Biomedical Engineering and Science, Graduate School of Medicine, Tokyo Women's Medical University, 8-1 Kawada-cho, Shinjuku-ku, Tokyo, 162-8666, Japan
Department of Neurosurgery, Neurological Institute, Tokyo Women's Medical University, 8-1 Kawada-cho, Shinjuku-ku, Tokyo, 162-8666, Japan
e-mail: ymuragaki@abmes.twmu.ac.jp

H. Iseki, M. Chernov, and K. Takakura
Faculty of Advanced Techno-Surgery, Institute of Advanced Biomedical Engineering and Science, Graduate School of Medicine, Tokyo Women's Medical University, 8-1 Kawada-cho, Shinjuku-ku, Tokyo, 162-8666, Japan
Department of Neurosurgery, Neurological Institute, Tokyo Women's Medical University, 8-1 Kawada-cho, Shinjuku-ku, Tokyo, 162-8666, Japan
International Research and Educational Institute for Integrated Medical Sciences (IREIIMS), Tokyo Women's Medical University, 8-1 Kawada-cho, Shinjuku-ku, Tokyo, 162-8666, Japan

M. Tanaka, C. Shinohara, T. Hori, and Y. Okada,
Department of Neurosurgery Neurological Institute, Tokyo Women's Medical University, 8-1 Kawada-cho, Shinjuku-ku, Tokyo, 162-8666, Japan

T. Suzuki, K. Yoshimitsu, and S. Ikuta
Faculty of Advanced Techno-Surgery, Institute of Advanced Biomedical Engineering and Science, Graduate School of Medicine, Tokyo Women's Medical University, 8-1 Kawada-cho, Shinjuku-ku, Tokyo, 162-8666, Japan

Introduction

Contemporary technological developments revolutionized surgical management of intraaxial brain tumors. Introduction of the intraoperative MRI (ioMRI) and related updated neuronavigation permitted for neurosurgeons to perform resection of the tumor under precise anatomical guidance. Moreover, at present it is possible to obtain intraoperatively not only structural, but functional and metabolic images. Comprehensive neurophysiological monitoring and intraoperative brain mapping by direct cortical and subcortical electrical stimulation, particularly performed during "awake craniotomy", allows precise localization of the cerebral functions and preservation of the functionally-important brain structures during removal of the tumor. Neurochemical navigation with 5-aminolevulinic acid (5-ALA) permits direct visualization of the residual neoplasm under the operating

M.N. Pamir et al. (eds.), *Intraoperative Imaging*, Acta Neurochirurgica Supplementum, Vol. 109,
DOI 10.1007/978-3-211-99651-5_11, © Springer-Verlag/Wien 2011

microscope and its differentiation from the peritumoral brain, whereas techniques of intraoperative histopathological diagnosis allow fast direct investigation of the pathological tissue for identification of the neoplastic cells. Incorporation of these adjuncts into surgical management of gliomas provides for the surgeon an opportunity to perform aggressive resection of the tumor with minimal risk of postoperative neurological morbidity. The present report highlights our experience with information-guided surgical management of gliomas using low magnetic field strength ioMRI with an emphasis on tumor resection rate and outcome.

Materials and Methods

From 2000 to 2009, 734 neurosurgical procedures with the use of ioMRI were performed in the intelligent operating theater of the Tokyo Women's Medical University. The vast majority of these surgeries (574 cases; 78.2%) were directed on biopsy or resection of gliomas using the concept of their information-guided surgical management. Nearly half of patients (263 cases; 45.8%) were followed more than 2 years after surgery.

Intelligent Operating Theater

Detailed information on the internal organization of the intelligent operating theater of the Tokyo Women's Medical University has been provided previously elsewhere [1, 2]. It equipped with an open ioMRI scanner (AIRIS II^{TM}, Hitachi Medical Co., Chiba, Japan) with magnetic field strength of 0.3 T, which has a hamburger-like shape with a 43 cm gantry gap and a permanent magnet producing vertical magnetic field with resonance frequency of 12.7 MHz. Low magnetic field strength creates narrow 5-gauss line, which extends 2 m from both sides, 2.2 m in front, 1.8 m backwards, and 2.5 m upwards. It permits for the surgeon to use some conventional surgical devices and instruments in the working space outside 5-gauss line. It should be specially marked, that this ioMRI scanner does not require a cooling system, which significantly reduce its operating costs by approximately 10,000 Japanese yen (around 100 US $) per month. Originally developed radiofrequency receiver coil integrated with Sugita head-holder (Head-holder coil; Mizuho Ltd., Tokyo, Japan) significantly improved the quality of intraoperative images. It provides an opportunity to perform MRI investigations with minimal distortion artifacts and maximum structure contrasting in any plane irrespectively to orientation of the object, which allows fixation of the patient head in the most desirable position for tumor removal. From the surgical point of view it allows use of any required approach including retrosigmoid and transtentorial. Moreover, use of the device provides an opportunity to perform intraoperatively not only volumetric, but diffusion-weighted imaging (DWI), MR angiography (MRA), and functional investigations, with sufficient quality of images comparable to those one obtained on scanners with higher magnetic field strength.

For facilitation of the tumor removal and detection of the neoplastic remnants we use previously developed navigator for photon radiosurgery system (PRS navigator; Toshiba, Tokyo, Japan), which allows fast and easy updating of the information obtained with ioMRI. It is based on a conventional infrared location-identification device, which shows the location of the suction tip and position of the suction tube in 3 sectional planes. The mislocalization errors of the device constitute 0.8 mm in average, 1.5 mm at maximum, and 0.5 mm at minimum, and typically do not exceed 1 mm [1]. The system permits co-registration, fusion and three-dimensional reconstruction of the various images, and provides easy-to-understand information.

If the tumor is located near or in the eloquent brain area, cortical mapping, neurophysiological monitoring, and/or stimulation of the cranial nerves are performed as appropriate before resection of the neoplasm for identification of the motor area, speech area, cranial nerves and their nuclei. "Awake craniotomy" was performed in 152 cases of the present series. Motor evoked potentials were investigated in 437 cases, whereas somatosensory evoked potentials were monitored routinely during surgery. Neurochemical navigation with 5-ALA and intraoperative histopathological investigation were done routinely, as appropriate.

Concept of the Information-Guided Surgical Management of Gliomas

Our concept of the information-guided surgical management of gliomas is based on the integration of various intraoperative anatomical, functional, and histological data with a purpose to attain maximal surgical resection of the tumor with minimal risk of postoperative neurological morbidity (Fig. 1). In our practice ioMRI investigations are usually performed when approach to the tumor is attained and then when the lesion is removed [2]. It permits assessment of completeness of the tumor resection and identification of the residual neoplasm or possible adverse effects, such as haemorrhage. If residual tumour is identified and considered suitable for additional resection the newly obtained ioMRI data are transferred to the neuronavigation device with subsequent resection of the neoplasm using this updated information.

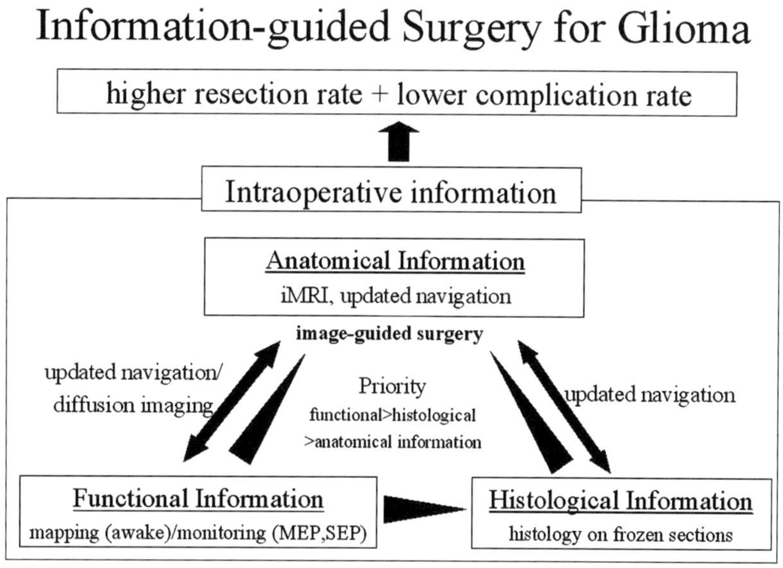

Fig. 1 Main principles of information-guided surgery for glioma. To maximize resection rate and minimize neurological morbidity various types of intraoperative information, namely anatomical, functional, and histological, are analyzed. All data are integrated with updated neuronavigation. In surgical decision-making the first priority is given to functional information provided by intraoperative brain mapping and comprehensive neurophysiological monitoring. *ioMRI* intraoperative MRI, *MEP* motor evoked potentials, *SEP* somatosensory evoked potentials

Whereas such anatomical data are used for removal of the bulk of the tumor, the resection of the residual neoplasm is based not only on the anatomical images, but on the results of the neurochemical navigation with 5-ALA and histopathological investigation of the walls of the surgical cavity.

It should be marked, that neither anatomical data obtained with ioMRI, nor histopathological information on presence of the residual neoplasm are sufficient for guidance of the tumor resection, especially if the lesion is located near or within functionally-important cerebral structures. In our opinion in any occasion the first priority in surgical decision-making should be given to functional information provided by the intraoperative brain mapping and comprehensive neurophysiological monitoring.

Results

ioMRI investigations provided informative images in 572 out of 574 cases (99.7%).

Maximal possible tumor resection was attained in 569 patients (99.1%). It included cases of radiologically complete tumor removal as well as subtotal removal leaving the residual neoplasm within the vital functionally-important brain areas detected with neurophysiological monitoring and/or brain mapping. In 3 cases aggressive tumor resection was not completed as planned due to lost of cooperation with the patient operated on in awake condition (2.0% of such cases).

The resection rate did not depend on the histopathological tumor grade and constituted, in median, 95%, 95%, and 98%, for WHO grade II, III, and IV gliomas, respectively (Fig. 2). Importantly, our low-field-strength ioMRI showed high sensitivity for detection of the residual glioma, which was confirmed by postoperative high-field-strength MRI investigations. In no one case of the present series unexpected residual tumor was disclosed.

Actuarial 5-year survival rate in patients who were followed more than 2 years after surgery was significantly worse in WHO grade IV gliomas (19%; $P<0.0001$), but did not differ significantly between WHO grade III and II tumors (69% vs. 87%; $P=0.0942$).

Illustrative Case

An 18-year-old man underwent information-guided surgery for left insular glioblastoma multiforme located adjacent to the compressed pyramidal tract medially and arcuate fasciculus associated with speech function, superiorly (Fig. 3). After craniotomy and dissecting of the Sylvian fissure baseline iMR images were obtained. Tumor removal was attained under awake condition of the patient. Incorporation of the DWI into neuronavigation device permitted for the surgeon to identify clearly the white matter bundle containing pyramidal tract and to perform anatomically controlled dissection of the neoplasm from this functionally important structure. Transitory motor weakness and aphasia were observed at the time of surgical manipulations in the vicinity to pyramical tract and superior longitudinal tract, respectively. Total *en bloc* removal of the contrast-enhanced tumor was attained and control ioMRI did not disclose residual neoplasm. Correspondingly, histopathological investigation of the wall of the resection cavity did not disclose neoplastic cells' clusters. The postoperative period was uncomplicated.

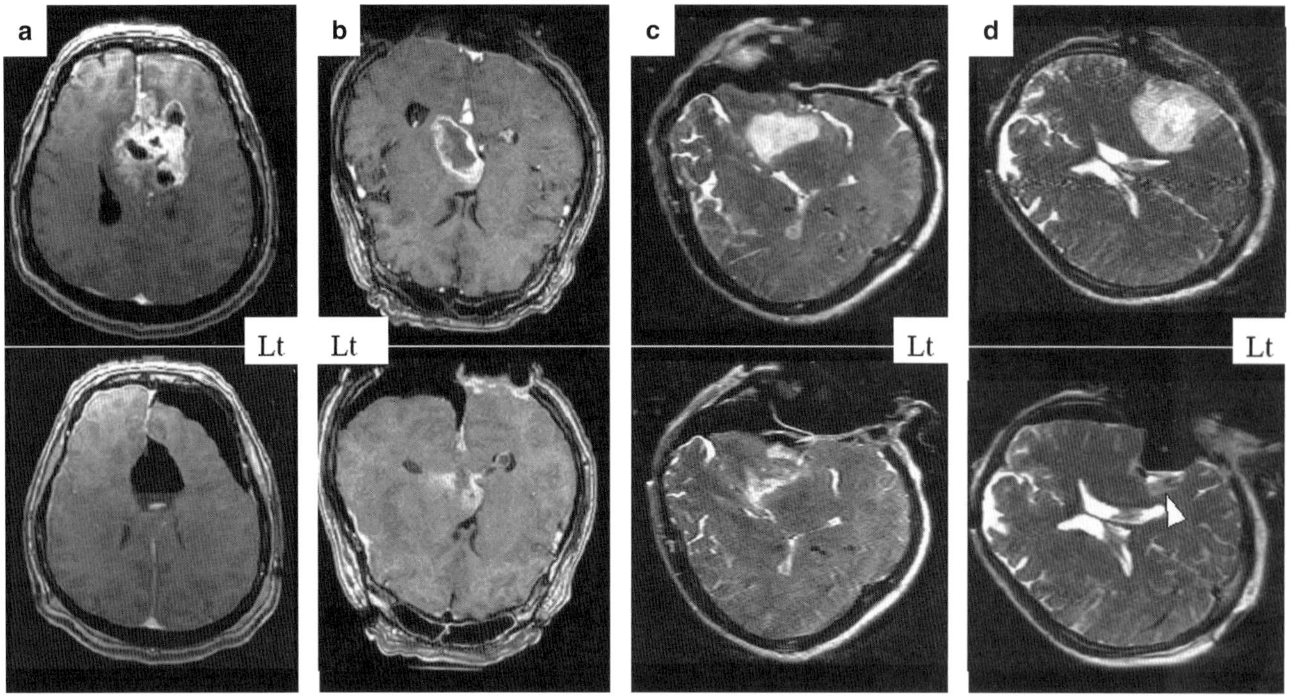

Fig. 2 Results of information-guided surgery for glioma using 0.3 T intraoperative MRI. Images before (*upper row*) and after (*lower row*) tumor removal are presented: (**a**) 100% resection of glioblastoma multiforme of the corpus callosum and both frontal lobes; (**b**) 85% resection of glioblastoma multiforme of the left thalamus; (**c**) 98% resection of the low-grade astrocytoma of the left basal ganglia and insula; (**d**) 98% resection of the anaplastic astrocytoma of the left parietal lobe with residual tumor left in the functionally important brain area (*arrowhead*)

Transitory intraoperative motor weakness and aphasia recovered completely and no neurological morbidity was observed after surgery.

Discussion

Introduction of ioMRI and updated neuronavigation into routine neurosurgical practice provided an opportunity to perform resection of gliomas under precise anatomical guidance. In our initial report use of ioMRI resulted in 93% average resection rate of gliomas, and 46% of total tumor removals [2]. Growing experience resulted in even better results presented herein. Maximal possible tumor resection, defined as radiologically complete tumor removal or subtotal removal leaving the residual neoplasm within the vital functionally-important brain areas, was attained in 99.1% of cases. While such aggressive tumor resection is frequently associated with increased rate of temporary postoperative neurological deterioration, the permanent neurological morbidity was noted just in 14% of cases [2]. Additionally, it seems that use of ioMRI reduces the risk of postoperative hemorrhagic complications, and does not increase the risk of infection despite prolonged operative time [2].

During the last decade there is a trend for introduction of ioMRI with high magnetic field strength of 1.5 T and 3 T [3, 4]. The advantages of such devices include high image quality, possibility to attain diffusion tensor and spectroscopic images, and short scanning time. However, increase of magnetic field strength is associated with greater possibility of image distortion artifacts. Additionally, the maintenance costs of such iMR scanners is high. In the same time latest technical achievements have permitted improvement of image quality of low-field-strength ioMRI [1, 5–7]. As it is shown herein, our open ioMRI scanner with magnetic field strength of just 0.3 T allows to attain not only standard T_1-weighted and T_2-weighted images of sufficient quality and resolution, but permits one to perform functional, DWI and MRA investigations. Further possibilities of fusion of preoperative high-field-strength and intraoperative low-field-strength MR images using deformable model within advanced computer software, can result in combining of the advantages of both techniques and may significantly diminish the need for ioMRI of high magnetic field strength.

It should be specially underlined, that in cases of intra-axial brain neoplasms anatomical data alone, even if obtained with ioMRI, are not sufficient for guidance of the resection. Precise histopathological information and, especially, use of comprehensive neurophysiological monitoring with cortical and subcortical brain mapping are absolutely necessary for attainment of the optimal results [2, 8]. Intraoperative integration of anatomical, histopathological and neurophysiological data constitutes the basis of our

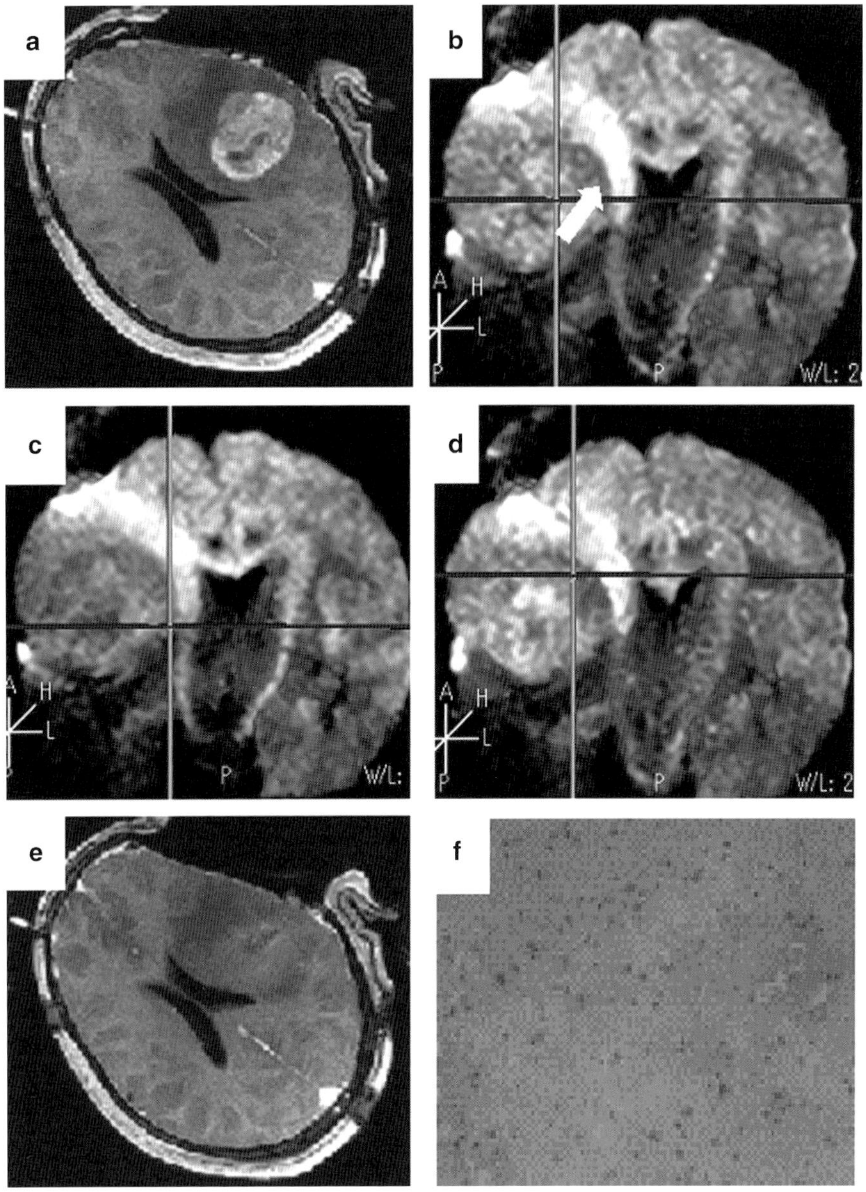

Fig. 3 Information-guided surgery for left insular glioblastoma multiforme in 18-year-old man. Contrast-enhanced T_1-weighted intraoperative MR image obtained after craniotomy and before tumor resection showed the tumor located in the left posterior insula (**a**). Incorporation of the intraoperative diffusion-weighted image into neuronavigation system permitted for the surgeon to identify white matter bundle containing pyramidal tract (**b**, *arrow*), and brain areas in which surgical manipulations resulted in transitory motor weakness (**c**) and aphasia (**d**). At the end of tumor removal no definite residual neoplasm could be seen on structural intraoperative MRI (**e**) and, correspondingly, histopathological investigation of the wall of the resection cavity did not disclose neoplastic cells' clusters (**f**)

concept of "information-guided surgery" with a goal of maximal possible tumor resection and minimal risk of post-operative neurological deterioration.

Meanwhile, the main question is still remains unanswered: whether total removal of the glial neoplasm, particularly high-grade one, is translated into longer survival of the patient? Published data on this important issue are unequivocal and result in a great controversy providing few reasonable arguments both for opponents and advocates of aggressive tumor resection. It seems, however, that the study of Stummer et al. [9] provides a high level of evidence in favor of total glioma removal. The authors adjusted biases of age and eloquent area location in the dataset of randomized study on use of neurochemical navigation with 5-ALA during resection of glioblastoma multiforme, and found that median overall survival after complete removal of the contrast-enhanced lesion (17 months) was significantly longer compared to cases with its incomplete removal (12 months). In concordance, in the report of van den Bent et al. [10] on EORTC 26951 randomized trial of combined chemotherapy for anaplastic gliomas, the overall survival was better after complete tumor removal compared to partial ones or to biopsy. The similar results were marked in the Brain Tumor Registry of Japan [11]. Analysis of 6,400 cases of WHO grade III and IV gliomas showed, that more than 90% tumor removal is associated with survival advantage, while such resection rate was attained in 6–10% of cases only.

Our current retrospective analysis could not be reliable for evaluation of the association between resection rate of glioma and patients' survival after surgery. Anyway, in the present series actuarial 5-year survival rate for patients with WHO grade II, III, and IV gliomas constituted 87%, 69%, and 19%, respectively. For comparison, according to the last edition of the Brain Tumor Registry of Japan [11] the same rates in general neurosurgical practice constitutes 75%, 40%, and 7%, respectively. Moreover, the finding of the similar long-term prognosis in our cases of WHO grade II and III gliomas seems intriguing. It can reflect the significance of survival advantage associated with aggressive resection of WHO grade III gliomas [12] and should be definitely investigated further.

In conclusion, information-guided surgical management of gliomas using low-field-strength ioMRI based on the intraoperative integration of anatomical, histopathological and neurophysiological data permits to perform maximal possible tumor resection with minimal risk of postoperative neurological morbidity, and may result in significant survival advantage, particularly in patients with WHO grade III gliomas.

Conflict of interest statement We declare that we have no conflict of interest.

Acknowledgements The authors are thankful to Drs. Osami Kubo, Ken'ichi Hirasawa, Takemasa Kawamoto, Kosaku Amano, Yuichi Kubota, Tatsuya Ishikawa, Atsushi Watanabe, and Ayako Horiba (Department of Neurosurgery, Tokyo Women's Medical University) for their help with the present study. This work was supported by the Industrial Technology Research Grant Program in 2000–2005 (A45003a) from the New Energy and Industrial Technology Development Organization of Japan (to Y. Muragaki). The research activities of Drs. H. Iseki, M. Chernov, and K. Takakura are supported by the Program for Promoting the Establishment of Strategic Research Centers, Special Coordination Funds for Promoting Science and Technology, Ministry of Education, Culture, Sports, Science and Technology (Japan).

References

1. Iseki H, Nakamura R, Muragaki Y, Suzuki T, Chernov M, Hori T, Takakura K (2008) Advanced computer-aided intraoperative technologies for information-guided surgical management of gliomas: Tokyo Women's Medical University experience. Minim Invasive Neurosurg 51:285–291
2. Muragaki Y, Iseki H, Maruyama T, Kawamata T, Yamane F, Nakamura R, Kubo O, Takakura K, Hori T (2006) Usefulness of intraoperative magnetic resonance imaging for glioma surgery. Acta Neurochir Suppl 98:67–75
3. Nimsky C, Ganslandt O, Von Keller B, Romstock J, Fahlbusch R (2004) Intraoperative high-field-strength MR imaging: implementation and experience in 200 patients. Radiology 233:67–78
4. Pamir MN, Ozduman K, Dincer A, Yildiz E, Peker S, Ozek MM (2010) First intraoperative, shared resource, ultrahigh-field 3-Tesla magnetic resonance imaging system and its application in low-grade glioma resection. J Neurosurg 112:57–69
5. Hadani M, Spiegelman R, Feldman Z, Berkenstadt H, Ram Z (2001) Novel, compact, intraoperative magnetic resonance imaging-guided system for conventional neurosurgical operating rooms. Neurosurgery 48:799–809
6. Ozawa N, Muragaki Y, Nakamura R, Iseki H (2008) Intraoperative diffusion-weighted imaging for visualization of the pyramidal tracts. Part II: clinical study of usefulness and efficacy. Minim Invasive Neurosurg 51:67–71
7. Senft C, Seifert V, Hermann E, Franz K, Gasser T (2008) Usefulness of intraoperative ultra low-field magnetic resonance imaging in glioma surgery. Neurosurgery 63(suppl 2):257–267
8. Ojemann JG, Miller JW, Silbergeld DL (1996) Preserved function in brain invaded by tumor. Neurosurgery 39:253–259
9. Stummer W, Reulen HJ, Meinel T, Pichlmeier U, Schumacher W, Tonn JC, Rohde V, Oppel F, Turowski B, Woiciechowsky C, Franz K, Pietsch T, ALA-Glioma Study Group (2008) Extent of resection and survival in glioblastoma multiforme: identification of and adjustment for bias. Neurosurgery 62:564–576
10. van den Bent MJ, Carpentier AF, Brandes AA, Sanson M, Taphoorn MJ, Bernsen HJ, Frenay M, Tijssen CC, Grisold W, Sipos L, Haaxma-Reiche H, Kros JM, van Kouwenhoven MC, Vecht CJ, Allqeier A, Lacombe D, Gorlia T (2006) Adjuvant procarbasine, lomustine, and vincristine improves progression-free survival but not overall survival in newly diagnosed anaplastic oligodendrogliomas and oligoastrocytomas: a randomized European Organisation for Research and Treatment of Cancer phase III trial. J Clin Oncol 24:2715–2722
11. The Committee of Brain Tumor Registry of Japan (2003) Report of brain tumor registry of Japan (1969–1996), 11th edition. Neurol Med Chir (Tokyo) 43(suppl):1–111
12. Shinohara C, Muragaki Y, Maruyama T, Shimizu S, Tanaka M, Kubota Y, Oikawa M, Nakamura R, Iseki H, Kubo O, Takakura K, Hori T (2008) Long-term prognostic assessment of 185 newly diagnosed gliomas: Grade III glioma showed prognosis comparable to that of Grade II glioma. Jpn J Clin Oncol 38:730–733

Implementation of the Ultra Low Field Intraoperative MRI PoleStar N20 During Resection Control of Pituitary Adenomas

Ruediger Gerlach, Richard du Mesnil de Rochemont, Thomas Gasser, Gerhard Marquardt, Lioba Imoehl, and Volker Seifert

Abstract *Objective*: To describe our experience with the application of an intraoperative ultra low field magnetic resonance imaging system (ioMRI) PoleStar N20, Medtronic Surgical Navigation Technologies, Louisville, USA during resection control of pituitary adenomas.

Methods: Forty-four patients were operated on a pituitary adenoma (1 microadenoma, 43 macroadenomas; mean size 26.0±9.7 mm). The ioMRI system was used for navigation and resection control after transseptal, transsphenoidal microsurgical tumour removal using standard instruments and standard microscope. If any accessible tumour remnant was suspected surgery was continued for navigation guided re-exploration and if necessary continued resection.

Results: The applications of the scanner integrated navigation system, with a 3-planar reconstruction of the coronal scan, enabled the surgeon to safely approach and remove the tumour. The quality of preoperative tumour visualization with the ultra low field ioMRI in patients with macroadenomas is very good and has a good congruency with the preoperative 1.5 T MRI. For microadenomas the preoperative visualization is poor and very difficult to interpret. In seven patients ioMRI resection control showed residual tumours leading to further resection. After final tumour resection the ioMRI scan documented adequate decompression of the optic pathway in all patients. However, the intraoperative image interpretation was equivocal in four patients in whom it was difficult to distinguish between small intrasellar tumour remnants and perioperative changes.

Conclusions: The PoleStar N20 is a safe, helpful and feasible tool for navigation guided pituitary tumour approach. Image interpretation is requires some experience, but decompression of the optic system can be reliable shown in cases with pituitary macroadenomas. This system is of limited value for resection control of pituitary microadenomas.

Keywords ioMRI · Pituitary adenoma · Suprasellar tumour · Surgery

Introduction

The estimation of tumour removal during microsurgical resection of pituitary adenomas can be intricate because of limited visualization of supra- and parasellar structures. Especially the proof of adequate decompression of the optic pathway is crucial in patients with large suprasellar tumour extension. To overcome this obvious problem intraoperative MRI (ioMRI) resection control [1–9] has been propagated. Intraoperative MRI systems differ with respect to scanner field strength (*low field* [1, 3, 4, 6, 8–15], *high field* [5, 7] or *3T* [16, 17]) and therefore require diverse perquisites for implementation into a surgical procedure. According to the field strength of the various systems the operation room or at least the ioMRI system needs (ultra low field system PoleStar N10 and N20) special shielding. To apply ioMRI either a patient or scanner movement is necessary, which needs different technical installation requirements of the scanner and/ or operating table, which has implications for the operative work flow.

It has been demonstrated that the rate of further resection of non secreting pituitary adenomas was increased after the implementation of low [1, 4] and high field ioMRI scanner systems [5, 7]. Furthermore the use of ioMRI increased the rate of resection and therefore endocrinological cure of patients with GH- secreting tumours [5].

The PoleStar N20 (Medtronic Surgical Navigation Technologies, Louisville, USA) is the second generation of a compact ultra low field ioMRI scanner. It represents a further developed system, which was at first introduced by Hadani et al. in 2001 [12].

R. Gerlach (✉), R. du M. de Rochemont, T. Gasser, G. Marquardt, L. Imoehl, and V. Seifert
Department of Neurosurgery and Neuroradiological Institute, Johann Wolfgang Goethe- University, Schleusenweg 2-16, 60528 Frankfurt/Main, Germany
e-mail: r.gerlach@em.uni-frankfurt.de

DOI 10.1007/978-3-211-99651-5_12,

In this report we discuss our experience wit this ultra low file intraoperative scanner type during microsurgical resection of pituitary adenomas.

Patients and Methods

The PoleStar N20 system was installed in the Department of Neurosurgery, Johann Wolfgang Goethe- University Frankfurt/ Main, Germany in September 2004. This scanner type is applicable either with the use of a mobile shielding device or in a shielded conventional operating room. In our department the complete operating room was shielded.

We report about 44 patients (24 male, 20 female; mean age 55.5±13.5 years) with pituitary macroadenomas (43) and one patient with microadenoma, which were partly included in a recent publication [11]. All patients had preoperative 1.5 T contrast enhanced MRI focused on the sellar region to diagnose the extent of tumour growth and invasion of the cavernous sinus.

A standard microsurgical procedure with a transseptal, transsphenoidal tumour resection was performed in all patients and the PoleStar N20 system was used for neuronavigation and preoperative tumour visualization and resection control. All anaesthesiological equipment was fully ioMRI compatible and used without any interference during the whole procedure. After introduction of general anaesthesia and supine positioning the patients head was fixed in a 3-point pin titanium head clamp (Odin, Medical Technologies Ltd; Yokneam, Israel) and a flexible surface radiofrequency (rf) head coil is placed around the head. For co-registration and navigation, a dynamic patient reference frame (PRF) was fixed to the head holder (Fig. 1). During the procedure the scanner is stored beneath the operating table. For data acquisition the magnets were elevated into the scan-position. To avoid any interfering during the scanning procedures and to achieve optimal image quality the power supplies of all electrical medical devices, which are not necessarily needed, were turned off during all scanning procedures using a main switch. The system offers the application of several T1 and T2 weighted sequences [14]. Selection of MRI sequences was described recently [11] after these sequences were evaluated the ioMRI was used with a defined protocol. The first scans were performed to proof the correct head position in the centre of the magnet. Therefore an axial ultra fast mixed T1/T2 weighted sequence (esteady: TR 11.00 ms, TE 3.00 ms, 24 s, 8 mm, Fig. 2) or a short T1 sequence (T1: TR 40.0 ms, TE 3.00 ms, 60 s, 8 mm) was used depending on the surgeons preference. To obtain best image quality it is crucial to position the patients head in the centre of the magnets. Moreover, for navigation purposes the field of view (FOV) should cover the nasal cavity besides

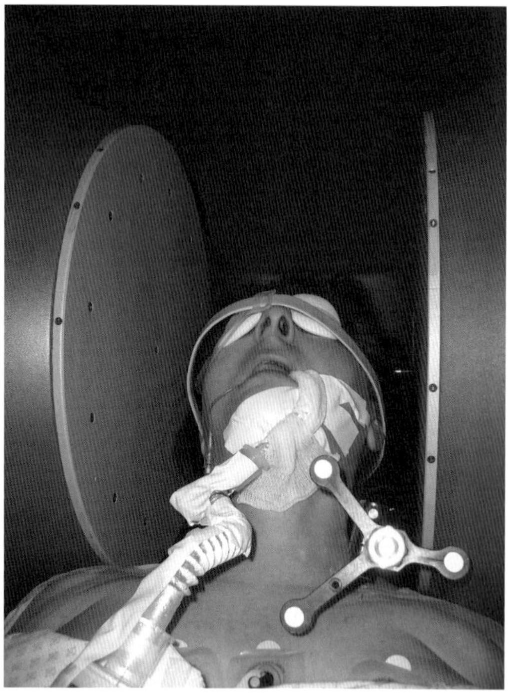

Fig. 1 Position of the patient within the magnet (PoleStar N20) from the patients left side. Because image quality strongly depends on a head centered within the magnet positioning is a crucial step during the procedure. Shoulders are pulled down to optimize head position. For head fixation a 3-point sharp pin non ferromagnetic head holder was used. The DRF is mounted on the head holder for navigation and the head coil is placed around the head

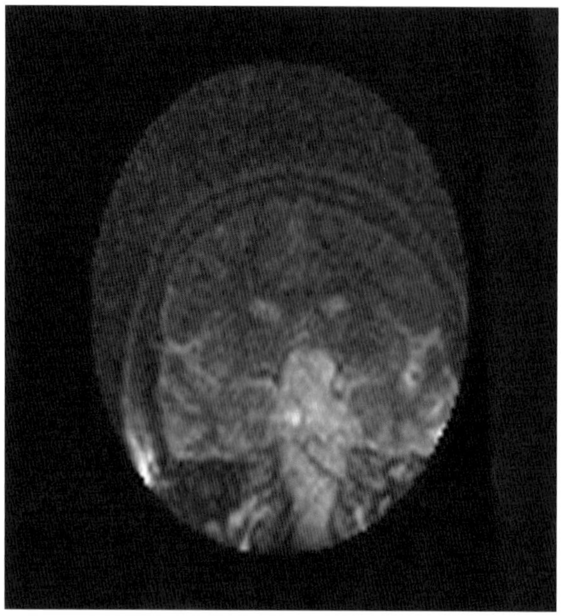

Fig. 2 Short ioMRI sequence used for head positioning control using an axial mixed T1/T2 sequence (esteady 24 s) showing the large intra and suprasellar tumour. Identification of correct head position is crucial for the image quality and can be performed in axial or coronal plane

the sellar region to facilitate reliable navigation during the transsphenoidal approach.

A coronal T1 weighted (TR 60.00 ms, TE 3.00 ms, 6.5 min, 3 mm) gadolinium-DTPA enhanced (0.4 ml Gd/kg body, Magnevist, Schering, Berlin; Germany) sequence was used for navigation with calculation of a 3-planar reconstruction (Fig. 3). After the pre- resection scans the operative field was prepared and sterile draped. To cover the magnet sterile plastic drapes were used. For Navigation we used the Odin navigation software during the first time and later on the stealth station (Vers.4.0; Medtronic Surgical Navigation Technologies, Louisville, USA). A standard surgical microscope (NC4, Karl Zeiss Medical, Oberkochen, Germany) and normal ferro magnetic instruments were used throughout the whole procedure.

When the surgeon considered the tumour to be completely removed or at least achieved the intended amount of tumour resection if the tumour had cavernous sinus invasion, a resection control scan was performed. The time from stopping surgery to start ioMRI resection control scanning ranges between 1 and 2 min. If an accessible tumour remnant was visible on the ioMRI scan navigation guided surgical resec-

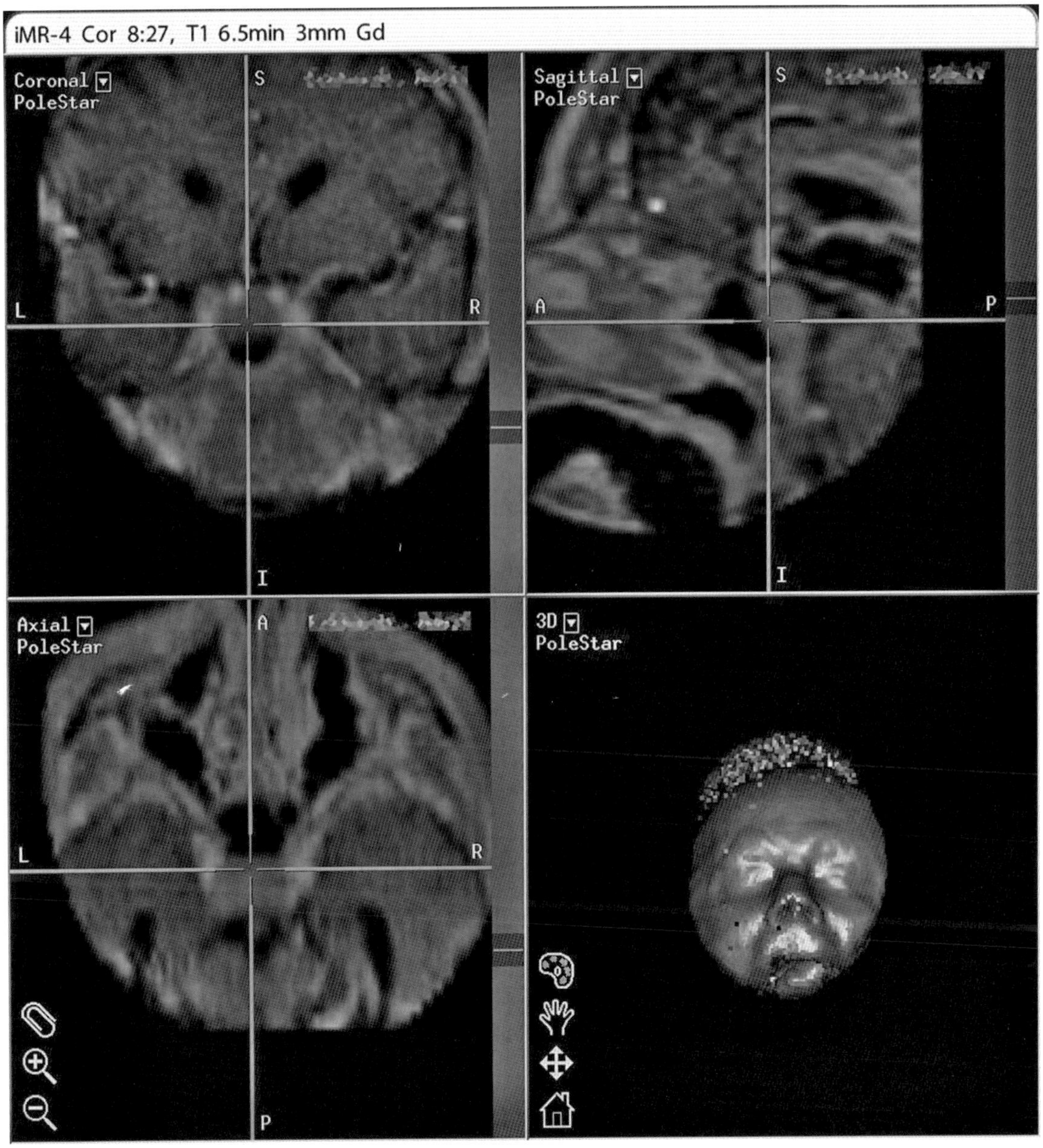

Fig. 3 A coronal T1 weighted Gd enhanced scan (3 mm) is used for neuronavigation. A triplanar reconstruction is calculated and displayed by the system. (**a**) The Odin system was used during the first 8 months, (**b**) the Stealth station which was used afterwards and offers a virtual tip extension for surgical guidance after application the navigation probe (**c**)

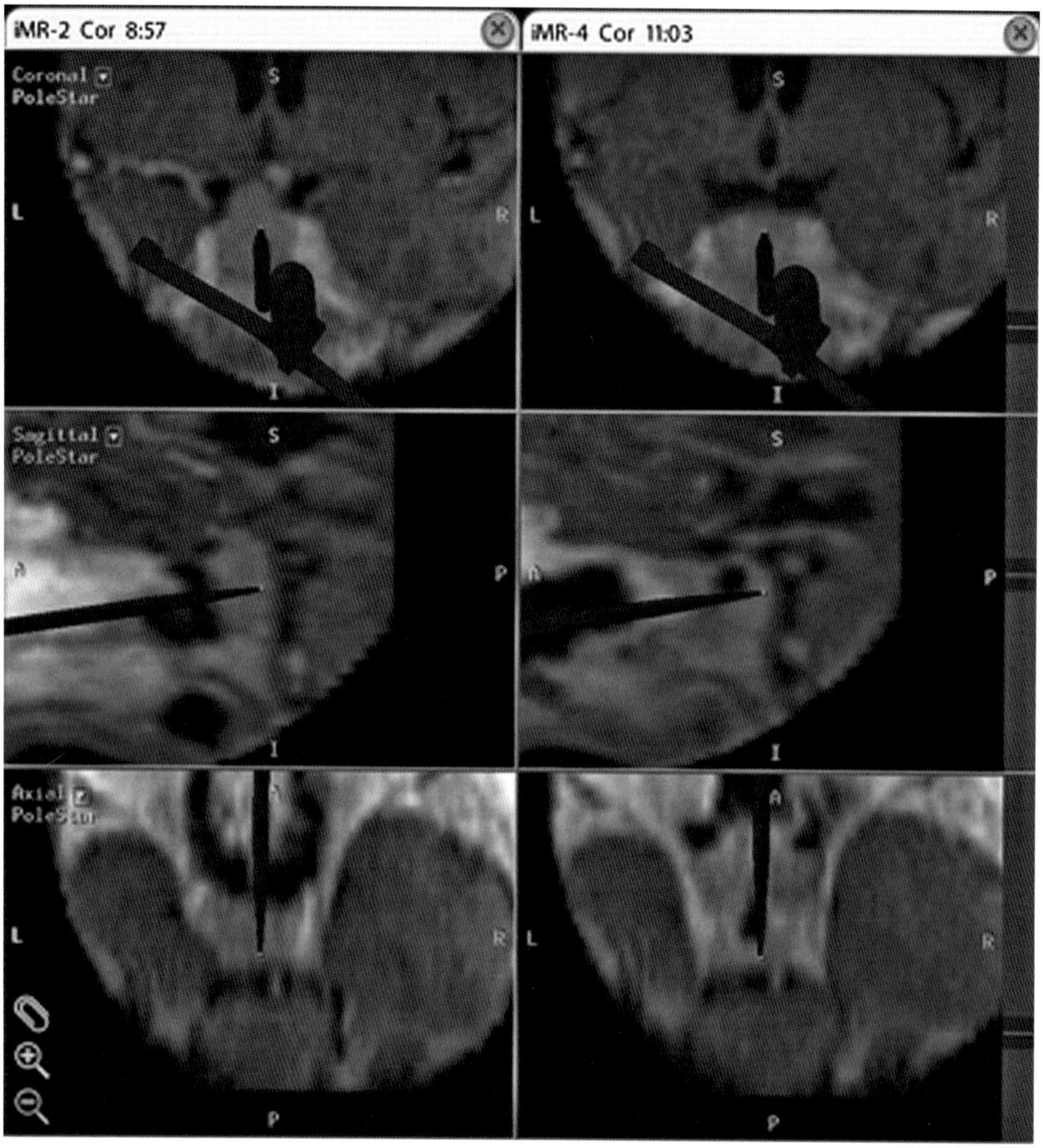

Fig. 4 Pre (*left*) and post resection (*right*) ultra low field ioMRI scan with 3-planar reconstruction for navigation guided (re-) exploration. The complete removal of the suprasellar tumour with adequate decompression of the optic system is demonstrated, while the interpretation of the intrasellar region is difficult due to oozing during obtaining the scan

tion was continued until further scan(s) documented complete resection or the accomplished intended resection goal (Fig. 4).

Results

Forty-four patients underwent transsphenoidal tumour resection with the use of the ioMRI system PoleStar N20. Forty-three patients had a macro- and one patient had a microadenoma. No adverse events related to the application of the intraoperative ioMRI system PoleStar N20 were observed. There were no accidents caused by the use of standard ferromagnetic instruments. No procedure related complications occurred, especially no infection or surgery related visual disturbance, or injury to the carotid artery.

Intraoperative imaging allowed an accurate localization of the sellar region and pituitary tumours as well as identification of pertinent parasellar structures, which was the prerequisite for safe and effective navigation guided resection (Fig. 3). Thus the navigation safely guided the surgeon providing detailed anatomic information, which was also possible for the two patients with previous surgery and operations for recurrent tumours.

PoleStar N20 resection controlled surgery was feasible in all patients with macroadenomas, while the visualization of small pituitary adenoma was limited and therefore patients with microadenomas were not further evaluated.

According to the ioMRI surgery was continued in a total of 7 out of all 44 patients (15.9%). A continued resection was possible in 1 of 15 patients (6.7%) with intended complete resection, but the majority of cases were patients with cavernous sinus invasion and therefore intended incomplete resection. Thus the PoleStar N20 was mainly helpful in detecting residual tumour in invasive tumour types, were the surgeons tend to be less aggressive during tumour resection.

The ophthalmologic status improved in all patients with visual impairment (n = 19) and bilateral hemianopia (n = 18) except for one patients with blindness on one eye deriving from previous surgery in another institution. Only one patient with intended incomplete resection and sticky tumour had a transient VIth nerve palsy, which completely recovered within 6 weeks after surgery. In four of eight patients with GH-secreting tumours and one patient with prolactinoma endocrinological cure was achieved. Three patients with acromegaly had very small tumour remnants at 3 months 1.5 T MRI, which could not be shown by ioMRI. One patient had no visible tumour in standard control MRI 3 months postoperatively, but slightly elevated IgF 1 levels thus consensus criteria were not met in this patient.

Intraoperative image interpretation was equivocal in four patients and unfortunately three of the four patients suffered from GH- secreting adenomas, including the one patient with continued surgery. Compared with the 3 months 1.5 T MRI a discrepancy in the images was found in these four cases were no clear residual intrasellar tumour was seen on ioMRI by the surgeon. Intraoperative interpretation was challenging and a tiny small remnant could not be distinguished from perioperative changes but was identified in 1.5 T MRI at 3 months. However, re-evaluation for comparison analysis of the ioMRI scans depicted residual tumour comparable to the 1.5 T MRI at the time of surgery. Therefore, this misinterpretation of the images was rather a problem of the surgeons, rather than the system itself.

Discussion

Although there are associated financial burden the distribution and implementation of intraoperative MRI systems has gained more and more acceptance. One of the most appreciated indications for ioMRI is the resection control of pituitary macroadenomas (Fig. 5).

Two different developmental trends of intraoperative MRI systems have emerged over the last years. The implementation of high field ioMRI systems on the one side offers the quality of diagnostic scanners during the operation, but has more limitations in the surgical work flow. On the other end the ultra low field system, PoleStar N20, enables the surgeon to integrate the system with only minimal changes in the surgical work flow, but offers the possibility to use standard instruments and microscope during the whole operation. We report our experience with an compact ultra low field

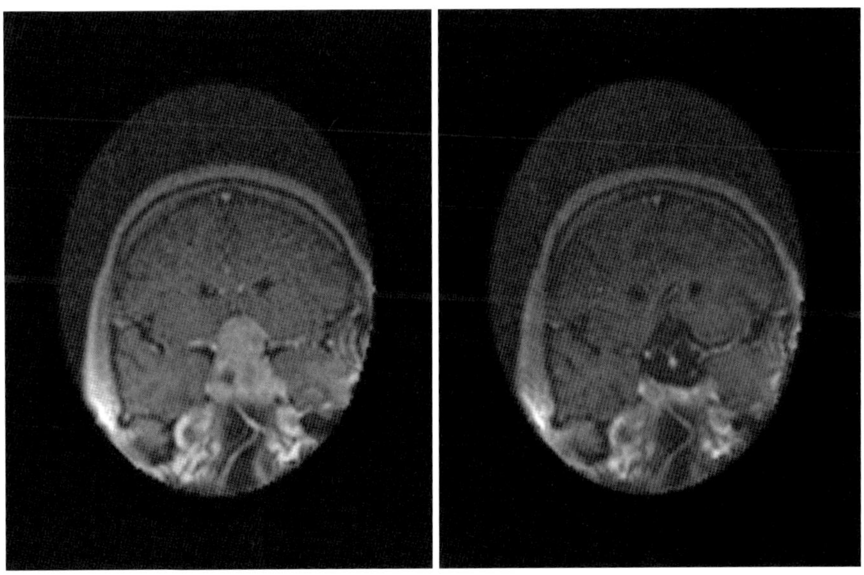

Fig. 5 Coronal T1 weighted contrast enhanced [0.15 T] scan before (*left*) and after (*right*) resection of a large intra and suprasellar adenoma (same patient as in Fig. 2). The intraoperative scan after resection demonstrates resection of the pituitary adenoma and a very good visualization of the suprasellar compartment with adequate decompression of the optic system and the pituitary stalk with a deviation to the left side is seen on the ultra low field ioMRI PoleSTar system

scanner, which is positioned underneath the operating table during surgery and can be easily and fast moved up for scanning purposes. This is the second generation of the compact ultra low field systems which demonstrates many refinements compared to the first scanner of this type, which was introduce by Hadani et al. [12]. A larger gap between the magnets eases patient positioning and the slightly higher field strength (0.15 T vs. 0.12 T) lead to improved image quality.

Similar to the N10 system no patient movement is necessary with the PoleStar N20 system when a resection control scan is required from the surgeon. Based on updated images acquired within minutes while surgery is paused remaining tumour can be removed by further navigation- guided resection. The ioMRI navigation was accurate as described by other groups [14, 18] and reliable to guide the surgeon during the procedure. Thus, beside a safe tumour approach – also in patients with residual tumour – the use of the PoleStar N20 integrated navigation system allows a precise intraoperative tracking of residual tumour.

However, the key question for ioMRI in pituitary surgery is whether or not the implementation of an ioMRI increases the amount of tumour resection and therefore the number of complete tumour removal, which is the precondition for endocrinological cure in patients with secreting tumours. Although not proven by randomized controlled trials the use of an ioMRI improved the rate of complete resection independent of the ioMRI system. This was demonstrated for both low and high field systems [1–8, 12, 14, 19].

Beside the above described advantages of the PoleStar N20 system there are also drawbacks associated with its use. This scanner type has an individually learning curve for image interpretation. The differentiation of small intrasellar tumour remnants can be very difficult as described in a recent series of patients with macroadenomas [11].

This uncertainty of intraoperative interpretation by the surgeon was due to difficulties in interpretation rather than a methodological problem of the ioMRI system and confirms that a high level of experience is necessary for adequate image interpretation. A comparative post surgery analysis comparing the intraoperative ultralow filed MR-images and the 1.5 T standard 3 months images showed these small residual tumours in the ultra low field obtained images. The image quality was significantly better for the suprasellar compartment compared to the intra- and parasellar compartment, which is important to assess the adequate decompression of the optic pathway and complete removal of suprasellar tumour parts. This is in accordance with the experience of other groups using various low field systems [1, 4, 6, 14, 19, 20]. Sufficient decompression of the chiasm is of paramount significance especially in patients with large invasive parasellar tumours, not accessible for complete resection.

Also, for small microadenomas the image quality has clear limitations and the benefit of intraoperative MRI scanning in those patients is low.

IoMRI resection control of pituitary macroadenomas significantly increases operation and total anaesthesia time, but the information of resection status and the chance for immediate re-exploration and continued resection outweighs the longer and operation time [11, 13]. The reliable assessment of the amount of resection increases the patients comfort and avoids any uncertainty about the grade of resection, which usually exists postoperatively up to 3 months until a routine 1.5 T MRI documents the actual extend of resection.

Conclusion

The 0.15 T ultra low field ioMRI PoleStar N20 offers immediate reliable resection control for suprasellar tumour parts, while image interpretation of intra- and parasellar tumours is difficult. Therefore the correct image interpretation of intrasellar compartment has an individually learning curve. After implementation of the PoleStar N20 System continued resection increased the amount of resected tumour especially in patients with intended subtotal tumour removal due to invasion of the cavernos sinus. The integrated navigation system displays accurate anatomic information also in patients with previous surgery.

Disclosure None of the authors has any financial interest in the methodology being advanced with the publication of our data. TG serves as a clinical consultant for Medtronic Surgical Navigation Technologies, Louisville, USA.

References

1. Bohinski RJ, Warnick RE, Gaskill-Shipley MF, Zuccarello M, van Loveren HR, Kormos DW, Tew JM Jr (2001) Intraoperative magnetic resonance imaging to determine the extent of resection of pituitary macroadenomas during transsphenoidal microsurgery. Neurosurgery 49:1133–1143
2. Darakchiev BJ, Tew JM Jr, Bohinski RJ, Warnick RE (2005) Adaptation of a standard low-field (0.3-T) system to the operating room: focus on pituitary adenomas. Neurosurg Clin N Am 16:155–164
3. De Witte O, Makiese O, Wikler D, Levivier M, Vandensteene A, Pandin P, Baleriaux D, Brotchi J (2005) Transsphenoidal approach with low field MRI for pituitary adenoma. Neurochirurgie 51:577–583
4. Fahlbusch R, Ganslandt O, Buchfelder M, Schott W, Nimsky C (2001) Intraoperative magnetic resonance imaging during transsphenoidal surgery. J Neurosurg 95:381–390

5. Fahlbusch R, Keller B, Ganslandt O, Kreutzer J, Nimsky C (2005) Transsphenoidal surgery in acromegaly investigated by intraoperative high-field magnetic resonance imaging. Eur J Endocrinol 153:239–248
6. Martin CH, Schwartz R, Jolesz F, Black PM (1999) Transsphenoidal resection of pituitary adenomas in an intraoperative MRI unit. Pituitary 2:155–162
7. Nimsky C, von Keller B, Ganslandt O, Fahlbusch R (2006) Intraoperative high-field magnetic resonance imaging in transsphenoidal surgery of hormonally inactive pituitary macroadenomas. Neurosurgery 59:105–114
8. Schwartz TH, Stieg PE, Anand VK (2006) Endoscopic transsphenoidal pituitary surgery with intraoperative magnetic resonance imaging. Neurosurgery 58:ONS44–ONS51
9. Steinmeier R, Fahlbusch R, Ganslandt O, Nimsky C, Buchfelder M, Kaus M, Heigl T, Lenz G, Kuth R, Huk W (1998) Intraoperative magnetic resonance imaging with the magnetom open scanner: concepts, neurosurgical indications, and procedures: a preliminary report. Neurosurgery 43:739–747
10. Black PM, Moriarty T, Alexander E III, Stieg P, Woodard EJ, Gleason PL, Martin CH, Kikinis R, Schwartz RB, Jolesz FA (1997) Development and implementation of intraoperative magnetic resonance imaging and its neurosurgical applications. Neurosurgery 41:831–842
11. Gerlach R, de RR Du Mesnil, Gasser T, Marquardt G, Reusch J, Imoehl L, Seifert V (2008) Feasibility of Polestar N20, an ultra-low-field intraoperative magnetic resonance imaging system in resection control of pituitary macroadenomas: lessons learned from the first 40 cases. Neurosurgery 63:272–284
12. Hadani M, Spiegelman R, Feldman Z, Berkenstadt H, Ram Z (2001) Novel, compact, intraoperative magnetic resonance imaging-guided system for conventional neurosurgical operating rooms. Neurosurgery 48:799–807
13. Kanner AA, Vogelbaum MA, Mayberg MR, Weisenberger JP, Barnett GH (2002) Intracranial navigation by using low-field intraoperative magnetic resonance imaging: preliminary experience. J Neurosurg 97:1115–1124
14. Schulder M, Salas S, Brimacombe M, Fine P, Catrambone J, Maniker AH, Carmel PW (2006) Cranial surgery with an expanded compact intraoperative magnetic resonance imager. Technical note. J Neurosurg 104:611–617
15. Wu JS, Shou XF, Yao CJ, Wang YF, Zhuang DX, Mao Y, Li SQ, Zhou LF (2009) Transsphenoidal pituitary macroadenomas resection guided by PoleStar N20 low-field intraoperative magnetic resonance imaging: comparison with early postoperative high-field magnetic resonance imaging. Neurosurgery 65:63–70
16. Hall WA, Galicich W, Bergman T, Truwit CL (2006) 3-Tesla intraoperative MR imaging for neurosurgery. J Neurooncol 77:297–303
17. Pamir MN, Peker S, Ozek MM, Dincer A (2006) Intraoperative MR imaging: preliminary results with 3 tesla MR system. Acta Neurochir Suppl 98:97–100
18. Salas S, Brimacombe M, Schulder M (2007) Stereotactic accuracy of a compact intraoperative MRI system. Stereotact Funct Neurosurg 85:69–74
19. Pergolizzi RS Jr, Nabavi A, Schwartz RB, Hsu L, Wong TZ, Martin C, Black PM, Jolesz FA (2001) Intra-operative MR guidance during trans-sphenoidal pituitary resection: preliminary results. J Magn Reson Imaging 13:136–141
20. Schulder M, Sernas TJ, Carmel PW (2003) Cranial surgery and navigation with a compact intraoperative MRI system. Acta Neurochir Suppl 85:79–86

Intraoperative MRI for Stereotactic Biopsy

Michael Schulder and David Spiro

Abstract This work aims at demonstrating the value of intraoperative magnetic resonance imaging (ioMRI) as a routine tool for stereotactic brain biopsy.

Biopsies were done using the PoleStar N-20 ioMRI (Medtronic Navigation, Louisville, Colorado, USA) under general anesthesia. Images were acquired after patient positioning and after insertion of an MRI-compatible biopsy cannula. A Navigus guide (Medtronic Navigation) was used to align and direct the cannula. Retargeting was done as necessary, to improve placement within the target and to avoid critical structures, using the system's integrated infrared navigation tool. Cannula placement was tracked using serial images.

ioMRI-guided biopsy was done in 39 patients, of whom 28 had neoplasms and 11 had non-neoplastic conditions. Additional OR time related to the use of ioMRI (including positioning of the patient and magnet, and imaging acquisition) averaged 1.1 h. In 53% of the surgeries the biopsy cannula was repositioned based on intraoperative imaging. A histologic diagnosis was obtained in all but one patient, with ioMRI confirming proper cannula placement in all cases. There were no significant hemorrhages on clinical or imaging grounds nor any other complications.

IoMRI can be routinely used for stereotactic biopsy in a regular neurosurgical operating environment. While general anesthesia is used and there is some additional time incurred from this technology the improved diagnostic yield and ability to avoid complications make ioMRI an ideal technical adjunct for brain biopsy.

Keywords Frameless stereotaxy · Intraoperative magnetic resonance imaging · Stereotactic brain biopsy

M. Schulder (✉) and D. Spiro
Department of Neurosurgery, North Shore LIJ, North Shore University Hospital, 9 Tower, Manhasset, NY 11030, USA
e-mail: Schulder@nshs.edu

Introduction

Techniques for brain biopsy have evolved in relation to the evolution of imaging methods. Until the advent of computed tomography (CT) stereotactic techniques, developed primarily for functional neurosurgical operations, were not applicable for morphologic targets except in rare cases. The advent of CT allowed for free-hand biopsies to be done with imaging control, but this approach lacked the ability for any stereotactic localization (except in the plane of a particular image) [1, 2]. The joining of CT to stereotactic frames in the mid-1980s allowed for the emergence of stereotactic biopsy as a routine procedure [3, 4]. Several years later magnetic resonance imaging (MRI) became available for this use. More recently, surgical navigation technology ("frameless stereotaxy") has become widely accepted. Comparison of stereotactic biopsy with a frame or frameless approach has shown equivalent efficacy and safety between these techniques.

Intraoperative MRI (ioMRI) was introduced by Black et al. at the Brigham and Women's Hospital in the mid-1990s [5]. The impetus behind this technological leap was to provide updated images that would account for the inevitable brain shift that renders information from preoperative images unreliable for safe navigation. In addition, images can of course be used for resection control and to rule out such complications as hemorrhage or stroke. The logic of adapting ioMRI for stereotactic biopsy lies in the ability to ensure accurate and safe placement of the sampling instrument, and to in essence make it an image controlled and not "blind" surgery. However, the effort and expense of using ioMRI for stereotactic biopsy – a procedure that is viewed (with reasonable accuracy) as routine and safe – may fairly be questioned.

We describe our experience with the PoleStar N20 (Medtronic Navigation, Louisville, Colorado, USA), a low field strength ioMRI, designed for use in a regular neurosurgical operating room (OR), for stereotactic brain biopsy.

M.N. Pamir et al. (eds.), *Intraoperative Imaging*, Acta Neurochirurgica Supplementum, Vol. 109,
DOI 10.1007/978-3-211-99651-5_13,

Surgical Technique

Patients selected for ioMRI-guided biopsy routinely undergo stereotactic MRI in advance of surgery. This allows confirmation that there has been no change in the lesion, for patients in whom the time between imaging and surgery is prolonged, and also provides a "hedge" should there be any technical difficulties with the ioMRI unit. In such an event surgery can proceed using "conventional" surgical navigation.

The PoleStar N20 ioMRI has been described in previous reports. It is the second generation of an innovative device designed by Hadani and colleagues [6, 7]. In brief, it is based on a mobile, 0.15 Tesla (T) permanent magnet. The system is stored in a cage in the back of the OR and brought out when needed. The OR is shielded against electrical interference from outside sources. During imaging, non-filtered electrical devices are shut off and unplugged. Anesthesia equipment is MRI-compatible. The magnet poles are separated by a 27 cm gap. An integrated infrared navigation tool is included in the system. The magnet is positioned under the OR table, raised as needed for imaging, and lowered again at other times. The low magnet field strength allows for the use of regular operating tools, including ferromagnetic ones, as long as the magnet poles are below the OR table.

General anesthesia is used, as patients require three-point head fixation in the MRI-compatible headholder that is part of the PoleStar system. Patients are positioned on a regular OR table. In our experience the prone position should be used when biopsy targets are located in the posterior half of the intracranial space; lateral positioning is possible but somewhat more cumbersome. A disposable, flexible MR receiving coil is positioned and draped out of the field; this avoids the need for coil replacement during surgery (Fig. 1).

After acquiring a 6.5 min T1 weighted image (with contrast as needed), a surgical plan is made using the desired target and entry points. If the surgeon wishes, the image may be exported to the StealthStation software, which resides as a separate program on the PoleStar computer. An incision long enough to accommodate the Navigus biopsy guide (Medtronic Navigation) is made, about 4 cm long. The burr hole and dural opening are done before seating the Navigus. The dedicated trackable probe is placed in the Navigus and aligned with the planned trajectory. A side-cutting MRI-compatible biopsy cannula is stopped at the appropriate length and inserted towards the target. The magnet is raised and short image sequences, between 24 s and 1 min, are acquired. If cannula position is adequate, then biopsies are taken at 2–3 levels if possible. A frozen section is requested.

The biopsy cannula is redirected if intraoperative imaging shows that it is not adequately placed within the lesion, or is too close to a critical structure such as a blood vessel. Imaging is repeated after each redirection. After taking the last specimen and removing the cannula a last image is acquired to rule out a hematoma.

Patient Data

IoMRI-guided stereotactic biopsies have been done on 39 patients. Their age ranged from 5 years to 86 years, with a mean of 49 years. There were 25 male and 14 female patients. Lesion locations, as in other series, reflected a typical distribution in the brain, including frontal [8], parietal [8], temporal [9], and occipital [10] lobes. Two patients had pineal lesions, two in the thalamus, and one each in the corpus callosum, suprasellar region, midbrain,

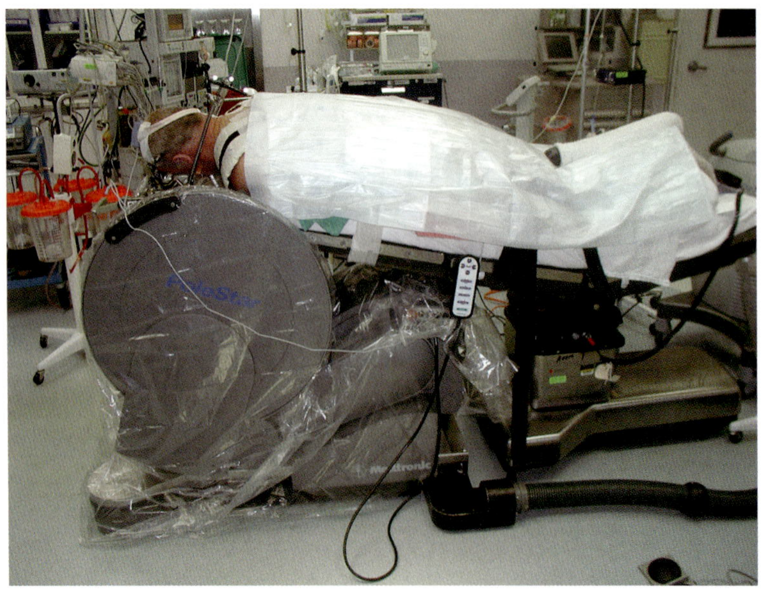

Fig. 1 Patient positioned prone for right parietal stereotactic biopsy in the PoleStar N20. Note that the flexible receive coil is positioned to allow for it to be draped out of the field. The reference frame for the infrared navigation tool is to the patient's left

hypothalamus, and cerebellum. The dominant hemisphere contained the target in 18 patients. The supine position was used in 28 patients, while 11 were turned prone.

Results

On one occasion the PoleStar N20 did not properly boot. As the patient had been referred specifically for ioMRI-guided biopsy, having had a nondiagnostic biopsy elsewhere, the procedure was aborted and rescheduled. The number of scanning sessions ranged from 2 to 9 (including multiple images as biopsies were obtained), with a mean of 3.5 per procedure. In 21 cases (53%) the intraoperative image led to replacement of the biopsy cannula. In 12 patients this change was made to improve cannula position in the target; in 4 patients, to avoid injury to a critical structure before taking a biopsy; and in 5 after an initial frozen section did not obviously show lesional tissue. The additional time needed for setup and use of ioMRI ranged from 0.5 to 2.0 h, with a men of 1.1 h. No significant hemorrhage was detected on final intraoperative images. All patients were neurologically stable after surgery. There were two deaths in the series due to progression of pre-existing disease – lymphoma in one and progressive multifocal leukoencephalopathy from AIDS in the other.

Diagnoses included high grade glioma in 15 patients, low grade glioma in 11, lymphoma in 1, and embryonal cell carcinoma in 1; and 10 patients had non-neoplastic lesions, including 3 bacterial abscesses. In one patient, although increased cellularity was seen, no definitive diagnosis was made. Intraoperative images showed the biopsy cannula to be within the enhancing component of the lesion (this patient remains neurologically intact, with stable MRI findings, 1 year later).

Case Illustrations

Patient 1. This 44 year old right handed man was transferred from another hospital, having come to the emergency room complaining of progressive headache and then left sided weakness. MRI showed a ring-enhancing lesion in the right thalamus, with some surrounding edema (Fig. 2a); symptoms improved on steroids. The preoperative diagnosis was high grade glioma. The patient was positioned supine for biopsy and a right coronal entry point was chosen (Fig. 2b). Imaging showed the biopsy cannula to be at the enhancing rim (Fig. 2c). Frozen section showed inflammatory tissue, and specimens for permanent pathology. Cultures were negative but pathology confirmed an abscess with gram positive cocci. The patient was treated with antibiotics and the lesion regressed.

Patient 2. This 70 year old right handed man presented with 2 weeks of left hemiparesis. Imaging revealed a ring-enhancing mass in the right insular cortex, with some involvement of the right Sylvian fissure. The medial aspect of the lesion was targeted to avoid injury to Sylvian vessels (Fig. 3a). Intraoperative imaging resulted in improved cannula placement (Fig. 3b, c). The patient proved to have a high grade glioma.

Discussion

The progress of neurosurgery over the last century has been marked by decreasing the need for guesswork. The practical beginning of minimally invasive approaches for brain biopsy came in the 1980s with the performance of freehand procedures done in CT scanners. A review of several CT-guided freehand biopsy series showed a diagnostic yield of 90% (range 79–97%) a mortality rate of 2.5% (0.5–4.7%) and morbidity rate of 7.8% [2]. For obvious technical reasons, these procedures were best reserved for patients with relatively large and superficial lesions.

The stereotactic frame, invented by Horsley and Clarke in 1908, was first adapted for human surgery in 1947 by Spiegel and Wycis [9]. For nearly 40 years thereafter, frames were used for functional neurosurgery, using ventriculography for guidance. The combination of the stereotactic concept with CT and then MRI allowed for surgery aimed at morphologic targets. Interestingly, the published experience with stereotactic biopsies yielded results that were grossly similar to those achieved with freehand approaches (although these series included targets that were smaller and deeper than those attempted before) [2]. With the advent of surgical navigation, sometimes called "frameless stereotaxy", similar results have been obtained – a diagnostic rate of slightly over 90%, with morbidity and mortality of 0.7 % and 3.5% [11].

Why then bother introducing a new technique for stereotactic biopsy? The answer lies in the continued incidence of non-diagnostic procedures and the complications, which can reflect unrecognized intracranial hemorrhage, injury to blood vessels, or unnecessary entry into critical brain areas. Intraoperative imaging offers several advantages in this regard (1) brain shifts that may occur with dural opening can be accounted for; (2) if a non-lesional frozen section is obtained, repeat imaging and targeting can be done during the same surgery; (3) the surgeon can ensure that the biopsy is taken from the area most likely to yield a diagnosis; (4) with serial imaging during biopsy, unnecessary penetrations with the

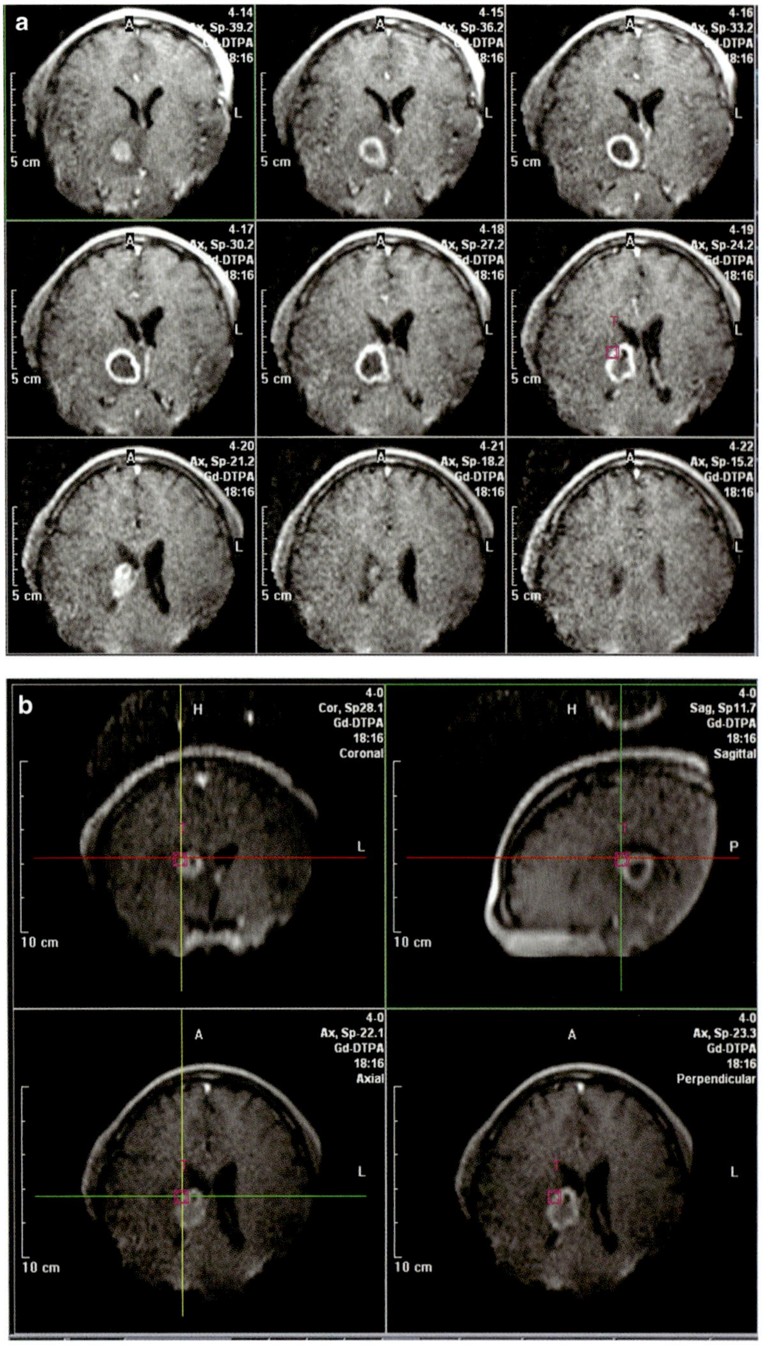

Fig. 2 (**a**) Preoperative ioMRI of a 44 year old man thought to have a right thalamic glioma. (**b**) Reconstructed triplanar views showing selected target on enhancing rim. (**c**) 24 s T2 ioMRI shows cannula at the target point. The lesion proved to be a bacterial abscess

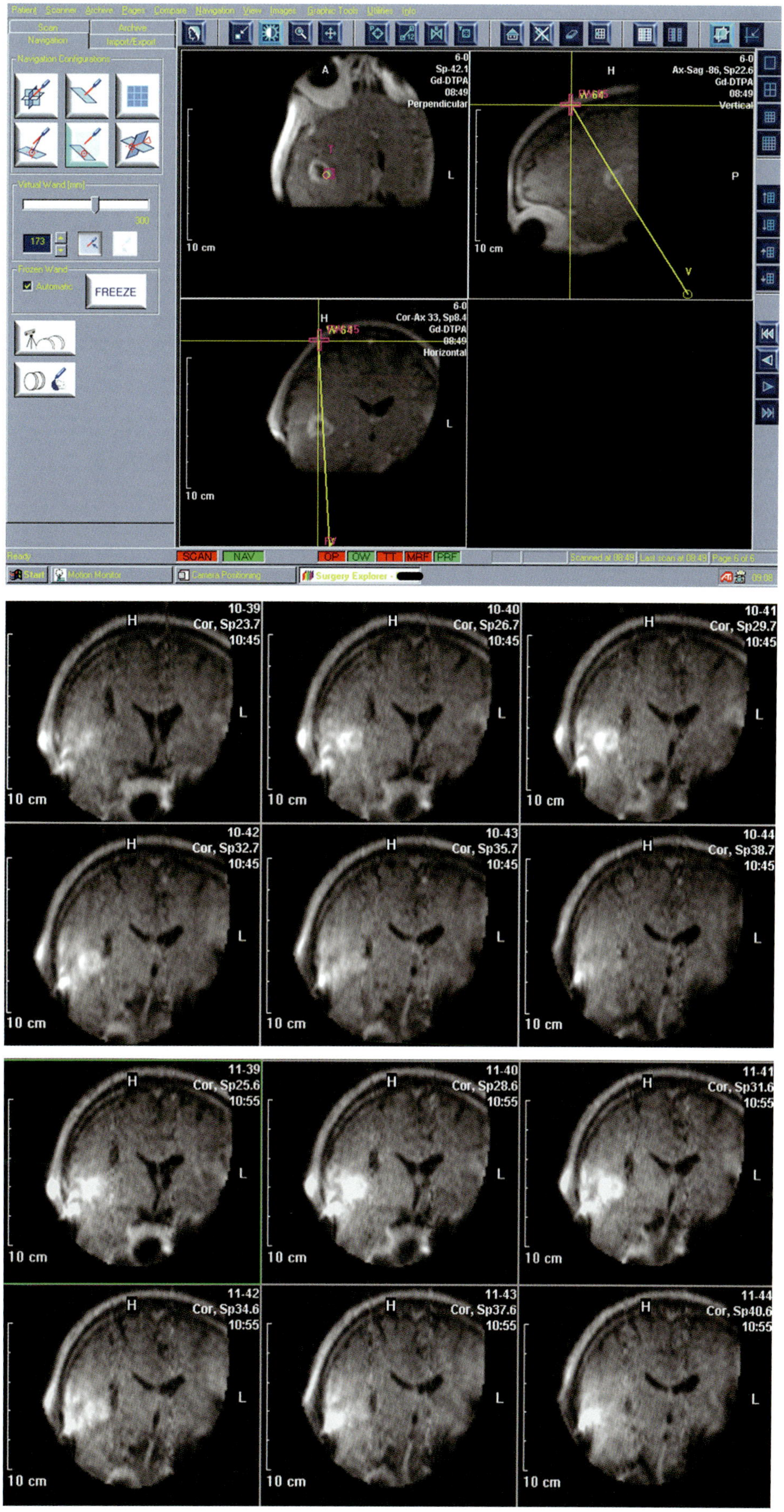

Fig. 3 70 year old man with mass in the right insula. (**a**) Targeting of the medial rim of the tumor, away from Sylvian vessels. (**b**) Image acquired after first pass of cannula. (**c**) Improved position of cannula to increase diagnostic yield, still avoiding Sylvian fissure. Frozen section and permanent pathology showed glioblastoma

cannula can be avoided; (5) hemorrhage can be ruled out at the end of the procedure.

For the foreseeable future brain imaging, intraoperatively or otherwise, will be best done with MRI. IoMRI-guided biopsy was first described by Black et al., using a 0.5 T magnet, in their pioneering article [5]. The authors reported a 100% diagnostic yield for brain biopsy; one patient was found to have an intracranial hemorrhage that required surgical evacuation. Bernays et al. reported a series devoted specifically to stereotactic biopsy, using a specially-designed, skull-mounted guide. In 113/114 patients a diagnosis was made; morbidity was 1.8% and mortality 0.9% [10]. Hall et al. performed biopsies in a diagnostic 1.5 MRI suite, modified for surgical use. The first 35 procedures were done freehand, and the following 40 with a device that evolved into the Navigus guide. The histological yield was 100%, with morbidity of 2.8% and mortality of 1.4% [12].

Ours is the first series to focus on use of a compact, low-field ioMRI for stereotactic biopsy. Several small series from groups using 0.2 T ioMRIs included diagnostic rates of 93–100%, with limited description of technique [8, 13, 14]. Kanner et al. reported their use of the PoleStar N10, which used a 0.12 T magnet [15]. Their overall experience included biopsies in 15 patients, all of which were diagnostic. As noted above, we made a histological diagnosis in all but one of our patients, but were able to confirm that the biopsy was taken from the area of interest. In addition, in this and in four other patients, the ability to image the cannula after receiving a non-lesional frozen section report allowed for retargeting as needed, without "poking the brain" based merely on a pre-operative image. While additional time (mean 1.1 h) was incurred with the use of ioMRI, this does not take into account the time saved by avoiding placement of a stereotactic frame and the subsequent imaging session in a diagnostic scanner. Additional time could be saved by eliminating the frozen section and relying on the images alone. We feel that the advantages of intraoperative pathology, which has been shown to increase the diagnostic yield of stereotactic biopsies, outweigh this small prolongation of surgery [16].

Advocates for the high field ioMRI approach note the improved resolution and the ability to acquire diffusion weighted imaging, MR spectroscopy or angiography, or functional images with these systems. It is not clear that these advanced capabilities, whatever their worth may be, would be required to perform what should be a routine procedure, namely, stereotactic biopsy. Compared to these other ioMRI devices, the PoleStar N20 offers some distinct advantages. These include the use of a regular OR table in a regular OR. This allows for patient positioning as dictated by the surgical approach, and causes minimal disruption to surgical routine. However, it must be noted that the incomplete field of view of the PoleStar N20 may limit imaging of targets in the posterior fossa.

Other objections that may be raised to this ioMRI-guided biopsy technique are the need for a bur hole and the longer incision needed to accommodate the Navigus guide. This is in contrast to frameless and especially frame-based approaches where a 5 mm incision and twist drill hole may suffice. In addition, the Navigus is a disposable device, whose use brings an added expense to the surgery. Finally, although intravenous sedation and local anesthetic may be considered for these cases, the need for 3-point head fixation and the added time of ioMRI use make general anesthesia far easier. This is a potential added source of morbidity compared to frame-based biopsies, which typically are done under local anesthesia.

Conclusions

Stereotactic brain biopsy can be done as a routine procedure in a low field ioMRI environment. Imaging enables the surgeon to compensate for brain shift, to re-image and re-target as necessary, and to rule out intracranial bleeding. With the increasing adoption of ioMRI at neurosurgical centers worldwide, we recommend that this be the method of choice for stereotactic biopsy.

Conflicts of interest statement We declare that we have no conflict of interest.

References

1. Greenblatt SH, Rayport M, Savolaine ER, Harris JH, Hitchins MW (1982) Computed tomography-guided intracranial biopsy and cyst aspiration. Neurosurgery 11:589–598
2. Wen DY, Hall WA, Miller DA, Seljeskog EL, Maxwell RE (1993) Targeted brain biopsy: a comparison of freehand computed tomography-guided and stereotactic techniques. Neurosurgery 32:407–412; discussion 412–413
3. Gildenberg PL (1983) Stereotactic neurosurgery and computerized tomographic scanning. Appl Neurophysiol 46:170–179
4. Heilbrun MP (1983) Computed tomography-guided stereotactic systems. Clin Neurosurg 31:564–581
5. Black P, Moriarty T, Alexander E 3rd, Stieg P, Woodard E, Gleason P, Martin C, Kikinis R, Schwartz R, Jolesz F (1997) Development and implementation of intraoperative magnetic resonance imaging and its neurosurgical applications. Neurosurgery 41:831–842; discussion 842–835
6. Hadani M, Spiegelman R, Feldman Z, Berkenstadt H, Ram Z (2001) Novel, compact, intraoperative magnetic resonance imaging-guided system for conventional neurosurgical operating rooms. Neurosurgery 48:799–807
7. Schulder M, Salas S, Brimacombe M, Fine P, Catrambone J, Maniker AH, Carmel PW (2006) Cranial surgery with an expanded compact intraoperative magnetic resonance imager. Technical note. J Neurosurg 104:611–617

8. Tronnier VM, Wirtz CR, Knauth M, Lenz G, Pastyr O, Bonsanto MM, Albert FK, Kuth R, Staubert A, Schlegel W, Sartor K, Kunze S (1997) Intraoperative diagnostic and interventional magnetic resonance imaging in neurosurgery. Neurosurgery 40:891–900; discussion 900–902
9. Gildenberg PL (1990) The history of stereotactic neurosurgery. Neurosurg Clin N Am 1:765–780
10. Bernays RL, Kollias SS, Khan N, Brandner S, Meier S, Yonekawa Y (2002) Histological yield, complications, and technological considerations in 114 consecutive frameless stereotactic biopsy procedures aided by open intraoperative magnetic resonance imaging. J Neurosurg 97:354–362
11. Woodworth GF, McGirt MJ, Samdani A, Garonzik I, Olivi A, Weingart JD (2006) Frameless image-guided stereotactic brain biopsy procedure: diagnostic yield, surgical morbidity, and comparison with the frame-based technique. J Neurosurg 104:233–237
12. Hall WA, Martin AJ, Liu H, Nussbaum ES, Maxwell RE, Truwit CL (1999) Brain biopsy using high-field strength interventional magnetic resonance imaging. Neurosurgery 44:807–813
13. Bernstein M, Al-Anazi AR, Kucharczyk W, Manninen P, Bronskill M, Henkelman M (2000) Brain tumor surgery with the Toronto open magnetic resonance imaging system: preliminary results for 36 patients and analysis of advantages, disadvantages, and future prospects. Neurosurgery 46:900–907; discussion 907–909
14. Fahlbusch R, Ganslandt O, Nimsky C (2000) Intraoperative imaging with open magnetic resonance imaging and neuronavigation. Childs Nerv Syst 16:829–831
15. Kanner AA, Vogelbaum MA, Mayberg MR, Weisenberger JP, Barnett GH (2002) Intracranial navigation by using low-field intraoperative magnetic resonance imaging: preliminary experience. J Neurosurg 97:1115–1124
16. Kim JE, Kim DG, Paek SH, Jung HW (2003) Stereotactic biopsy for intracranial lesions: reliability and its impact on the planning of treatment. Acta Neurochir (Wien) 145:547–554; discussion 554–555

The Evolution of ioMRI Utilization for Pediatric Neurosurgery: A Single Center Experience

Thomas M. Moriarty and W. Lee Titsworth

Abstract From its inception intraoperative magnetic resonance imaging (ioMRI) was envisioned to have significant applications in neurosurgery in general and pediatrics specifically. Over the last 9 years we have noted a dramatic shift in our ioMRI usage from intracranial tumors to cerebrospinal fluid management and complex cysts. Here we present seven selected cases to illustrate lessons learned from our operative experience within the GE Signa SP/I open-configuration "double-doughnut" MRI. These cases including a ganglioglioma, ependymoma, and pilocytic astrocytoma tumor resection, as well as arachnoid cysts, complex cyst, and microabscess drainage reflect our current use of ioMRI in pediatric neurosurgical cases. Namely that ioMRI is optimal for (1) resection of small tumors with poorly differentiated tumor margins, (2) large tumors with mass effect, and (3) shunt or catheter placement requiring either extreme accuracy or intraoperative confirmation of catheter placement. We also comment on the legitimate limitations of this technology in certain operations. Additionally emphasized are cases in which ioMRI imaging drives operative decision making, highlighting the unique and unequaled abilities of this technology for a subset of pediatric neurosurgical cases.

Keywords Catheter · CSF diversion · Ependymoma · Ganglioglioma · Interventional MRI · Intracranial abscesses · Intracranial tumors · Neurosurgery · Pediatric neurosurgery · Subarachnoid cyst

T.M. Moriarty (✉)
Kosair Children's Hospital, Norton Neuroscience Institute, 210 E Gray St.Suite 1105, Louisville, KY 40202, USA
e-mail: Thomas.Moriarty@nortonhealthcare.org

W.L. Titsworth
Department of Anatomical Sciences and Neurobiology, University of Louisville School of Medicine, Louisville, KY 40202, USA

Introduction

The first intraoperative MRI system (ioMRI) was a collaborative product between researchers at the Brigham and Women's Hospital in Boston, MA, and General Electric Medical Systems first implemented in 1996 [1]. The first ioMRI pediatric neurosurgery was performed on a small cerebellar tumor soon after. From its inception, ioMRI was seen as a tool most suited to neurosurgical application and was anticipated to have particular utility in tumor, epilepsy, hydrocephalus, cystic lesions, and potential for minimally invasive surgery [1, 2]. This subset of cases predicted that ioMRI would hold particular value in pediatric neurosurgery. Here we present a review of the ioMRI usage from 2000 to 2009 from a pediatric neurosurgery perspective using the GE double doughnut system.

There are currently three basic ioMRI concepts which can be categorized as either low, mid, or high-field systems. Low-field ioMRI consists of a 0.12-T magnet mounted directly on the OR table. When not in use the two 40-cm diameter discs, located 25 cm apart, are kept under the table. This device, which was originally designed by Odin, is available now through Medtronic as the Polestar [3]. While offering a lower startup cost, this product has significantly poorer image quality and limited MR capabilities. In contrast, mid-field ioMRI, originally developed by GE, consists of a "double-doughnut" design in which the surgeon operates while imaging. The physical design utilizes two superconducting magnets spaced 58 cm apart. This system offers the advantage of good quality images in a timely manner; however ergonomics and the requirement of special instrumentation limit its application in some surgeries. High-field systems utilize either a 1.5-T magnet that comes to and from the patient or requires moving the patient in and out of a stationary magnet [2, 4, 5]. These systems offer the advantage of improved images and the use of ferromagnetic instrumentation during portions of the operation but transport time limits the speed of image acquisition. Some recent versions of this configuration are the IMRIS, BrainSUITE,

M.N. Pamir et al. (eds.), *Intraoperative Imaging*, Acta Neurochirurgica Supplementum, Vol. 109,
DOI 10.1007/978-3-211-99651-5_14,

GE Amiga, and the Phillips system. A more thorough discussion of each system can be found elsewhere [6]. While pediatric neurosurgery has been performed on each of these configurations, this discussion will be limited to our experience with the GE double doughnut ioMRI.

Historical Use of ioMRI in One Institution

From 2000 to 2009 we utilized a Signa SP/I open-configuration "double-doughnut" MRI (GE Medical Systems, Milwaukee, WI, USA). Our ioMRI suit is a fully functional operating room located in the adult surgical facility with direct access to the pediatric hospital. Over the last 9 years we have preformed 610 neurosurgical cases, 282 of which were pediatric neurosurgery, with a majority of cases being craniotomies (44%), cyst management (25%), or CSF diversion (16%). Within our pediatric caseload we noticed a shift in usage over this time. During the first 2 years of service 76% of pediatric cases were craniotomies for the removal of masses while only 24% were either cyst drainage or CSF diversions. In contrast, over the last 2 years only 35% of pediatric cases were craniotomies while 65% were now complex cysts or shunts. This shift occurred secondary to our recognition of this systems strengths and limitations. Particularly we realized that not all tumors were ideally suited for ioMRI and secondly this technology is unrivaled in targeting small foci because it provided stereotaxis with instant real-time feedback and no discordance between reality and the virtual construct.

ioMRI Utilization in Tumors

During the initial days of our ioMRI usage we attempted a broad range of tumor operations within the ioMRI suit. Over time it became clear that ioMRI facilitated the removal of supratentorial tumors but had ergonomic challenges in posterior fossa tumors operations. However, it remained a good tool for posterior fossa stereotaxy as the following cases will illustrate. Traditionally low-grade gliomas are particularly difficult to remove since neoplastic tissue so closely resembles normal tissue in these lesions [7, 8]. However, patients who underwent subtotal resection are 1.4 times more like to have disease recurrence and have almost 5 times the risk of death relative to patients who underwent gross total resection [9]. In cases such as these, ioMRI is an ideal tool for removal of all necessary malignancy while maximally sparing native tissue. Case #1 is a 14 year old male who presented with a seizure disorder and was subsequently found to have a right temporal low grade ganglioglioma (WHO I) (Fig. 1a–c). While preoperative T1 sequence showed little abnormality, T2 images demonstrated a clear unifocal lesion suggesting the possibility of gross total resection [8]. Intraoperative T2 weighted sequences allowed proper localization of the lesion and a clean resection of a woody mass was achieved without disturbing normal tissue. Repeat imaging at 2 years showed no residual tumor and the patient remained seizure free.

In contrast to diminutive lesions, ioMRI also shows advantages over static stereotaxy in large intracranial masses. Case #2 is an 11 year old male with a $6 \times 5.7 \times 4.6$ cm^3 anaplastic ependymoma (WHO III) with marked surrounding edema

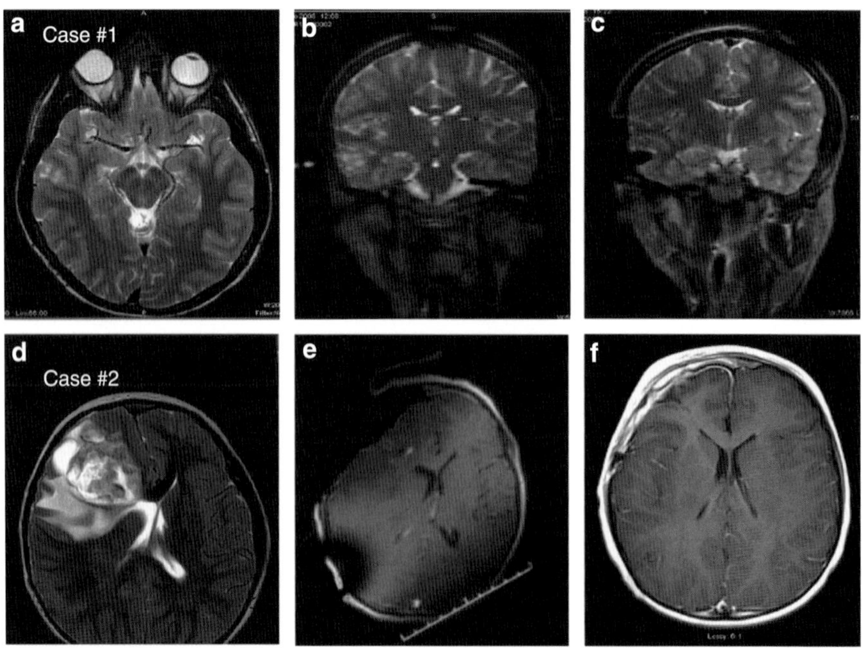

Fig. 1 *Case #1:* Low grade Ganglioglioma. T2 weighted preoperative (**a**) and intraoperative (**b**, **c**) images. Note the pointer in (**b**) used for localization. *Case #2:* Anaplastic ependymoma. Preoperative (**d**), intraoperative (**e**), and 5 month postoperative images (**f**). Note significant surrounding edema and mass effect (**d**)

(Fig. 1d–f). Again subtotal resection of these tumors has been shown to affects outcomes [10, 11]. ioMRI allowed access to the tumor via the most direct pathway similar to what is achieved with static stereotaxy. Next the small cystic component of the tumor was decompressed. However, frequent intraoperative imaging was used to quickly debulk the tumor. We were then able to remove the lesion along a clear plane. Five month postoperative images showed a barely perceptible surgical cavity. Four and a half years later the patient remains free from recurrence. The challenge of this operation in regards to image guided surgery was twofold. First, after craniotomy the shifting of intracranial contents rendered all preoperative images useless. Secondly, the surrounding edema so distorted normal tissue so as to obscure the tumor margins. Using ioMRI to quickly debulk the tumor allowed decompression of the surrounding tissue and brought into view a natural tissue plane.

However, this technology is not well suited to all tumors. First, we have learned through experience that ioMRI holds little advantage over the standard operating facilities for the resection of tumors with clear margins. Additionally the limited operative environment in the "double doughnut" design actually hinders this systems application in posterior fossa approaches. This is demonstrated by Case #3 in which a 5 year old female who presented with a posterior fossa pilocytic astrocytoma (Fig. 2a–c). Due to the 58 cm of operative space in the "double doughnut" system this approach can only be achieved by moving the prone patient superiorly while the surgeon is forced to abut the inferior magnet (see Fig. 2d, e). In this case, even with repositioning, the most superior portion of the tumor, which was clearly visible on ioMRI, remained unseen from the surgeon's viewpoint. Due to the potential spontaneous regression of these benign tumors the decision was made not to retrieve the unseen residual tumor and follow the patient with serial scans, a treatment option which has been well described by Hayward and colleges [12]. While we found posterior fossa approaches particularly challenging in the "double doughnut" system it should be noted that successful posterior fossa operations have been achieved with other ioMRI designs that allow more surgical freedom, such as the low-field Polestar [13] and the high-field systems.

However posterior fossa stereotactic procedures are unencumbered by the limited operative space within the double doughnut since catheter or probe placement does not require direct visualization by the surgeon. The advantage of utilizing ioMRI in these cases is the continually updated image information allows more precision when operating near eloquent anatomy of the brain stem. Case #4 is a 5 year old female who presented with increasing problems piano playing, gait changes, vision changes, and mild facial droop. Subsequent imaging revealed a cystic astrocytoma of the midbrain. Chemotherapy was initiated however the enlarging cyst was causing obstructive hydrocephalus and worsening of symptoms. Therefore it was decided to place a catheter through the right cerebellar hemisphere into the cystic component using ioMRI. Following placement of the catheter and confirmation in three planes by ioMRI, 15 cc of fluid was removed and a Rickham reservoir was attached and secured. The patient then continued her chemotherapy regimen without incident. Follow-up imaging showed incremental improvements until no sign of tumor or enhancement remained at 2 years postoperatively. She has remained free from recurrence for 8 years.

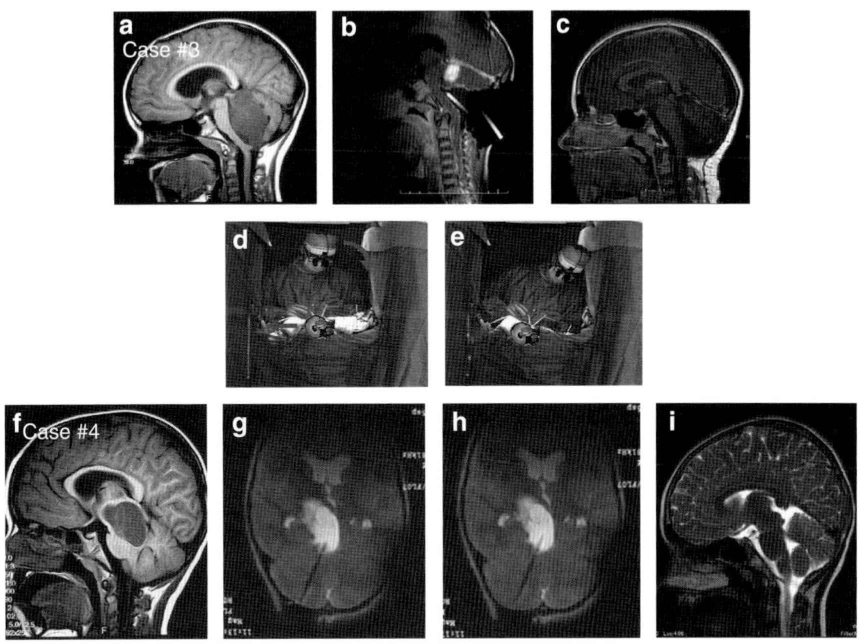

Fig. 2 *Case #3:* Cerebellary pilocytic astrocytoma. Preoperative (**a**), intraoperative (**b**), and 5 year postoperative image following resection (**c**). Surgical position inside "double doughnut" ioMRI (**d**, **e**). Posterior fossa operations are made significantly more challenging by requiring placement of the patient superiorly and rotation of the surgeon inferiorly (**d**). *Case #4:* Midbrain cystic astrocytoma. Note close proximity to midbrain structures. Preop (**f**), intraop (**g**, **h**) and 5 year postop images (**i**)

ioMRI Utilization in Cyst Management and CSF Diversion

Time has also shown ioMRI to be particularly effective in surgeries requiring precise localization. In our pediatric neurosurgical experience this has been most appreciated in difficult CSF diversions, complex cysts drainage, and placement of catheters near areas of eloquent anatomy. While most static frameless stereotactic guidance systems which rely on preoperative images can aid in surgical planning, these systems can not verify proper placement intraoperatively. Additionally static stereotaxy does not offer a dynamic view of operative changes (i.e. hemorrhage [14]) or guidance during the actual placement of the catheter because they lack real-time image revision. In contrast, ioMRI offers all three. An example of ioMRI driving surgical decision making in shunt placement is Case #5, a 3 year old who presented with pseudotumor cerebri, small ventricles, and intracranial hypertension (Fig. 3a–d). Using ioMRI, we easily and precisely place a catheter into the ventricles on the first pass. In addition to CSF return, accurate placement of the shunt was confirmed in the operating room prior to closure. Within this ioMRI system spatial coordinate experiments reveal a mean overall error in acquisition of only 0.2 mm [14–16].

The accuracy of ioMRI is similarly illustrated by cases such as that pictured in Fig. 3e–g. Case #6 is a 13 year old female with a seizure disorder who was admitted for increasing seizure activity, right-sided weakness, and pneumonia. She was subsequently discovered to have multiple brain abscesses. When obtaining culture material we elected to use the ioMRI facility due to the small size of these abscesses. With each catheter pass we could feel the tip hit the lesion and then slide off. With confirmation from intraoperative imaging the accuracy of our trajectory was not in question. Therefore we felt confident in attempting more invasive measures to perforate the abscesses wall. We enlarged the burr hole slightly, followed the tract with bipolar cautery and a #5 sucker, and entered the tense abscess rim exposing purulent material. Cultures obtained during this procedure grew streptococcus intermedius. Six month follow up imaging showed almost no sign of pathology.

As stated before, ioMRI is most useful when its real-time images drive surgical decision making. This is a function that cannot be duplicated by static frameless stereotaxis which relies on preoperative images. This is no truer than while shunting loculated cysts. Case #7 is a 9 year old male who presented with signs and symptoms of increased intracranial pressure. Subsequent imaging showed a complex cyst in the posterior right lateral ventricle (Fig. 3h–k). The septa can be clearly appreciated on the preoperative images (Fig. 3h). On the initial catheter placement CSF was obtained. However, after reviewing the intraoperative images, it was clear that the catheter had deviated medially, deflecting off the cysts (Fig. 3i). During a second attempt the shunt can be seen piercing the septa as it traverses the cyst and enters the left lateral ventricle, which was confirmed in three plains (Fig. 3j). ioMRI, while substantially more expensive that endoscopy, holds several key advantaged for catheter placement as illustrated by this case. First, the

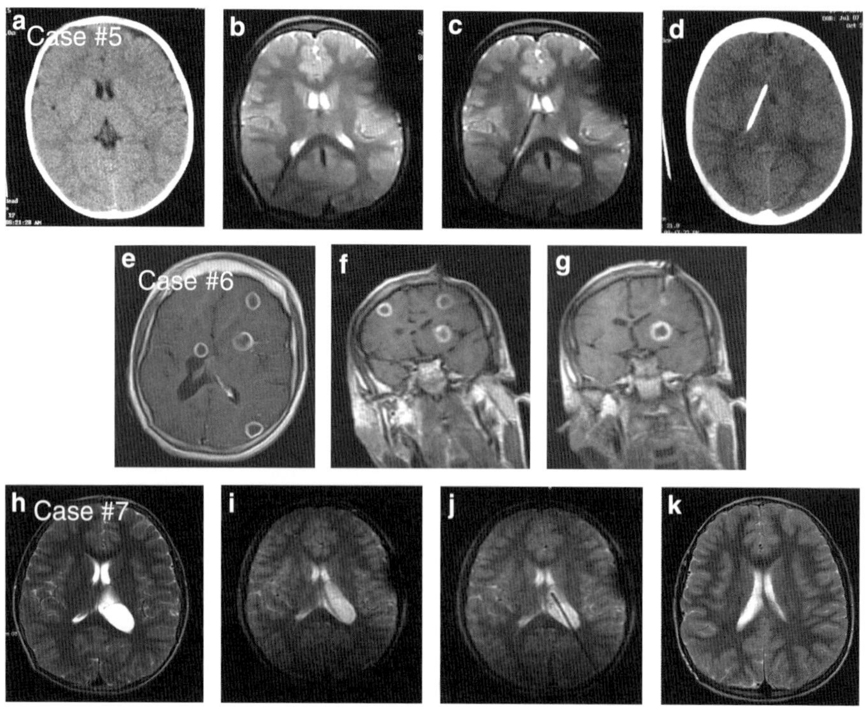

Fig. 3 *Case #5:* Intracranial Hypertension with Slit Ventricles. Preoperative CT (**a**), intraoperative MRI showing stent placement on first pass (**b**, **c**), and post operative CT images (**d**). *Case #6:* Abscess Drainage. Preoperative image (**e**) showing patient with multiple small strep positive abscesses. Intraoperative imaging immediately prior to and following abscess drainage (**f**, **g**). *Case #7*: Multiloculated Intraventricular Cyst. Preoperative (**h**) and intraoperative images showing a missed first pass (**i**) and a successful fenestration (**j**). Postoperative image showing decreased left lateral ventricle

altered anatomy of a complex cyst can be confusing. This often results in the surgeon having to pierce tissue plains blindly without knowledge of which cavity or structures they might be entering. Secondly, endoscopic views are often obscured by blood or debris rendering the endoscope useless. Third, as with shunt placement, endoscopy only provides feedback once a cavity has been pierced while ioMRI allows guidance through parenchyma as well as within fluid filled spaces. Fourth, ioMRI allows verification of shunt placement and allows assurance that all loculi have been violated prior to closure.

In 1996 the few ioMRI systems under development were predominantly housed within research universities. In 2009 over 100 systems are now in operation with a significant number in large clinical centers, thus indicating a shift in ioMRI from predominantly research applications to more widespread clinical usage. Additionally, while only 3% of United States hospitals have access to ioMRI facilities, 17 of the 170 children's hospitals have access, further indicating ioMRI's usefulness in pediatric neurosurgical cases. Additionally, private conversations within the field indicate that many other pediatric institutions plan to acquire this technology soon.

Summary

The general advantages of ioMRI have been explained elsewhere [15, 17, 18]. In brief the major advantages offered are continually updated dynamic images with a high level of accuracy in a timely manner [14]. However, here we present lessons learned in 9 years of ioMRI utilization in relation to pediatric neurosurgery. In short, within this population ioMRI is ideal for ...

1. Small, discrete tumors with poor normal/abnormal differentiation.
2. Large tumors with surrounding edema that ...
   (a) Obscures the normal/abnormal differentiation, or
   (b) Causes a mass effect that will alter the anatomy significantly from preoperative images after craniotomy.
3. Catheter/CSF diversion when the target ...
   (a) Is small
   (b) Is surrounded by eloquent anatomy, or
   (c) Verification of shunt placement and not merely CSF return is required (i.e. multiloculated or intraventricular cysts).

The only relative contraindication that we have discovered in this particular system is the posterior fossa approach. As a result of these observations, the number of pediatric ioMRI cases in our institution has actually decreased over the last 10 years due to more selective use of this technology. However, while a majority of pediatric neurosurgical cases can be performed in standard operating room; select cases, such as those detailed above, are made distinctly easier and safer by utilizing ioMRI. This suggests that certain cases will remain within the purview of this technology. Also given the ever expanding capabilities of MR the abilities of ioMRI will only continue to expand [19].

Conflicts of Interest Statement We declare that we have no conflict of interest.

References

1. Black PM, Moriarty T, Alexander E, Stieg P, Woodard EJ, Gleason PL, Martin CH, Kikinis R, Schwartz RB, Jolesz FA (1997) Development and implementation of intraoperative magnetic resonance imaging and its neurosurgical applications. Neurosurgery 41:831–842, Discussion 842–845
2. Tronnier VM, Wirtz CR, Knauth M, Lenz G, Pastyr O, Bonsanto MM, Albert FK, Kuth R, Staubert A, Schlegel W, Sartor K, Kunze S (1997) Intraoperative diagnostic and interventional magnetic resonance imaging in neurosurgery. Neurosurgery 40:891–900, Discussion 900–902
3. Schulder M, Jacobs A, Carmel PW (2001) Intraoperative MRI and adjuvant radiosurgery. Stereotact Funct Neurosurg 76:151–158
4. Hall WA, Martin AJ, Liu H, Pozza CH, Casey SO, Michel E, Nussbaum ES, Maxwell RE, Truwit CL (1998) High-field strength interventional magnetic resonance imaging for pediatric neurosurgery. Pediatr Neurosurg 29:253–259
5. Sutherland GR, Louw DF (1999) Intraoperative MRI: a moving magnet. CMAJ 161:1293
6. Mutchnick IS, Moriarty TM (2005) Neurosurgical uses for intraprocedural magnetic resonance imaging. Top Magn Reson Imaging 16:383–395
7. Shaw EG, Berkey B, Coons SW, Bullard D, Brachman D, Buckner JC, Stelzer KJ, Barger GR, Brown PD, Gilbert MR, Mehta M (2008) Recurrence following neurosurgeon-determined gross-total resection of adult supratentorial low-grade glioma: results of a prospective clinical trial. J Neurosurg 109:835–841
8. Talos IF, Zou KH, Ohno-Machado L, Bhagwat JG, Kikinis R, Black PM, Jolesz FA (2006) Supratentorial low-grade glioma resectability: statistical predictive analysis based on anatomic MR features and tumor characteristics. Radiology 239:506–513
9. Claus EB, Horlacher A, Hsu L, Schwartz RB, Dello-Iacono D, Talos F, Jolesz FA, Black PM (2005) Survival rates in patients with low-grade glioma after intraoperative magnetic resonance image guidance. Cancer 103:1227–1233
10. Maksoud YA, Hahn YS, Engelhard HH (2002) Intracranial ependymoma. Neurosurg Focus 13:e4
11. Robertson PL, Zeltzer PM, Boyett JM, Rorke LB, Allen JC, Geyer JR, Stanley P, Li H, Albright AL, McGuire-Cullen P, Finlay JL, Stevens KR Jr, Milstein JM, Packer RJ, Wisoff J (1998) Survival and prognostic factors following radiation therapy and chemotherapy for ependymomas in children: a report of the Children's Cancer Group. J Neurosurg 88:695–703
12. Gunny RS, Hayward RD, Phipps KP, Harding BN, Saunders DE (2005) Spontaneous regression of residual low-grade cerebellar pilocytic astrocytomas in children. Pediatr Radiol 35:1086–1091

13. Schulder M, Sernas TJ, Carmel PW (2003) Cranial surgery and navigation with a compact intraoperative MRI system. Acta Neurochir Suppl 85:79–86
14. Moriarty TM, Quinones-Hinojosa A, Larson PS, Alexander E 3rd, Gleason PL, Schwartz RB, Jolesz FA, Black PM (2000) Frameless stereotactic neurosurgery using intraoperative magnetic resonance imaging: stereotactic brain biopsy. Neurosurgery 47:1138–1145, discussion 1145–1146
15. Moriarty TM, Kikinis R, Jolesz FA, Black PM, Alexander E 3rd (1996) Magnetic resonance imaging therapy. Intraoperative MR imaging. Neurosurg Clin N Am 7:323–331
16. Schenck JF, Jolesz FA, Roemer PB, Cline HE, Lorensen WE, Kikinis R, Silverman SG, Hardy CJ, Barber WD, Laskaris ET et al (1995) Superconducting open-configuration MR imaging system for image-guided therapy. Radiology 195:805–814
17. Vitaz TW, Hushek S, Shields CB, Moriarty T (2003) Intraoperative MRI for pediatric tumor management. Acta Neurochir Suppl 85:73–78
18. Woodard EJ, Leon SP, Moriarty TM, Quinones A, Zamani AA, Jolesz FA (2001) Initial experience with intraoperative magnetic resonance imaging in spine surgery. Spine 26:410–417
19. Jolesz FA (2005) Future perspectives for intraoperative MRI. Neurosurg Clin N Am 16:201–213

Intraoperative MRI - High Field Systems

Implementation and Preliminary Clinical Experience with the Use of Ceiling Mounted Mobile High Field Intraoperative Magnetic Resonance Imaging Between Two Operating Rooms

Michael R. Chicoine, Chris C. H. Lim, John A. Evans, Amit Singla, Gregory J. Zipfel, Keith M. Rich, Joshua L. Dowling, Jeffrey R. Leonard, Matthew D. Smyth, Paul Santiago, Eric C. Leuthardt, David D. Limbrick, and Ralph G. Dacey

Abstract *Objective*: Intraoperative magnetic resonance imaging (ioMRI) provides immediate feedback and quality assurance enabling the neurosurgeon to improve the quality of a range of neurosurgical procedures. Implementation of ioMRI is a complex and costly process. We describe our preliminary 16 months experience with the integration of an IMRIS movable ceiling mounted high field (1.5 T) ioMRI setup with two operating rooms.

Methods: Aspects of implementation of our ioMRI and our initial 16 months of clinical experience in 180 consecutive patients were reviewed.

Results: The installation of a ceiling mounted movable ioMRI between two operating rooms was completed in April 2008 at Barnes-Jewish Hospital in St. Louis. Experience with 180 neurosurgical cases (M:F – 100:80, age range 1–79 years, 71 gliomas, 57 pituitary adenomas, 9 metastases, 11 other tumor cases, 4 Chiari decompressions, 6 epilepsy resections and 22 other miscellaneous procedures) demonstrated that this device effectively provided high quality real-time intraoperative imaging. In 74 of all 180 cases (41%) and in 54% of glioma resections, the surgeon modified the procedure based upon the ioMRI. Ninety-three percent of ioMRI glioma cases achieved gross/near total resection compared to 65% of non ioMRI glioma cases in this time frame.

Conclusion: A movable high field strength ioMRI can be safely integrated between two neurosurgical operating rooms. This strategy leads to modification of the surgical procedure in a significant number of cases, particularly for glioma surgery. Long-term follow up is needed to evaluate the clinical and financial impact of this technology in the field of neurosurgery.

Keywords Brain tumors · Gliomas · High field intraoperative magnetic resonance imaging · ioMRI · Neurosurgery · Pituitary adenomas

Introduction

Improvements in the operating theatre have been advancing for centuries [1], but never at such a rate seen in recent years. Applications of technological advancements are perhaps more apparent in neurosurgery than in any other surgical specialty. Over the past decade advancements in frameless stereotaxy and ioMRI have enhanced the neurosurgeon's capability to navigate the complex anatomy of the central nervous system, improve on safety and efficacy of neurosurgical procedures and optimize patient outcomes for many diseases affecting the brain [2–12].

A variety of ioMRI devices (high/low field, fixed/movable magnets) can be implemented in neurosurgical operating rooms. IoMRIs have been shown to improve the extent of resection especially in gliomas and pituitary adenomas and this translates into improved patient outcomes and survivals [9, 13–18].

The newest generation of high-field strength ioMRIs offers potential for improvements yet to be realized by the earlier generations of these devices. Through collaboration between Washington University, Barnes-Jewish Hospital, St. Louis Children's Hospital and IMRIS (Winnipeg, Manitoba, Canada) installation was completed of one of the first movable ceiling mounted high field strength ioMRI devices in the world that can be accessed and utilized from either of the two operating rooms (Fig. 1a). Integration of ioMRI into the operating room is a complex and costly process. We describe the process of integration of this ioMRI device

M.R. Chicoine (✉), C.C.H. Lim, J.A. Evans, A. Singla, G.J. Zipfel, K.M. Rich, J.L. Dowling, J.R. Leonard, M.D. Smyth, P. Santiago, E.C. Leuthardt, D.D. Limbrick, and R.G. Dacey
Department of Neurological Surgery, Washington University School of Medicine, Campus Box 8057, 660 S. Euclid Avenue, St. Louis, MO 63110, USA
e-mail: chicoinem@wudosis.wustl.edu

DOI 10.1007/978-3-211-99651-5_15, © Springer-Verlag/Wien 2011

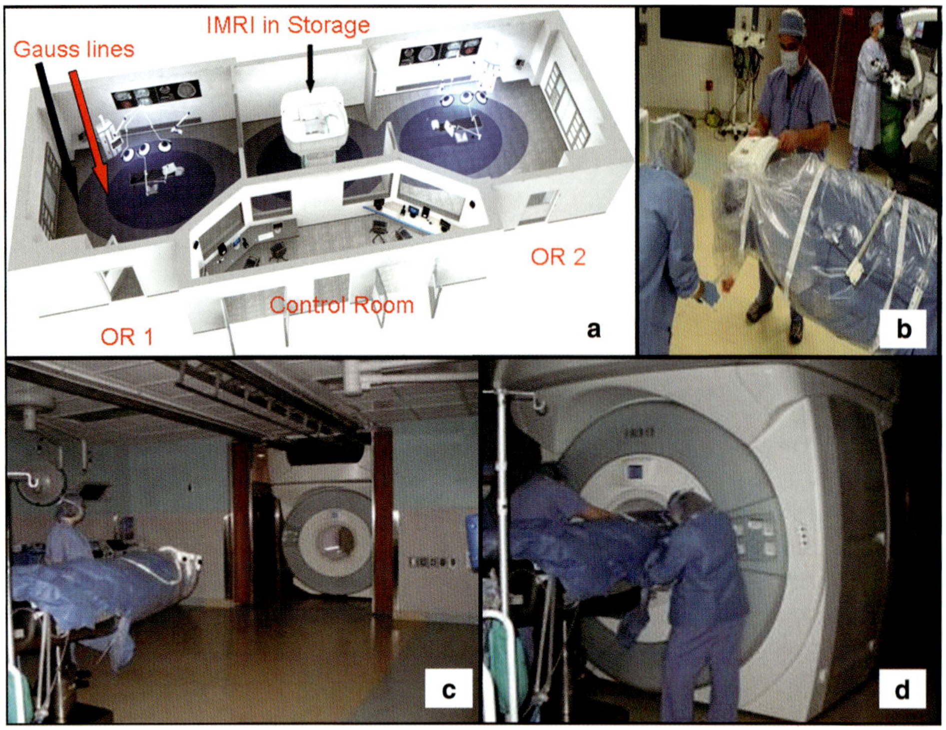

Fig. 1 (**a**) Line drawing depicting the IMRIS 2-room ioMRI model. Patient entry bore of the magnet is rotated to face either operating rooms within the storage bay prior to moving out from storage to its final position. Gauss lines depicted (50G line (*red*) and 5G line (*black*)) when the ioMRI is in final imaging position (image courtesy of IMRIS); (**b**) sterile "C-arm" drape covering patient and operating table with upper portion of 8-channel ioMRI coil in place; (**c**) opening doors to the magnet bay in preparation for moving ioMRI device to the patient for imaging (note the ceiling mounted tracts); (**d**) after 90 s ioMRI device is in its final position for acquisition of images

into our operating rooms and our initial 16 months experience with 180 cases.

Methods

A review was made of the financial, architectural, engineering, and marketing aspects of planning for and implementation of an IMRIS ceiling mounted movable ioMRI device situated between two multi-purpose neurosurgical operating rooms.

A prospective database has been established and maintained with approval of the Washington University Human Studies Institutional Review Board to monitor outcomes for all patients undergoing ioMRI procedures. A retrospective analysis of the database was performed to assess the clinical attributes, the impact on the surgeon's decision-making process, workflow issues and the preliminary outcomes of the 180 cases performed in the initial 16 months of experience.

Results

MRI Installation and Integration

Preparation for installation of an ioMRI included analysis of the commercially available ioMRI devices and our team visited other facilities internationally to assess these devices (Phillips and Hitachi open MRI, Medtronic Odin, BrainLab BrainSuite and the IMRIS ceiling mounted ioMRI) and to see them in use. High-field magnets provided better image resolution and more versatility for current and future imaging modalities, but with greater associated costs and more complex implementation issues. The BrainSuite offered appealing features including integration of surgical planning technology and high-resolution imaging. The IMRIS ioMRI device is ceiling mounted and movable, the operating table and patient remain in a fixed position and the device moves to the patient. This feature in our view enhances safety in terms of airway control, monitoring and head fixation. Also for our high volume center, two-room ioMRI access would add flexibility in terms of scheduling and room utilization. Standard surgical instruments could be used and these fully equipped operating rooms can be adapted to serve as multi-purpose operating rooms for any surgical case when the ioMRI is not in use.

The installation of an ioMRI was associated with complex architectural, engineering and safety issues and this was integrated into a major renovation project encompassing over 60 operating rooms with an estimated budget of US $100 million over a 2 year period. Alternative solutions including installation into the department of radiology were impractical with respect to workflow, efficiency and safety.

The integration of ioMRI into our current neurosurgical armamentarium was intended to improve the precision, efficacy and safety of neurosurgical procedures. Within the current coding system, direct billing and reimbursement for the addition of the ioMRI is rather limited. A shared diagnostic and intraoperative model could help reimburse the cost from diagnostic revenues generated but was not feasible in our setup. Economic reimbursement stems from the potential marketing impact. As one of the first centers worldwide to employ this latest state of the art technology, it uniquely strengthens our position to offer improved patient care at local, regional, national, and international level.

Upon completion of the project, rigorous training programmes and simulations were instituted for all personnel involved to improve safety and efficiency. Access to the ioMRI area is restricted through ioMRI security protected doors. As a fully functional 1.5 T MRI device with a large patient-entry bore (70 cm), the Siemens Espree MRI scanner integrated into our IMRIS ioMRI suite offers full MRI capability in a wide range of clinical and research utilization.

Some modifications of the surgical environment were necessary with the ioMRI. The IMRIS operating table has the ability to elevate, rotate, flex and had allowed us to perform our operations (146 supine, 27 prone and 7 lateral cases) in almost any surgical position. The 3-pin ioMRI head holder is made to hold the lower half of the MRI coil and attaches to the operating table in a novel fashion. It has required some minor adjustments in order to incorporate it into routine use. The ioMRI compatible anesthesia machine perhaps does not have all of the capabilities of a standard anesthesia machine but has been more than adequate for even complex surgical procedure so far.

We have also incorporated the Medtronic Stealth frameless stereotaxy and endoscopy systems with large high definition flat panel wall and touch screen monitors with tracking cameras on ceiling mounted booms into our ioMRI rooms which facilitate work flow well.

When the ioMRI is required, appropriate patient draping and safety checks are completed (Fig. 1b). All equipment, surgical instruments, and ferromagnetic objects are moved outside the 5 Gauss line (delineated with colored floor tiling). A floor space in excess of 850 sq ft for each operating room enables us to move the equipment to a safe distance without having to remove the equipment from the room. The ioMRI device moves from storage to imaging position in 90 s (Fig. 1c, d).

Initial 16 Months Clinical Experience

Between April 2008 and August 2009, 187 ioMRI cases were performed. Seven cases were excluded (four planning MRI only, one image distortion from ET tube, one large body habitus and one technical failure). Of the remaining 180 patients (M:F – 100:80, age range 1–79 years, median 44 years), 71 were gliomas, 57 pituitary adenomas, 9 metastases, 5 craniopharyngiomas, 2 clival chordomas, 2 meningiomas, 3 hemangioblastomas, 1 medulloblastoma, 1 trigeminal schwannoma, 6 resections for epilepsy, 4 Chiari decompressions and 19 other procedures for cyst aspiration/resection, biopsy or catheter placement. On 23 occasions, both of the operating rooms were used simultaneously for 46 ioMRI-guided procedures. In 74 of 180 cases (41%) the surgeon modified the surgical procedure based upon the findings of ioMRI.

Gliomas: For the 71 glioma patients (34 high/37 low grade), tumor resections were performed in 68 cases (32 high/36 low grade) and the remainder underwent two biopsies and one cyst aspiration. Awake techniques were incorporated into eight of these resections (six high/two low grades). Thirty-seven of 68 resections (54%) had additional tumor resected after ioMRI (Fig. 2). For the subset of 36 low-grade gliomas (World Health Organization, WHO I–II), additional tumor was resected in 15 cases (42%). Twenty-two of the 32 (69%) high-grade glioma (WHO II–IV) patients had further resections. Pathological analysis of post ioMRI resection materials revealed tumor in 23 of the 29 specimens received (79%). Six specimens were negative for tumor and additional eight specimens were not analyzed.

Pituitary Adenoma: Fifty-seven resections were performed (55 transphenoidal, 2 transcranial) in 56 patients. IoMRI revealed possible residual tumor in 37 cases (65%) (Fig. 3). Nineteen cases were not re-explored as it was felt unsafe. Thirteen of the 18 explored had further resection, 4 had no tumor visualized and 1 had tumor encasing the carotid. Of the nine post ioMRI resection pathology specimens received, eight were positive for tumor.

Metastases: For the nine resections of brain metastases performed, ioMRI after initial tumor resection suggested residual tumor in five cases (56%). Four cases were explored and histology revealed tumor in two.

Chiari Malformations: IoMRI was completed after suboccipital craniotomy and C-1 laminectomy with dural band release without durotomy in four cases. In all cases ioMRI (anatomical) did not convincingly demonstrate adequate decompression and therefore duraplasties were performed. Post duraplasty ioMRI showed improved decompression in all cases.

Aspiration/Biopsy: The ioMRI has been used in 19 cases to guide and assess the adequacy of biopsies, catheter insertions and cyst aspirations/resections but did not lead to any modifications of the procedures.

Epilepsy Resections: Six cases used ioMRI to assess the extent of resection for an epileptogenic focus. IoMRI confirmed accurate localization of resection in all. Three of six cases lead to additional surgical resection.

Wound Infections and Safety: Due to the increased duration of surgery and the additional sterile draping and undraping procedures necessary to perform an ioMRI, one

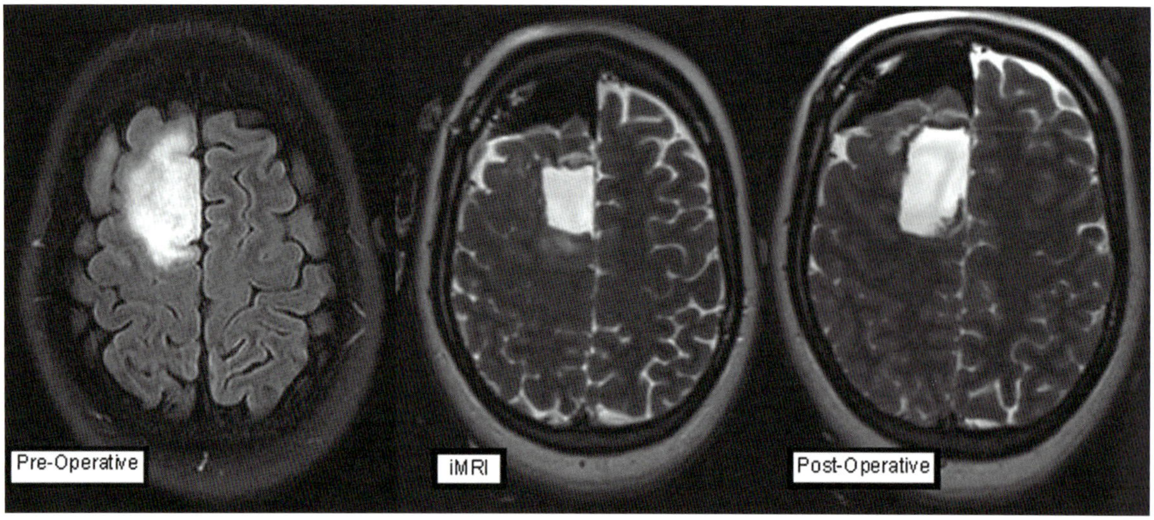

Fig. 2 Sample glioma case. (**a**) Preoperative MRI (*left*) of right frontal anaplastic oligodendroglioma prior to surgery. (**b**) ioMRI (*middle*) after initial resection demonstrated residual tumor at the posterior margin of the resection cavity which prompted further resection of tumor. (**c**) Postoperative MRI (*right*) demonstrating resection of the residual tumor identified on ioMRI

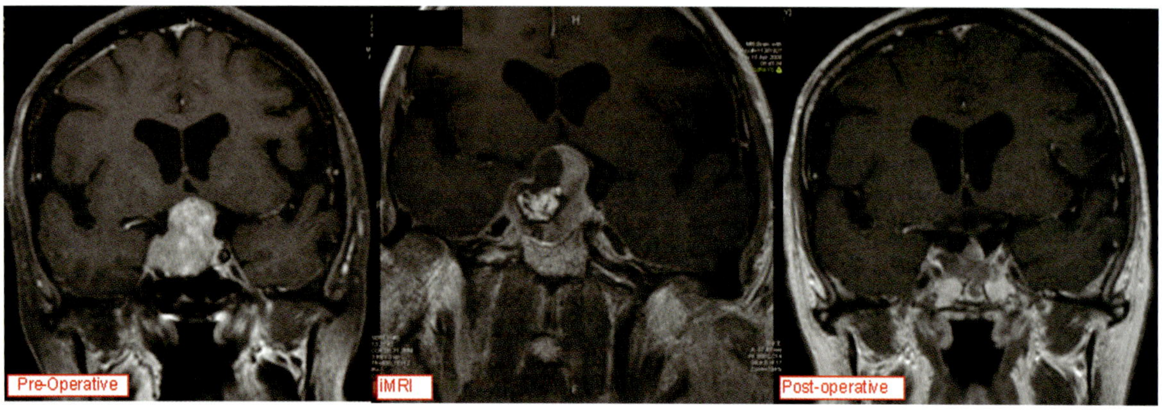

Fig. 3 Sample pituitary adenoma case. (**a**) Preoperative MRI (*left*) of large non-functioning pituitary macro-adenoma with suprasellar extension. (**b**) ioMRI (*middle*) demonstrated evidence of residual tumor on the left side which prompted further resection of tumor. There is evidence of the autologous adipose graft in the right aspect of the sella. (**c**) Postoperative MRI (*right*) demonstrating resection of the residual tumor identified on the ioMRI

might predict an increased risk of surgical infection. Thus far no surgical wound infections have been identified for the 180 procedures that have been completed to date. Using a rigid set of safety guidelines, instrument counting and other checklist strategies, no projectile objects or other safety issues have been identified thus far with the use of this movable high field ioMRI device.

Time intervals and workflow: Preparation time for ioMRI averaged 21 min (7–66 min). Scanning time averaged 41 min (15–104 min). Post ioMRI time averaged 16 min (3–63 min) to the start of further resection or wound closure.

Total operating room (OR) times were calculated for the two largest subgroups, namely glioma (resection and non-awake cases) and pituitary adenoma (transphenoidal) to determine if delay occurs when ioMRI cases were carried out in two rooms simultaneously. When two rooms were used in tandem, total OR time averaged 466 min for glioma (n=16) and 398 min for pituitary adenoma (n=17), compared to 485 min for glioma (n=44) and 423 min for pituitary adenoma (n=38) when one room was used.

Discussion

An IMRIS ioMRI suite consisting of two operating rooms on either side of a movable high field strength 1.5 T magnet was successfully installed in April 2008. Barnes-Jewish Hospital is one of the few facilities in the world to have this advanced intraoperative imaging capability with access from two adjacent operating rooms. The concept of ioMRI has been available for over a decade, but recent advances make this technique more versatile than ever before. Intraoperative MRI offers immediate feedback to the surgeon so that the extent of resection might be determined. Increasingly evidence indicates that a more complete surgical resection is associated with increased survival for both low and high-grade gliomas, and that the extent of resection can be improved with the use of ioMRI [14, 16, 17, 19, 20, 24].

Our preliminary experience with 68 glioma resections indicates that the MRI device enabled the neurosurgeon to improve the extent of resection in 54% of cases, including 42% for low-grade gliomas and 69% of high-grade gliomas. Ninety-three percent (n=71) of ioMRI cases achieved gross/near total resection compared to 65% (n=53) of non ioMRI cases in this time frame based on MRI scans within 72 h post-op. Continued monitoring of these patients will provide information on the impact of ioMRI upon survival.

Maximal safe resection is typically the goal for pituitary surgery. Most lesions are adequately assessed via the transphenoidal route, but there are limitations to visualization because of the depth of the surgical approach and the limited corridor that can be establish through the anterior face of the sella. The endoscope circumvents some of these limitations by providing a more panoramic view especially when coupled with contemporary high definition/3D video equipments. Nonetheless, unintentional incomplete resection of pituitary adenomas through the transphenoidal approach remains a potential issue. Previous reports have shown residual adenoma in 39–66% leading to additional resection in 22–66% of cases [9, 13]. Our initial experience with 57 cases is consistent with prior reports in that ioMRI showed evidence of probable residual tumor in 37 cases (65%). Eighteen of these were explored (32%) and 13 had further resections, 4 were not visible and 1 found encasing the carotid artery. With the continued evolution of surgical techniques for pituitary tumors in recent years including the application of surgical navigation and endonasal endoscopy, the precise role and benefit of ioMRI remains to be defined.

Surgical resection of brain metastases is well established, particularly for solitary lesions. Metastatic tumors typically appear well encapsulated and readily resectable yet surgery alone is associated with significant rates of local recurrence. Because of this, post-operative radiation is typically recommended [21–23]. IoMRI in our small series showed suspicious areas in five of the nine patients, yet histopathological evidence of tumor is verified in only two of the four cases explored. The role of ioMRI for resection of brain metastases and the significance of the intraoperative MRIs needs further refinement.

The number of cases in the remainder of this review is too few to draw hard conclusions. These cases do show that ioMRI can be used effectively for a wide range of neurosurgical procedures but the full potential of application of this technology in the neurosurgical operating room remains to be seen.

The two-room model serves us well. There was no significant workflow delay noted when the two ioMRI rooms were used in tandem.

Conclusion

A movable high field strength ioMRI can be integrated into neurosurgical practice and provide real time high quality imaging to guide the surgical treatment of brain tumors and other diseases. This technique provides immediate feedback to assess the adequacy of surgery. This strategy leads to modification of the surgical procedure in a significant number of cases, particularly glioma surgery in which ioMRI may suggest need for additional resection in every second case. Long-term follow up is needed to evaluate the clinical and financial impact of this technology in the field of neurosurgery.

Conflicts of interest statement Dr. Chicoine has received an unrestricted educational grant from IMRIS, Winnepeg, Canada for maintenance of a database.

References

1. Liu CY, Apuzzo MLJ (2003) The genesis of neurosurgery and the evolution of the neurosurgical operative environment: Part I – Prehistory to 2003. Neurosurgery 52:3–19
2. Adeolu AA, Sutherland GR (2006) Intraoperative magnetic resonance imaging and meningioma surgery. West Afr J Med 25 (3):174–178
3. Black PM, Alexander E 3rd, Martin C, Moriarty T, Nabavi A, Wong TZ, Schwartz RB, Jolesz F (1999) Craniotomy for tumor treatment in an intraoperative magnetic resonance imaging unit. Neurosurgery 45(3):423–431, discussion 431–433
4. Black PM, Moriarty T, Alexander E 3rd, Stieg P, Woodard EJ, Gleason PL, Martin CH, Kikinis R, Schwartz RB, Jolesz FA (1997) Development and implementation of intraoperative magnetic resonance imaging and its neurosurgical applications. Neurosurgery 41 (4):831–842, discussion 842–845
5. Buchfelder M, Fahlbusch R, Ganslandt O, Stefan H, Nimsky C (2002) Use of intraoperative magnetic resonance imaging in tailored temporal lobe surgeries for epilepsy. Epilepsia 43(8):864–873
6. Kelly JJ, Hader WJ, Myles ST, Sutherland GR (2005) Epilepsy surgery with intraoperative MRI at 1.5 T. Neurosurg Clin North Am 16(1):173–183
7. Lee MW, De Salles AA, Frighetto L, Torres R, Behnke E, Bronstein JM (2005) Deep brain stimulation in intraoperative MRI environment – comparison of imaging techniques and electrode fixation methods. Minim Invasive Neurosurg 48(1):1–6
8. Mittal S, Black PM (2006) Intraoperative magnetic resonance imaging in neurosurgery: the Brigham concept. Acta Neurochir Suppl 98:77–86
9. Nimsky C, von Keller B, Ganslandt O, Fahlbusch R (2006) Intraoperative high-field MRI in transsphenoidal surgery of hormonally inactive pituitary macroadenomas. Neurosurgery 59(1):105–114

10. Tirakotai W, Sure U, Benes L, Krischek B, Bien S, Bertalanffy H (2003) Image guided transsylvian transinsular approach for insular cavernomas. Neurosurgery 53:1299–1305
11. Tyler D, Mandybur G (1999) Interventional MRI-guided stereotactic aspiration of acute -subacute intracerebral hematomas. Stereotact Funct Neurosurg 72(2–4):129–135
12. Walker DG, Talos F, Bromfield EB, Black PM (2002) Intraoperative magnetic resonance for the surgical treatment of lesions producing seizures. J Clin Neurosci 9(5):515–520
13. Bohinski RJ, Warnick RE, Gaskill-Shipley MF, Zuccarello M, van Loveren HR, Kormos DW, Tew JM Jr (2001) Intraoperative magnetic resonance imaging to determine the extent of resection of pituitary macroadenomas during transsphenoidal microsurgery. Neurosurgery 49(5):1133–1143, discussion 1143–1144
14. Claus EB, Horlacher A, Hsu L, Schwartz RB, Dello-Iacono D, Talos F, Jolesz FA, Black PM (2005) Survival rates in patients with low-grade glioma after intraoperative magnetic resonance image guidance. Cancer 103(6):1227–1233
15. Martin CH, Schwartz R, Jolesz F, Black PM (1999) Transsphenoidal resection of pituitary adenomas in an intraoperative MRI unit. Pituitary 2(2):155–162
16. Nimsky C, Ganslandt O, von Keller B, Fahlbusch R (2003) Preliminary experience in glioma surgery with intraoperative high-field MRI. Acta Neurochir Suppl 88:21–29
17. Schneider JP, Trantakis C, Rubach M, Schulz T, Dietrich J, Winkler D, Renner C, Schober R, Geiger K, Brosteanu O, Zimmer C, Kahn T (2005) Intraoperative MRI to guide the resection of primary supratentorial glioblastoma multiforme – a quantitative radiological analysis. Neuroradiology 47(7):489–500
18. Vitaz TW, Hushek S, Shields CB (2003) Moriarty T. Intraoperative MRI for pediatric tumor management. Acta Neurochir Suppl 85:73–78
19. Hirschberg H, Samset E, Hol PK, Tillung T, Lote K (2005) Impact of intraoperative MRI on the surgical results for high-grade gliomas. Minim Invasive Neurosurg 48(2):77–84
20. Stummer W, Reulen HJ, Meinel T, Pichlmeier U, Schumacher W, Tonn JC, Rohde V, Oppel F, Turowski B, Woiciechowsky C, Franz K, Pietsch T (2008) ALA-Glioma Study Group. Extent of resection and survival in glioblastoma multiforme: identification of and adjustment for bias. Neurosurgery 62(3):564–576
21. Limbrick DD, Lusis EA, Chicoine MR, Rich KM, Dacey RG, Dowling JL, Grubb RL, Filiput EA, Dryzmala RE, Mansur DB, Malyapa R, Simpson JR (2009) Combined surgical resection and stereotactic radiosurgery for treatment of cerebral metastases. Surg Neurol 71(3):280–288, discussion 288–289
22. Patchell RA, Tibbs PA, Regine WF et al (1998) Postoperative radiotherapy in the treatment of single metastases to the brain: a randomized trial. JAMA 280(17):1485–1489
23. Patchell RA, Tibbs PA, Walsh JW et al (1990) A randomized trial of surgery in the treatment of single metastases to the brain. N Engl J Med 322(8):494–500
24. Oh DS, Black PM (2005) A low-field intraoperative MRI system for glioma surgery: is it worthwhile? Neurosurg Clin North Am 16 (1):135–141

High-Field ioMRI in Glioblastoma Surgery: Improvement of Resection Radicality and Survival for the Patient?

H. Maximilian Mehdorn, Felix Schwartz, Stefan Dawirs, Jürgen Hedderich, Lutz Dörner, and Arya Nabavi

Abstract Since the first patients underwent intracranial tumor removal with the radicality control of intraoperative MRI (ioMRI) in September 2005 in our department, the majority of operations performed in the ioMRI room have been indicated for high grade gliomas. In order to elucidate the role of ioMRI scanning in patients harboring high-grade gliomas (HGG) on their survival, one hundred ninety three patients with gliomas WHO grades III and IV were operated either in a standard microsurgical neuronavigated fashion or using additionally ioMRI and were included in a follow-up study. The series started with surgeries from September 2005 until October 2007. Patient attribution to the two groups was based on the logistical availability of the ioMRI on a scheduled surgery day, and on the assumed "difficulty" of the surgery based on the location of the glioma in or near to an eloquent area. Surgery was intended to be as radical as possible without reduction of quality of life.

First surgery was performed in 103 patients (75 WHO IV and 28 WHO III) and will be the main topic of this paper. In 60 patients, ioMRI was used, while in 43 patients standard microsurgical neuronavigated resection techniques were applied.

Patients were followed in regular intervals mostly until death. Statistical analysis showed a median survival time for patients in whom ioMRI had been used of 20, 37 months compared to 10, 3 months in the cohort who had undergone conventional microsurgical removal.

Major influencing concomitants were WHO grades and age which were balanced in both groups.

Keywords High-grade glioma · Intraoperative magnetic resonance imaging · Karnofsky performance score · Microsurgery · Survival

H.M. Mehdorn (✉), F. Schwartz, S. Dawirs, J. Hedderich, L. Dörner, and A. Nabavi
Dept of Neurosurgery, University Clinics of Schleswig-Holstein Campus Kiel, Arnold Heller Street 41, 24105, Kiel, Germany
e-mail: mehdorn@nch.uni-kiel.de

Introduction

The value of aggressive cytoreduction in gliomas has been discussed and established in recent years [1–12], yet, the use of intraoperative magnetic resonance imaging (ioMRI) has been questioned in the context of high-grade glioma WHO grades III and IV (HGG) surgery. Several publications have stressed the value of ioMRI in low grade gliomas (LGG) [13–15], but only one group has published long-term results [13]. Therefore we undertook to collect and follow our glioma patients series from the start of our clinical use of a 1.5 T Philips Intera MRI machine [16, 17], short bore, integrated into a new operating room fully equipped with microsurgical and neuronavigation (BrainLAB) facilities adjacent to other neurosurgical operating rooms with identical microsurgical and neuronavigation (BrainLAB) facilities [18]. ioMRI should add to the benefit of neuronavigation [19].

Since first surgical brain tumor resection using intraoperative MRI (ioMRI) control in September 2005 an additional 425 procedures have been performed in the Dept. of Neurosurgery at Kiel University Medical Center until late May 2009. The majority of patients (N=282) being treated for gliomas, this report will focus on the benefit and discuss some pitfalls encountered in this type of surgery.

Material and Methods

Out of 426 operations performed in the period of September 2005 until late May 2009, 76% of the operations were performed for gliomas, seventeen percent for transsphenoidal surgery including pituitary adenomas, craniopharyngeomas and clival chordomas. In the glioma group, fifty percent of the patients harbored a WHO grade IV glioma, 21% presented with a WHO grade III glioma and only 9% with a grade II glioma.

The patients were taken to the operating room with the head fixed into a MRI compatible Mayfield three-pin head

DOI 10.1007/978-3-211-99651-5_16,

holder attached to the sliding and rotating operating table derived from a Philips Medical Systems angiography table.

The intraoperative imaging protocol evolving over time included (1) preop T2fast images MRI scans to check for optimal head positioning within the magnetic field and any abnormalities that might interfere with the later intraoperative scans e.g. MRI incompatible pins, undetected metals etc. (2) Next, the patient is brought to the operating position by approximately 30° rotation of the table, draped in a regular manner, and surgery is performed as usual using regular neurosurgical instruments including neuronavigation and operating microscope. Stepwise tumor removal is controlled by repeated switch from white light to fluorescent light incorporated in our microscopes, using ALA fluorescence [20] nearly routinely for HGG surgery. When no more fluorescence is seen the patient's operating field is draped in such a fashion that he can be brought back into the scanning position. T2 W images are obtained in three dimensions, and depending on the dignity of the tumor these images may serve to re-reference for neuronavigation and further tumor resection, or T1 W images without and with contrast medium as well as DWI are additionally obtained. Depending on the progress and difficulty of surgery, additional intermediate studies are performed or a final scan is obtained prior to dural and wound closure.

In order to study the effect of ioMRI onto the clinical evolution of HGG patients, a study was performed analysing, early in the clinical use of our ioMRI setting, patients who underwent surgery with ioMRI and comparing them to patients operated, in the same time, without ioMRI, using only regular microsurgical neuronavigated tumor removal. In the time interval between September 2005 until October 2007, a group of 193 patients were operated in our dept for HGG. Follow up for these patients was continued until March 2009. Patients are usually regularly seen as outpatients or follow up phone calls were made to the patients, their families or physicians. Among patients undergoing first surgery, 28 patients harbored a WHO grade III glioma, and 75 patients presented with a WHO grade IV glioma. All patients underwent subsequent radiochemotherapy with temozolamide (TMZ). A multivariate analysis was performed concerning WHO grade, use +/− of ioMRI, radical resection of tumor as seen on 24 h postoperative MRI scan, awake craniotomy (which was used in 42 patients with tumors in eloquent areas), carmustine implants and others as age and sex.

Table 1 Extent of resection of gliomas WHO grades III and IV

		No ioMRI	ioMRI
Radical resection – intention preop	No	16	20
	Yes	27	40
Radical resection seen on postop MRI	No	21	23
	Yes	22	37

Results

Comparing the extent of resection in combined grads III and IV gliomas, Table 1 shows that radical resection – if intended – is more often achieved using ioMRI than not using it. This indicates that ioMRI has been able to guide and help the surgeon to a more radical surgical approach.

Of course the question came up whether this more radical approach would result in a more frequent reduction of quality of life as assessed by Karnofsky performance score (KPS). This was evaluated by comparing the KPS preoperatively to the KPS at 2 weeks postop. Figure 1 shows that there is indeed a reduction of KPS 2 weeks after surgery but for both groups of patients although slightly more prominent in the ioMRI group.

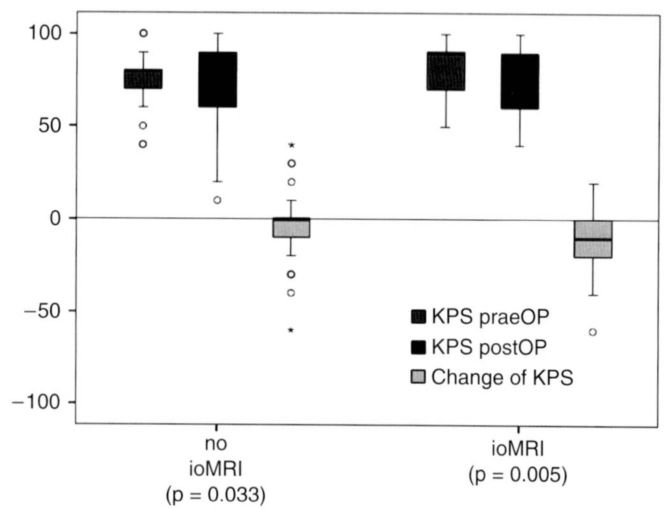

Fig. 1 Karnofsky performance score pre- and 2 weeks postop

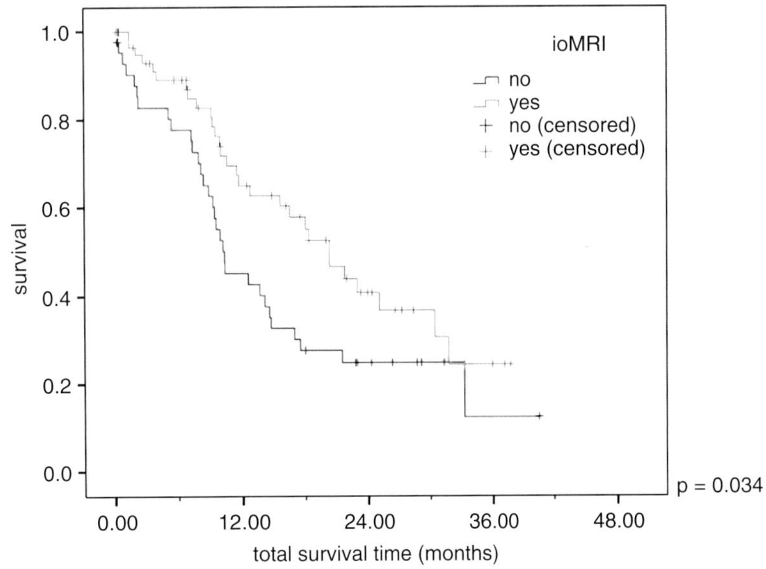

Fig. 2 Survival curves – all primary high-grade gliomas (N= 103)

Survival for both groups of patients was evaluated calculating Kaplan–Meier survival curves. Figure 2 shows the combined curves for all 103 HGG patients. It is evident that using ioMRI improves survival statistically (p=0.034) while (not shown) survival is still slightly better even in WHO grade IV patients operated using ioMRI but no more statistically different from patients operated without ioMRI.

Discussion

The data presented here show that by adding ioMRI into the armamentarium of modern neurosurgery it is possible to improve overall survival measured in median survival time even for HGG patients. Due to the protocol implied in this group of patients using if possible both ALA-fluorescence and ioMRI it is formally impossible to differentiate the benefit of each of the two adjuncts to radical glioma surgery. This would obviously be interesting but rather on an academic or economical point of view. Further studies are under way in this regard.

In the longterm follow up after 32 months, the survival curves approach each other. This confirms data obtained e.g. in the ALA studies [20] and points to the fact that additional therapy is required to further improve the longterm survival in these patients.

The data are important since they are derived from an unselected cohort of patients from a primary university referral center favoring aggressive surgery even in patients when other centers might have adopted a rather conservative approach. Attribution to one of the two treatment groups was performed rather on a logistical than on a randomized basis: this means that patients thought to harbor a "difficult" HGG in or close to an eloquent area underwent surgery using ioMRI while "simple" gliomas were operated in a standard fashion. This also explains why we have so far used quite frequently, in 34 patients, combined awake with ioMRI in order to prevent additional neurological deficits to occur [21, 22].

So far in the series, no patient has suffered from adverse events when using ioMRI, although some have complained discomfort when undergoing awake craniotomy and ioMRI [23]. On-the-spot interpretation of ioMRI images by the surgeon requires a certain knowledge related to contrast media dynamics [24], particularly when performing repeat T1W examinations. Some help is provided by computer programs which our group has evaluated on a larger scale and uses now frequently to detect minor tumor remnants [25]. The benefit of answering the question of brain shift by using ioMRI is evident [26]. The socio-economic question, however, of using ioMRI cannot be addressed here since it touches the treatment of malignant tumors generally spoken. In the same sense, every dept. has to carefully decide whether it can take the burden of implementing a high-field ioMRI into its budget [27, 28]. Other options besides dedicated neurosurgical ioMRI machines are certainly possible. On the other hand, the possibility to work around such a dedicated machine offers additional research incentives () to better understand the brain, its anatomy and treatment options.

Conflicts of Interest Statement We declare that we have no conflict of interest.

References

1. Durmaz R, Erken S, Arslantaş A, Atasoy MA, Bal C, Tel E (1997) Management of glioblastoma multiforme: with special reference to recurrence. Clin Neurol Neurosurg 99(2):117–123

2. Hall WA (2004) Extending survival in gliomas: surgical resection or immunotherapy? Surg Neurol 61(2):145–148
3. Jeremic B, Grujicic D, Antunovic V, Djuric L, Stojanovic M, Shibamoto Y (1994) Influence of extent of surgery and tumor location on treatment outcome of patients with glioblastoma multiforme treated with combined modality approach. J Neurooncol 21 (2):177–185
4. Knauth M, Wirtz CR, Tronnier VM, Aras N, Kunze S, Sartor K (1999) Intraoperative MR imaging increases the extent of tumor resection in patients with high- grade gliomas. Am J Neuroradiol 20(9):1642–1646
5. Laws ER, Parney IF, Huang W, Anderson F, Morris AM, Asher A, Lillehei KO, Bernstein M, Brem H, Sloan A, Berger MS, Chang S, Investigators GO (2003) Survival following surgery and prognostic factors for recently diagnosed malignant glioma: data from the Glioma Outcomes Project. J Neurosurg 99(3):467–473
6. Rostomily RC, Spence AM, Duong D, McCormick K, Bland M, Berger MS (1994) Multimodality management of recurrent adult malignant gliomas: results of a phase II multiagent chemotherapy study and analysis of cytoreductive surgery. Neurosurgery 35 (3):378–388
7. Salcman M (1988) Surgical resection of malignant brain tumors: who benefits? Oncology 2(8):47–56
8. Shinoda J, Sakai N, Murase S, Yano H, Matsuhisa T, Funakoshi T (2001) Selection of eligible patients with supratentorial glioblastoma multiforme for gross total resection. J Neurooncol 52(2):161–171
9. Stark AM, Nabavi A, Mehdorn HM, Blömer U (2005) Glioblastoma multiforme-report of 267 cases treated at a single institution. Surg Neurol 63(2):162–169
10. Stark AM, Hedderich J, Held-Feindt J, Mehdorn HM (2007) Glioblastoma–the consequences of advanced patient age on treatment and survival. Neurosurg Rev 30(1):56–66
11. Vuorinen V, Hinkka S, Färkkilä M, Jääskeläinen J (2003) Debulking or biopsy of malignant glioma in elderly people – a randomised study. Acta Neurochir 145(1):5–10
12. Yoshida J, Kajita Y, Wakabayashi T, Sugita K (1994) Long-term follow-up results of 175 patients with malignant glioma: importance of radical tumour resection and postoperative adjuvant therapy with interferon, ACNU and radiation. Acta Neurochir 127(1–2):55–59
13. Claus EB, Horlacher A, Hsu L, Schwartz RB, Dello-Iacono D, Talos F, Jolesz FA, Black PM (2005) Survival rates in patients with low-grade glioma after intraoperative magnetic resonance image guidance. Cancer 103(6):1227–1233
14. Fahlbusch R, Ganslandt O, Nimsky C (2000) Intraoperative imaging with open magnetic resonance imaging and neuronavigation. Childs Nerv Syst 16(10–11):829–831
15. Nimsky C, Ganslandt O, Von Keller B, Romstöck J, Fahlbusch R (2004) Intraoperative high-field-strength MR imaging: implementation and experience in 200 patients. Radiology 233(1):67–78
16. Hall WA, Martin AJ, Liu H, Pozza CH, Casey SO, Michel E, Nussbaum ES, Maxwell RE, Truwit CL (1998) High-field strength interventional magnetic resonance imaging for pediatric neurosurgery. Pediatr Neurosurg 29(5):253–259
17. Martin AJ, Hall WA, Liu H, Pozza CH, Michel E, Casey SO, Maxwell RE, Truwit CL (2000) Brain tumor resection: intraoperative monitoring with high-field-strength MR imaging-initial results. Radiology 215(1):221–228
18. Nabavi A, Dörner L, Stark AM, Mehdorn HM (2009) Intraoperative MRI with 1.5 Tesla in neurosurgery. Neurosurg Clin North Am 20(2):163–171
19. Wirtz CR, Albert FK, Schwaderer M, Heuer C, Staubert A, Tronnier VM, Knauth M, Kunze S (2000) The benefit of neuronavigation for neurosurgery analyzed by its impact on glioblastoma surgery. Neurol Res 22(4):354–360
20. Stummer W, Pichlmeier U, Meinel T, Wiestler OD, Zanella F, Reulen HJ, ALA-Glioma Study Group (2006) Fluorescence-guided surgery with 5-aminolevulinic acid for resection of malignant glioma: a randomised controlled multicentre phase III trial. Lancet Oncol 27(5):392–401
21. Nabavi A, Goebel S, Doerner L, Warneke N, Ulmer S, Mehdorn M (2009) Awake craniotomy and intraoperative magnetic resonance imaging: patient selection, preparation, and technique. Top Magn Reson Imaging 19(4):191–196
22. Pinsker MO, Nabavi A, Mehdorn HM (2007) Neuronavigation and resection of lesions located in eloquent brain areas under local anesthesia and neuropsychological-neurophysiological monitoring. Minim Invasive Neurosurg 50(5):281–284
23. Goebel S, Nabavi A, Schubert S, Mehdorn HM (2010) Patient perception of combined awake brain tumour surgery and intraoperative 1.5-T-MRI: The Kiel experience. Neurosurgery
24. Knauth M, Wirtz CR, Aras N, Sartor K (2001) Low-field interventional MRI in neurosurgery: finding the right dose of contrast medium. Neuroradiology 43(3):254–258
25. Ulmer S, Helle M, Jansen O, Mehdorn HM, Nabavi A (2009) Intraoperative dynamic susceptibility contrast weighted magnetic resonance imaging (iDSC-MRI) – Technical considerations and feasibility. Neuroimage 45(1):38–43
26. Nimsky C, Ganslandt O, Cerny S, Hastreiter P, Greiner G, Fahlbusch R (2000) Quantification of, visualization of, and compensation for brain shift using intraoperative magnetic resonance imaging. Neurosurgery 47(5):1070–1079
27. Oh DS, Black PM (2005) A low-field intraoperative MRI system for glioma surgery: is it worthwhile? Neurosurg Clin N Am 16(1): 135–141, Review
28. Schneider JP, Trantakis C, Schulz T, Dietrich J, Kahn T (2003) [Intraoperative use of an open mid-field MR scanner in the surgical treatment of cerebral gliomas]. Z Med Phys 13(3): 214–218

Image Guided Aneurysm Surgery in a Brainsuite® ioMRI Miyabi 1.5 T Environment

R.W. König, C.P.G. Heinen, G. Antoniadis, T. Kapapa, M.T. Pedro, A. Gardill, C.R. Wirtz, T. Kretschmer, and T. Schmidt

Abstract

Objective: Current literature only gives sparse account of aneurysm surgery in an intraoperative MRI environment. After installation of a BrainSuite® ioMRI Miyabi 1.5 T at our institution the aim of the present preliminary study was to evaluate feasibility, pros and cons of aneurysm surgery in this special setting.

Material and Methods: Since February 2009, during a 3 months period we performed elective image guided aneurysm surgery in 4 ACM and 1 ACOM aneurysm (four patients) in this ioMRI setting. The patients' heads were rigidly fixed in the Noras 8-Channel OR Head Coil. Our imaging protocol included MP-RAGE, T2-TSE axial, TOF-MRA and diffusion-/perfusion-imaging immediately before surgery and after clip application. Presurgical 3D-planning was performed using the iPlan-Software.

Results: All five aneurysms were operated without temporary clipping. There were no intra- or postoperative complications. Patient positioning and head fixation with the integrated Noras Head Clamp was feasible, but there were significant limitations particularly with regard to more complex approaches and patient physiognomy. Image quality especially TOF-MRA was good in 4, insufficient in 1 aneurysm. Presurgical planning especially vessel extraction from TOF-MRA was possible but certainly needs significant future improvement. Diffusion- and perfusion weighted examinations yielded good image quality.

Conclusion: Our limited experience is encouraging so far. Further improvement particularly concerning flexibility of patient positioning and presurgical 3D-planning for vascular procedures is most necessary. As a future perspective image guided aneurysm surgery in an ioMRI-environment may be helpful especially in complex aneurysms and provide neurosurgeons and neuroanaesthesiologists with additional information about cerebral haemodynamics and perfusion pattern in the vascular territory distal to the target vessel.

Keywords Aneurysm clipping · BrainSuite · Image guidance · ioMRI · Intraoperative imaging

Introduction

After its introduction intraoperative MRI (ioMRI) rapidly became the imaging modality of choice for central nervous system pathology, particularly with regard to resection control in glioma and pituitary surgery [1–5]. Additionally numerous articles published till now discuss various aspects of image guidance in aneurysm surgery [6–9].

Sutherland [10] was the first who reported about one case of elective clipping of an ACOM aneurysm in an ioMRI environment especially accentuating the significance of MRA and diffusion weighted imaging.

This is the first study reporting about elective aneurysm surgery in four patients in a fully integrated neurosurgical OR (BrainSUITE® ioMRI Miyabi 1.5 T; BrainLAB, Germany) combining image guidance with intraoperative imaging particularly diffusion and perfusion weighted imaging. The aim of the present study was to highlight the aspects of *feasibility* and *diagnostic relevance* of *MR-TOF-Angiography* and *Perfusion Weighted Imaging (PWI)* before and after clip application in our special setting.

Materials and Methods

The fully integrated single-room BrainSUITE® ioMRI Miyabi consists of a 1.5 T Siemens MAGNETOM Espree scanner combined with the Miyabi table concept. Hereby the

R.W. König (✉), C.P.G. Heinen, G. Antoniadis, T. Kapapa, M.T. Pedro, A. Gardill, C.R. Wirtz, and T. Schmidt
Department of Neurosurgery, University of Ulm, Ludwig-Heilmeyer-Str. 2, 89312, BKH, Guenzburg, Germany
e-mail: ralph.koenig@uni-ulm.de
T. Kretschmer
Department of Neurosurgery, Ev. Krankenhaus, Oldenburg, Germany

M.N. Pamir et al. (eds.), *Intraoperative Imaging*, Acta Neurochirurgica Supplementum, Vol. 109,
DOI 10.1007/978-3-211-99651-5_17, © Springer-Verlag/Wien 2011

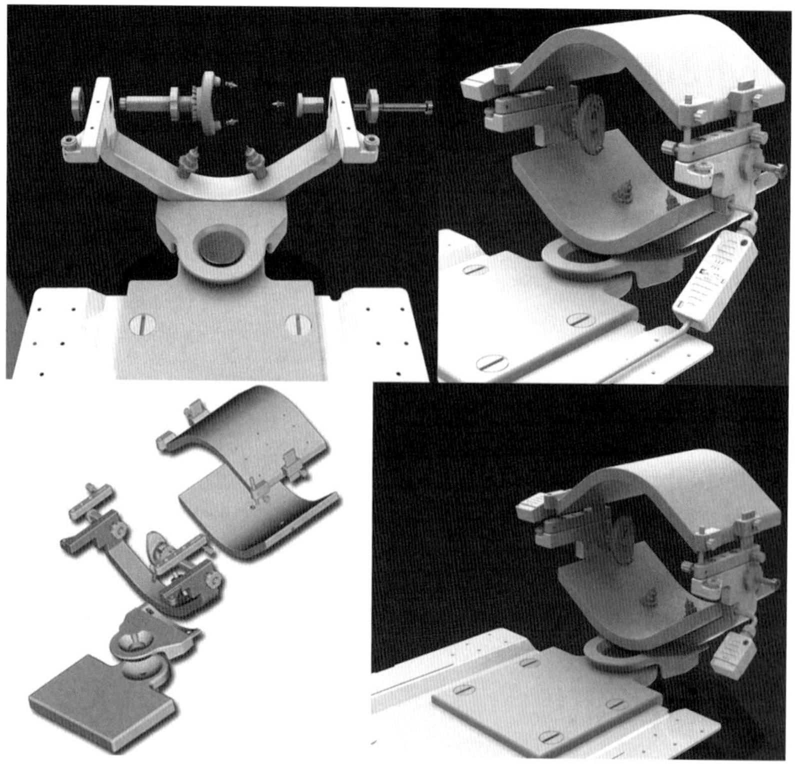

Fig. 1 Noras 8-Channel OR Head Coil with integrated head holder (with permission of Noras MRI products GmbH, Germany)

patient is positioned on the specially designed Miyabi shell, which is mounted to a regular Trumpf Jupiter OR table (TRUMPF Medizinsysteme, Germany). The layout chosen allows the neurosurgeon to use conventional surgical instruments beyond the 5-G line. The patient's head is rigidly fixed in a head holder integrated in the Noras 8-Channel OR Head Coil (NORAS MRI products GmbH, Germany). In contrast to the BrainSUITE® ioMRI rotating table a height adjustable fixation of the head coil is not possible, the coil is mounted to the Miyabi shell with a semi-spherical joint (Fig. 1).

Since February 2009, during a 3 months period we performed elective image guided aneurysm surgery in 4 ACM and 1 ACOM aneurysm (four patients). The imaging protocol included MP-RAGE, T2-TSE axial, TOF-MRA and diffusion-/perfusion-imaging immediately before surgery and after clip application. Presurgical planning was performed using the iPlan®-Software (BrainLAB AG, Germany).

Results

Patient Outcome: Management of all five aneurysms was uneventful without any temporary clipping. As expected the overall procedure time was extended (average additional time 105 min) due to scanning before surgery and after clipping and because of some limitations in patient positioning. Infections as possible consequence of prolonged surgical procedures did not occur.

Feasibility: All patients were operated via a standard frontolateral approach. As a consequence patient positioning was feasible but needed some additional preparation time before surgery. Flexibility of head fixation (tilting, vertex down positioning) is markedly restricted primarily due to the fixation of the head coil with the Miyabi shell, which allows only a limited range of movement. Due to missing height adjustment in the fixation of the head coil neurosurgical procedures in prone position (so far no experience in aneurysm surgery, only in AVM surgery) are feasible but need elaborate padding under the breast of the patient. Obese patients and those with unfavourable physiognomy (short neck, broad shoulders) should not be considered as surgical candidates in the ioMRI environment described.

Diagnostic relevance of MR-TOF-Angiography Before and After Clip Application

We used MR-TOF-Angiography as basis of image guided aneurysm surgery (Fig. 2). The image quality was excellent

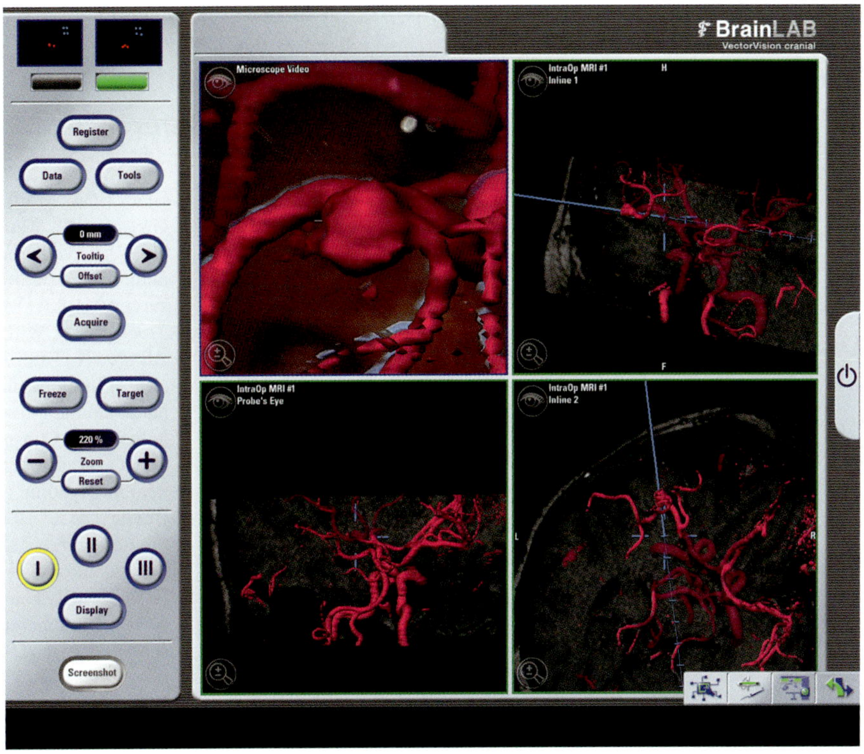

Fig. 2 Image guided surgery of left sided MCA bifurcation aneurysm

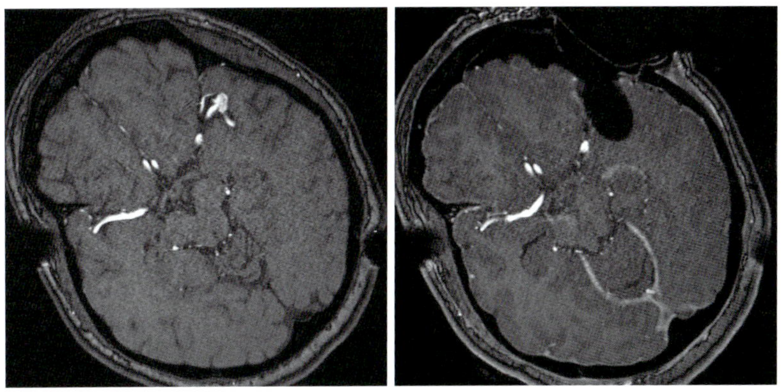

Fig. 3 TOF-MRA before and after clipping of a left sided MCA bifurcation aneurysm

in 3 MCA and one ACOM aneurysms correlating very well with preoperative 3D-CT-angiographic studies (3D-CTA) and intraoperative findings. On the other hand TOF-MRA underestimated size and configuration of one left sided MCA bifurcation aneurysm. The main aneurysm sac (1.2 cm) projected mainly downward and therefore out of the vector of the main blood flow, therefore TOF-MRA demonstrated the inflow zone of the aneurysm at its neck but not the complete lesion.

Intraoperative MRA after clip application revealed significant susceptibility artefacts around the clip (Fig. 3a, b). Hence judgement of aneurysm remnants or clip stenosis will not be possible without significant reduction of these artefacts. Patency of the efferent vessels distal to the clipping site could be demonstrated in all cases.

Perfusion Weighted Imaging Before and After Clip Application

Image quality of PWI before and after clip application was good. Besides the clip-induced artefact PWI could demonstrate normal haemodynamics and perfusion of both hemispheres, especially in the vascular territory distal to the aneurysm. In one patient after uneventful clipping of a MCA aneurysm there was a slight delay in time to peak and mean transit time in the territory of the posterior parietal artery. Recovery of the patient was normal and follow-up studies did not reveal any infarctions.

Discussion

To our knowledge this is the first study reporting about elective aneurysm surgery in a fully integrated neurosurgical OR (BrainSUITE® ioMRI Miyabi 1.5 T; BrainLAB, Germany) combining image guidance with advanced intraoperative imaging particularly diffusion and perfusion weighted imaging.

The pioneer study of Sutherland [10] already demonstrated feasibility of elective aneurysm surgery in an ioMRI environment with a ceiling mounted moveable 1.5 T magnet. Image guidance was not integrated. The study especially stressed the diagnostic relevance of MRA and intraoperative diffusion weighted imaging. Reduction of image distorsions caused by the aneurysm clip is one big issue discussed there. We believe that further decrease of MR image artefacts aiming at judgement of probable aneurysm remnants or vessel stenosis after clipping will be hard to achieve. But this intraoperative diagnostic flaw can easily be compensated by adding e.g. microscope integrated near infrared indocyanine green video angiography [11].

The combination of different advanced intraoperative imaging modalities like ioMRI (TOF, PWI, DWI, arterial spin labelling) and ICG-videoangiography might be helpful in selected aneurysm cases. On the other hand there are some disadvantages especially concerning patient positioning which have to be balanced with the potential advantages achieved by performing aneurysm surgery in an ioMRI environment.

Conflicts of interest statement We declare that we have no conflict of interest.

References

1. Black PM, Moriarty T, Aleander E III, Stieg P, Woodard EJ, Gleason PL, Martin CH, Kikinis R, Schwartz RB, Jolest FA (1997) Development and implementation of intraoperative magnetic resonance imaging and its neurosurgical applications. Neurosurgery 41:831–842
2. Tronnier VM, Wirtz CR, Knauth M, Lenz G, Pastyr O, Bonsanto MM, Albert FK, Kuth R, Staubert A, Schlegel W, Sartor K, Kunze S (1997) Intraoperative diagnostic and interventional magnetic resonance imaging in neurosurgery. Neurosurgery 40:891–900
3. Nimsky C, Ganslandt O, Kober H, Buchfelder M, Fahlbusch R (2001) Intraoperative magnetic resonance imaging combined with neuronavigation: a new concept. Neurosurgery 48:1082–1089
4. Bradley WG (2002) Achieving gross total resection of brain tumors: intraoperative MR imaging can make a big difference. Am J Neuroradiol 23:348–349
5. Fahlbusch R, Ganslandt O, Buchfelder M, Schott W, Nimsky C (2001) Intraoperative magnetic resonance imaging during transsphenoidal surgery. J Neurosurg 95:381–390
6. Albert FK, Wirtz CR, Forsting M, Jansen O, Polarz H, Mittermaier G, Kunze S (1998) Image guided excision of a ruptured feeding artery "pedicle aneurysm" associated with an arteriovenous malformation in a child. Case report. Comput Aided Surg 2:5–10
7. Schmid-Elsaesser R, Muacevic A, Holtmannspötter M, Uhl E, Steiger HJ (2003) Neuronavigation based on CT angiography for surgery of intracranial aneurysms: primary experience with unruptured aneurysms. Minim Invasive Neurosurg 46:269–277
8. Pirotte B, Wikler D, David P, Lefranc F, Brotchi J, Levivier M (2004) Magnetic resonance angiography image guidance for the microsurgical clipping of intracranial aneurysms: a report of two cases. Neurol Res 26:429–34
9. Raabe A, Beck J, Rohde S, Berkefeld J, Seifert V (2006) Three-dimensional rotational angiography guidance for aneurysm surgery. J Neurosurg 105:406–411
10. Sutherland G, Kalibara T, Wallace C, Boguslaw T, Richter M (2002) Intraoperative assessment of aneurysm clipping using magnetic resonance angiography and diffusion-weighted imaging: technical case report. Neurosurgery 50:893–898
11. Raabe A, Beck J, Gerlach R, Zimmermann M, Seifert V (2003) Near-infrared indocyanine green video angiography: a new method for intraoperative assessment of vascular flow. Neurosurgery 52:132–139

From Intraoperative Angiography to Advanced Intraoperative Imaging: The Geneva Experience

Karl Schaller, Marc Kotowski, Vitor Pereira, Daniel Rüfenacht, and Philippe Bijlenga

Abstract *Objective*: We aimed at the integration of recent flat panel technology in a joint interventional suite for neurosurgeons and neuroradiologists.

Methods: A Flat Panel system, allowing for intraoperative performance of 2D and 3D DSA, for automated segmentation of vascular structures, and for performance of computed tomography, was connected with a surgical microscope and neuronavigation. All surgical and neurointerventional cases were monitored and stored in a prospective data base.

Results: N=99 patients were treated neurosurgically: N=63 aneurysm clippings in n=51 patients; n=12 resections of arteriovenous malformations (AVM); n=6 clippings/excisions of dural AV fistulae (dAVF); n=3 EC-IC bypass procedures; n=10 resections of skull base tumours; n=17 spine procedures. All patients had intraoperative imaging for angiographic control and/or for anatomical allocation. Intraoperative 3D-rotational angiography was performed n=54 times in n=42 patients in <15 min each, with repositioning of aneurysm clips in n=9 patients.

Conclusion: This hybrid neuro-interventional suite opens a new avenue for intraoperative imaging by the provision of highly resoluted angiographic or CT images, which may be co-registered with a navigation system. In addition, the workflow in treatment of aneurysmal SAH can be improved, as all diagnostic and therapeutic measures can be taken without having to move the patient to other facilities.

K. Schaller (✉), M. Kotowski, V. Pereira, D. Rüfenacht, and P. Bijlenga
University of Geneva Medical Center, Faculty of Medicine, University of Geneva, Rue Gabrielle-Perret Gentil 4, 1211 Geneva, Switzerland
e-mail: karl.schaller@hcuge.ch

Keywords Flat panel · Intraoperative angiography · Intraoperative CT · Intraoperative imaging · Vascular neurosurgery

Introduction

Neurosurgeons deal with intracranial and spinal vascular, bony, and soft tissue pathologies, or with a combination of those. Due to its strength for the visualization of soft-tissue properties, intraoperative MRI (ioMRI) has become an important tool for resection control in surgery of intra-axial brain tumours, and in pituitary surgery [1]. It requires large and expensive equipment, however, and its use is still not very intuitive in a strictly surgical sense. Intraoperative CT (ioCT) scanning requires large equipment as well, and interferes with the natural course of surgery as the patient needs to be moved into the gantry [2]. Furthermore, vascular imaging does not allow for dynamic visualization of blood flow.

Recent Flat Panel (FP) technology allows for imaging of vascular structures at high spatial and temporal resolution with up to 100 images/s. In addition, it allows for bone imaging at high spatial resolution, e.g. precise visualization of the human skull base, or of trabecular bone of the human spine. The hardware itself is smaller than previously used X-ray machines, and it can be ceiling-mounted, or attached to robotic arms. This technology may represent an interesting alternative to the above-mentioned modalities, ioMRI and ioCT due to its flexibility and due to the fact that it allows for dynamic vascular imaging, as well as for flat panel derived computed tomography as well. In addition, adaptation of image-guidance could allow for co-registration of the various image modalities – taking advantage of each of those. It was our ambition to develop and to evaluate a joint hybrid neuroradiological and neurosurgical interventional suite, based on FP technology (Figs. 1–3).

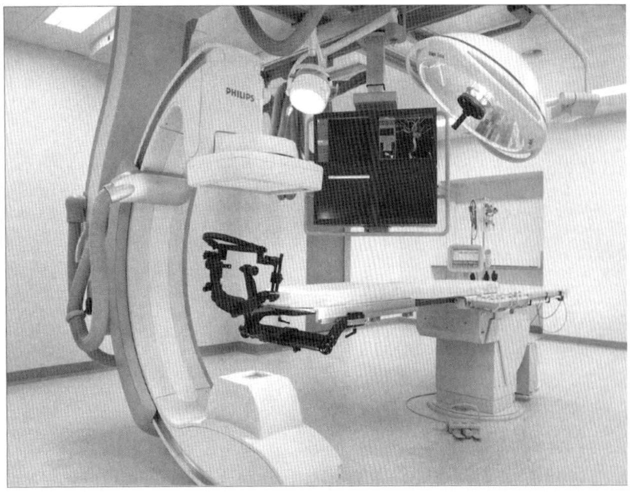

Fig. 1 Illustration of basic setup in the hybrid room. The Flat Panel system, including table with radiolucent headholder, and overhead monitors. Not in the figure: Surgical microscope and neuronavigation, which are coupled with the FP system. 3D screen and Neuromonitoring system

Materials and Methods

Infrastructure

The hybrid interventional room is located between diagnostic radiological facilities, such as MRIs, the emergency surgical suites of the hospital, and the urological operating rooms. It can be entered from three sides. The assigned interventional room surface was restricted to 65 m^2 for local architectural reasons. In addition, there is a control room with all monitors and computer workstations, shielded by protecting glass towards the interventional suite, and a small storage room with a scrubbing facility – adding to another 25 m^2. Local bioengineers have evaluated the hygienical aspects, as the room was intended for use in diagnostic and in open surgical interventions. Therefore, a vertical laminar air flow system had to be installed at the foot end of the interventional table.

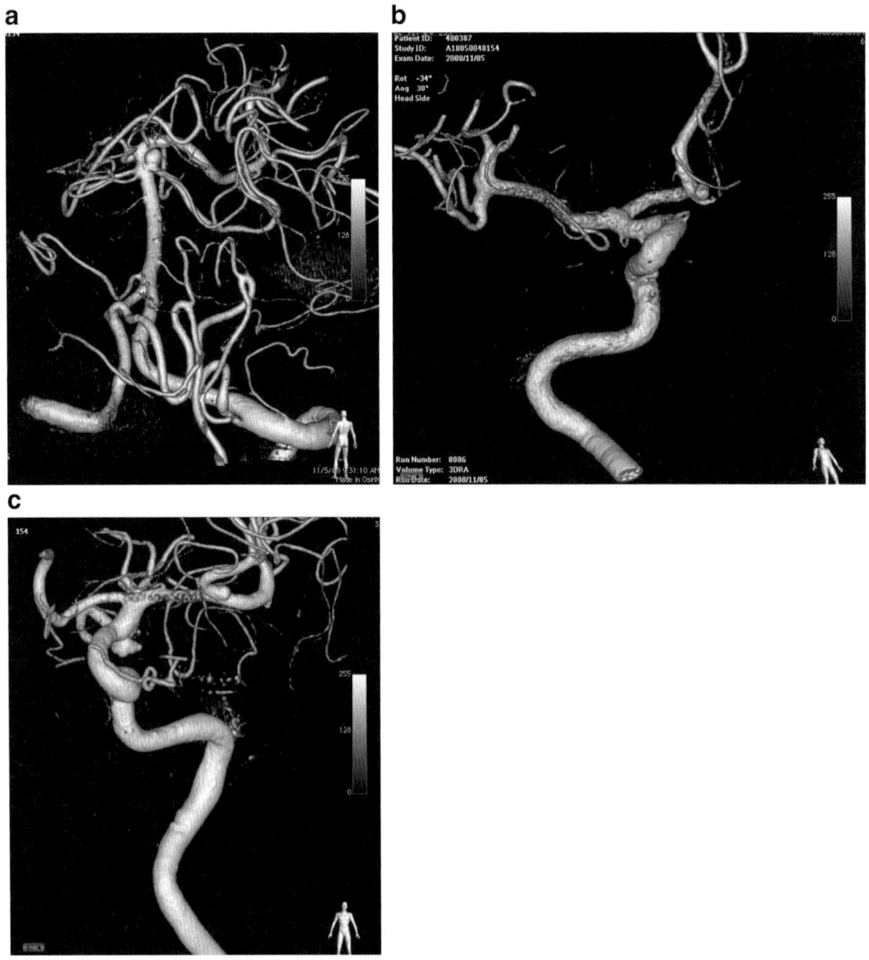

Fig. 2 Example of joint neurosurgical–neuroradiological intervention. Sixty-eight-year old woman with incidentally found aneurysms of her right superior cerebellar (SCA) (**a**), anterior communicating (Acom) (**b**), left middle cerebral (MCA) (**c**), and left posterior communicating (Pcom) (**c**) arteries. All aneurysms were treated the same day, on the same table, during the same session. Interventional neuroradiologists started with coil occlusion of the right SCA aneurysm. These images underscore the quality of the 3D angiographic images

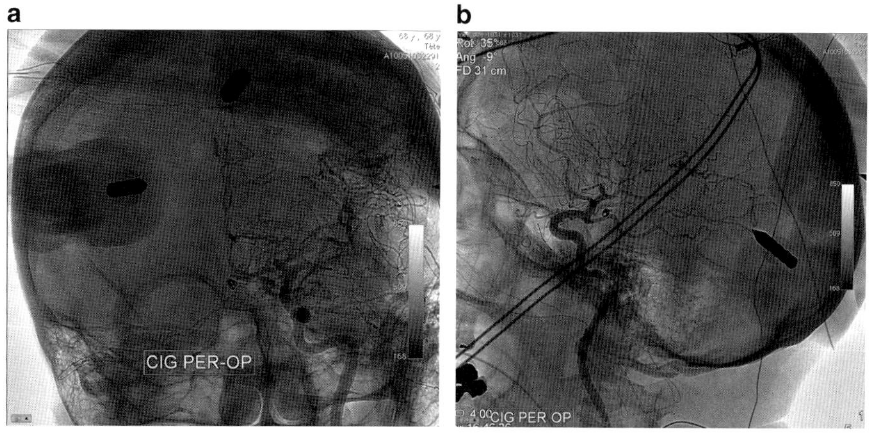

Fig. 3 Intra-operative angiographic control, showing complete occlusion of all aneurysms (2D DSA) in anterior–posterior (**a**) and lateral (**b**) view. Please note the limited artefacts of the headholder

Equipment

A monoplane Philips Allura FD20 system (≤620 projections along 240° in 8–10 s, rotational speed: 30°/55°/s, 30 frames/s), allowing for automated segmentation of vascular structures was installed (Philips Medical systems, Best, Netherlands). This system allows for dynamic imaging (e.g. angiography), as well as for CT imaging. The accompanying (angio-)table can be adjusted in height only in its present version. A special adapter for the radiolucent head clamp (Doro, Promedics, Düsseldorf, Germany) was constructed.

A BrainLAB neuronavigation system (VV^2; BrainLAB, Heimstetten, Germany) was installed in addition, and a recent surgical microscope (Zeiss Pentero; Zeiss, Oberkochen, Germany) including an Indocyanine green (ICG) videoangiography unit completed the basic equipment. The microscope is navigable, and the navigation system was adapted for integration and co-registration of FP-derived images (angiography and CT) with conventional imaging data sets.

All surgical and neuroradiological and joint interventions were prospectively stored in a data base.

All patients had intra-operative imaging for anatomical allocation (e.g. FP CT scanning for resection control in skull base tumours) or for angiographic control (e.g. of clipped aneurysms). Co-registration of intraoperatively acquired imaging data (either angiographic, or FP CT) with the navigation system was performed when considered useful for the intervention.

Results

Open Neurosurgical Patients

A total of n=99 patients were treated neurosurgically within a 19-month period of time (February 2008 – September 2009). This includes n=63 aneurysm clippings in n=51 patients, n=12 resections of arteriovenous malformations (AVMs), n=6 clippings/excisions of dural AV fistulae (dAVF), n=3 EC-IC bypass procedures, n=10 resections of skull base tumours, and n=17 complex spine procedures.

Intraoperative 3D-rotational angiography was performed in all vascular patients in <15 min each. It allowed for direct control of aneurysm-clipping and displayed incomplete clipping (n=7) or vascular compromise (n=2). Direct repositioning of aneurysm clips was performed in n=9 patients. Thereby, intraoperative 3D angiography had stipulated clip correction in 14.3% of aneurysms, thus allowing complete aneurysm occlusion in 100%. Intraoperative FP-based CT scanning was performed in skull base tumours. It was particularly helpful, where a far lateral transcondylar approach had to be used in a recurrent foramen magnum meningioma, and in a partially calcified clival chordoma (see Figs. 4 and 5). The respective intraoperative data sets were co-registered with preoperative images on the navigation system. However, soft tissue properties could not be visualised with the same quality as with extraoperative CT – and certainly not as with MRI.

Two patients of the whole series developed locally confined decubitus following prolonged lateral positioning.

Neuroradiological Patients

Within the same period, a total of n=147 diagnostic and n=106 interventional (neuroradiological) procedures were performed (n=51 coilings, n=28 stentings, n=13 AVM- or AVF-embolizations, n=14 vertebroplasties). In addition, n=364 percutaneous infiltrations were performed.

Discussion

In the same way, neurosurgeons are eager to perform resection control in case of intrinsic brain tumours by intraoperative MRI, they are looking for innovative ways of

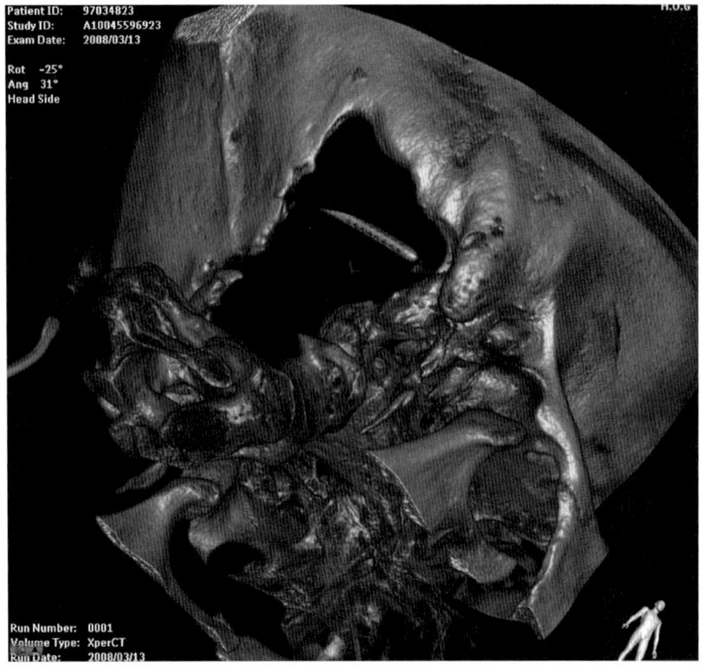

Fig. 4 Intra-operative 3D skull radiography during extended far lateral approach for a skull base tumour. These images can be transferred and co-registered with the navigation station

intraoperative visualization in neurovascular surgery, in surgery around the skull base, and for spine surgery. That goal should be accomplished in an intuitive manner, and whatever methodology applied – it should not interfere too much with the surgical workflow. As the physical properties of the tissues neurosurgeons are dealing with are so different from each other, it is very unlikely to achieve this goal with a single imaging modality in the near future.

As far as it concerns vascular imaging, the dynamics of intravascular flow have to be considered in addition. Whereas ioMRI is steadily advancing, e.g. in the field of glioma and pituitary surgery, there have not been reasonable approaches for vascular and skull base surgery so far [1, 3, 4]. Spatial resolution and lack of practicability of conventional angiographic tools did not promote their application in a surgical environment, despite the clear advantage of e.g. having the opportunity to perform direct control of surgical clipping in cerebral aneurysm surgery [5, 6]. Thus, some surgical groups perform direct post-operative angiographic control with the patients still anesthetized, in order to take them back to surgery directly in case of incomplete aneurysm clipping or inadvertent clipping of a parent vessel [7]. Indocyanine green videoangiography has become a very important tool in microneurosurgical routine [8]. Its particular value concerns the visualisation of small and perforating vessels, whereas vessels, which are not directly visible though the microscope may escape microangiographic analysis [8]. It should be seen as an excellent complementary tool to advanced intraoperative 3D DSA as this is possible with our proposed concept for integration of FP technology in a hybrid operating room. Another approach is the use of intra-operative CT scanners, the most recent of which do even allow for intraoperative performance of angio-CT scanning in addition [9]. These scanners are large, however, fairly static, and it thus seems reasonable to combine the technical and physical flexibility of recent Flat Panel technology in order to overcome the shortcomings of standard 2D DSA and CT scanning.

Whereas the direct advantage of such a hybrid interventional environment may not be as obvious for surgery of intracranial tumours, it has to be stated that the integration of such a joint neurosurgical–neuroradiological suite may change and improve the overall in-house management and workflow of neurovascular emergencies: E.g., currently, one has to transfer a patient with acute SAH from the emergency department to the CT scanner, then to the ICU, or to the OR for placement of an external drainage, then to the angiography suite for further diagnostics, and finally – to the operating room, if free at the time. Control angiography has to be scheduled separately in the conventional setup. The proposed hybrid concept allows for completion of all diagnostic and interventional/surgical activities, including CT, DSA, and open, or endovascular aneurysm treatment – plus immediate control of aneurysm occlusion. All can be done in the same room, on the same table, and even jointly (e.g. preparation for arteriography and placement of external ventricular drainage). Unfortunately, two patients developed locoregional – and reversible – decubitus after having been placed in the lateral position for several hours. It is quite clear that the present solution with a modern yet standard angiography table is not sufficient for use in an important number of neurosur-

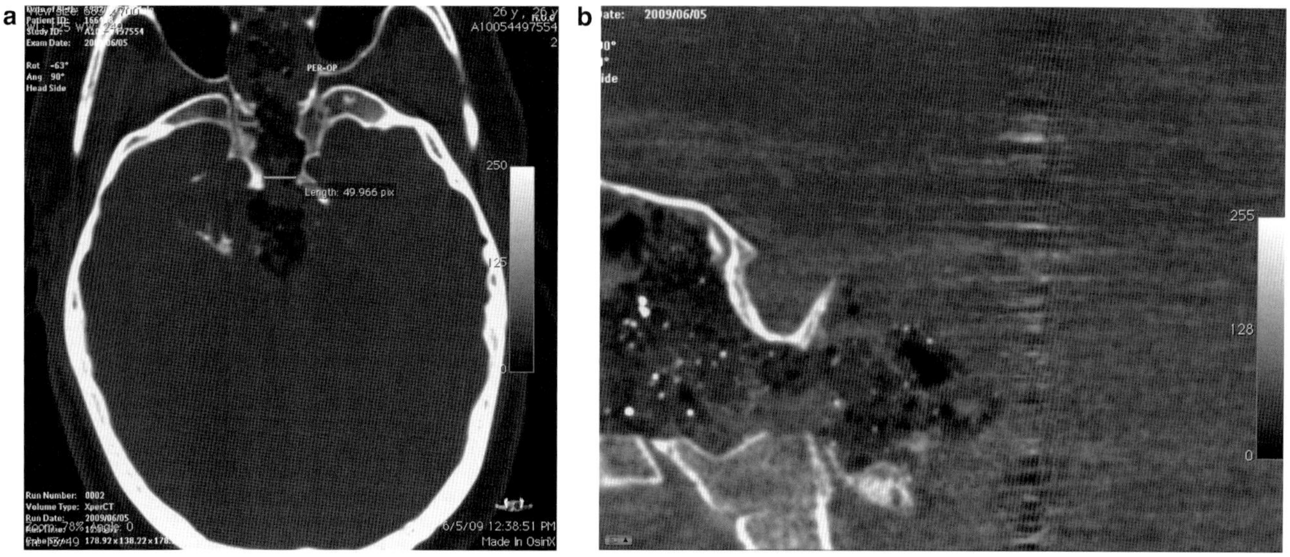

Fig. 5 Intra-operative CT-images, obtained with Flat Panel system, for resection control in case of large calcified clival chordoma, which was approached via the sublabial transsphenoidal route. Remnants of the calcified tumour can still be appreciated on axial images (**a**), as well as inferiorly on sagittal reconstructions (**b**)

gical pathologies. The next evolutionary step of such a hybrid room should concern the development of a specifically adapted carbon table, which can be adjusted like any other operating table.

Conclusion

The new neuro-interventional suite opens a new avenue for intraoperative imaging by the provision of highly resoluted CT or angiographic images, which may be co-registered with a commercially available navigation system. High temporal resolution of vascular diagnostics may assist in developing better virtual and customized treatment plans for patients suffering from aneurysms and vascular malformations. In addition, the workflow in treatment of aneurysmal subarachnoid hemorrhage can be improved significantly, as all diagnostic and therapeutic measures can be taken without having to move the patient to other facilities. In addition, due to high resolution of bony structures and the connection with image guidance, there is good potential concerning skull base and spinal surgery. The further development of a fully-functioning carbon-made surgical table is recommended.

Conflicts of interest statement The project to develop this experimental joint interventional suite benefitted from the following: BrainLAB supported the project by the one-year cost-free use of a navigational system and Philips Medical Systems provided regular cost-free upgrades of software.

References

1. Nimsky C, von Keller B, Schlaffer S, Kuhnt D, Weigel D, Ganslandt O, Buchfelder M (2009) Updating navigation with intraoperative imaging data. Top Magn Reson Imaging 19:197–204
2. Matula C, Rössler K, Reddy M, Schindler E, Koos WT (1998) Intraoperative computed tomography guided neuronavigation: concepts, efficiency, and work flow. Comput Aided Surg 3:174–182
3. Gerlach R, du Mesnil de Rochemont R, Gasser T, Marquardt G, Reusch J, Imoehl L, Seifert V (2008) Feasibility of Polestar N20, an ultra-low-field intraoperative magnetic resonance imaging system in resection control of pituitary macroadenomas: lessons learned from the first 40 cases. Neurosurgery 63:272–284
4. Jankovski A, Francotte F, Vaz G, Fomekong E, Duprez T, Van Boven M, Docquier MA, Hermoye L, Cosnard G, Raftopoulos C (2008) Intraoperative magnetic resonance imaging at 3-T using a dual independent operating room-magnetic resonance imaging suite: development, feasibility, safety, and preliminary experience. Neurosurgery 63:412–426
5. Alexander TD, Macdonald RL, Weir B, Kowalczuk A (1996) Intraoperative angiography in cerebral aneurysm surgery: a perspective study of 100 craniotomies. Neurosurgery 39:10–18
6. Raabe A, Beck J, Rohde S, Berkefeld J, Seifert V (2006) Three-dimensional rotational angiography guidance for aneurysm surgery. J Neurosurg 105:406–411
7. Meyer B, Urbach H, Schaller C, Baslam M, Nordblom J, Schramm J (2004) Immediate postoperative angiography after aneurysm clipping – implications for quality control and further guidance of management. Zentralbl Neurochir 65:49–56
8. De Oliveira JG, Beck J, Seifert V, Teixeira MJ, Raabe A (2007) Assessment of flow in perforating arteries during intracranial aneurysm surgery using intraoperative near-infrared indocyanine green videoangiography. Neurosurgery 61(3 Suppl):63–73
9. Uhl E, Zausinger S, Morhard D, Heigl T, Scheder B, Rachinger W, Schichor C, Tonn J (2009) Intraoperative computed tomography with integrated navigation system in a multidisciplinary operating suite. Neurosurgery 64(5 Suppl 2):231–240

Intraoperative MRI – Ultra High Field Systems

Intraoperative Magnetic Resonance Imaging

Walter A. Hall and Charles L. Truwit

Abstract Neurosurgeons have become reliant on image-guidance to perform safe and successful surgery both time-efficiently and cost-effectively. Neuronavigation typically involves either rigid (frame-based) or skull-mounted (frameless) stereotactic guidance derived from computed tomography (CT) or magnetic resonance imaging (MRI) that is obtained days or immediately before the planned surgical procedure. These systems do not accommodate for brain shift that is unavoidable once the cranium is opened and cerebrospinal fluid is lost. Intraoperative MRI (ioMRI) systems ranging in strength from 0.12 to 3 Tesla (T) have been developed in part because they afford neurosurgeons the opportunity to accommodate for brain shift during surgery. Other distinct advantages of ioMRI include the excellent soft tissue discrimination, the ability to view the surgical site in three dimensions, and the ability to "see" tumor beyond the surface visualization of the surgeon's eye, either with or without a surgical microscope. The enhanced ability to view the tumor being biopsied or resected allows the surgeon to choose a safe surgical corridor that avoids critical structures, maximizes the extent of the tumor resection, and confirms that an intraoperative hemorrhage has not resulted from surgery. Although all ioMRI systems allow for basic T1- and T2-weighted imaging, only high-field (>1.5 T) MRI systems are capable of MR spectroscopy (MRS), MR angiography (MRA), MR venography (MRV), diffusion-weighted imaging (DWI), and brain activation studies. By identifying vascular structures with MRA and MRV, it may be possible to prevent their inadvertent injury during surgery. Biopsying those areas of elevated phosphocholine on MRS may improve the diagnostic yield for brain biopsy. Mapping out eloquent brain function may influence the surgical path to a tumor being resected or biopsied. The optimal field strength for an ioMRI-guided surgical system and the best configuration for that system are as yet undecided.

Keywords Brain activation · Brain neoplasms · Intraoperative magnetic resonance imaging · Magnetic resonance imaging

W.A. Hall (✉)
Department of Neurosurgery, SUNY Upstate Medical University, 750 East Adams Street, Syracuse, NY 13210, USA
e-mail: hallw@upstate.edu

C.L. Truwit
Departments of Radiology, Hennepin County Medical Center, University of Minnesota, Minneapolis, MN, USA

Introduction

Neurosurgeons have used magnetic resonance imaging (MRI) for more than 20 years to visualize the brain because of the ability to view the brain in three dimensions with excellent soft tissue discrimination. Other technological advances that have accompanied MRI over the same time period include frame-based stereotaxy, frameless neuronavigation, and most recently, intraoperative MRI (ioMRI)-guided neurosurgery. Intraoperative MRI-guidance in the operating room has the advantage over the other technical advancements in that it allows for the surgeon to visualize the surgical site during the procedure in near-real time. This capability provides the neurosurgeon with valuable information that will help to guide the surgical procedure to its successful completion primarily by allowing for the compensation of brain shift which occurs after the cranium is opened and cerebrospinal fluid (CSF) is lost [1].

As ioMRI-guided neurosurgery continues to disseminate to more and more academic health centers and community hospitals, it has become uncertain which magnetic field strength is best suited for surgical use. Since the first utilization of this technology in 1994, multiple MRI systems of varying field strengths have been developed for surgical use ranging from 0.12 Tesla (T) to 3 T [1, 2]. The first ioMRI system was a mid-field 0.5 T double coil design (SIGNA SP, General Electric Medical Systems, Milwaukee, WI) that was installed at Brigham and Women's Hospital in Boston, MA.

M.N. Pamir et al. (eds.), *Intraoperative Imaging*, Acta Neurochirurgica Supplementum, Vol. 109,
DOI 10.1007/978-3-211-99651-5_19, © Springer-Verlag/Wien 2011

With this MRI system, the surgeon operated between the coils and image updates could be obtained continuously during surgery (Fig. 1). Low field MRI systems have ranged from 0.12 to 0.23 T and high field systems are either 1.5 or 3 T in magnet strength. As image quality and MRI functionality is proportional to field strength, many diagnostic imaging techniques such as MR angiography (MRA), MR venography (MRV), MR spectroscopy (MRS), diffusion-weighted imaging (DWI), and brain activation studies considered functional MRI (fMRI) can be obtained at 1.5 T or higher field strength.

Being able to image patients intraoperatively provides the neurosurgeon with information that will allow him or her to alter the surgical treatment plan resulting in improved patient safety and the assurance of successful completion of the procedure. Each field strength ioMRI system has distinct advantages and disadvantages which are considered by neurosurgeons as they determine whether the various imaging capabilities provided by each will address their surgical needs. The surgical applications for each ioMRI system will be the focus of this contribution.

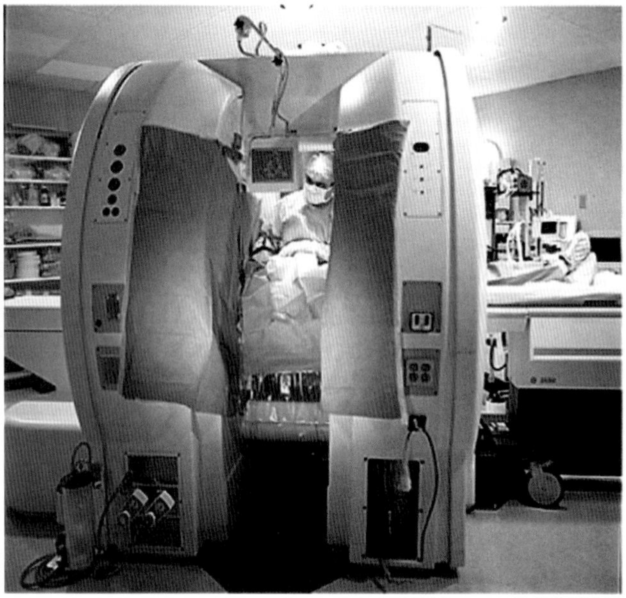

Fig. 1 General Electric Signa SP double coil 0.5 T magnetic resonance imaging scanner design that was installed at Brigham and Woman's Hospital in Boston in 1994. The surgeon is standing directly within the scanner and imaging updates can be obtained continuously during the procedure

Materials and Methods

Low Field ioMRI Systems

The very low field strength 0.12 T ioMRI system (Medtronic Navigation, Minneapolis, MN) has recently had an increase in its field strength to 0.15 T (Polestar N20). With this system the magnets are maintained below the surgical operating table until imaging is required at which time they are elevated to each side of the surgical field (Fig. 2). Imaging with this system affords incomplete visualization of the head due to limitations on field of view, but does allow for the surgical field of view to be seen. Surgery can be performed entirely within the magnetic field using standard surgical instrumentation. This ioMRI system allows for considerable access to the patient although there are technical limitations due to the distance between the magnetic poles that delimit which patients can be treated. Another advantage of this system is that the surgeon does not need to

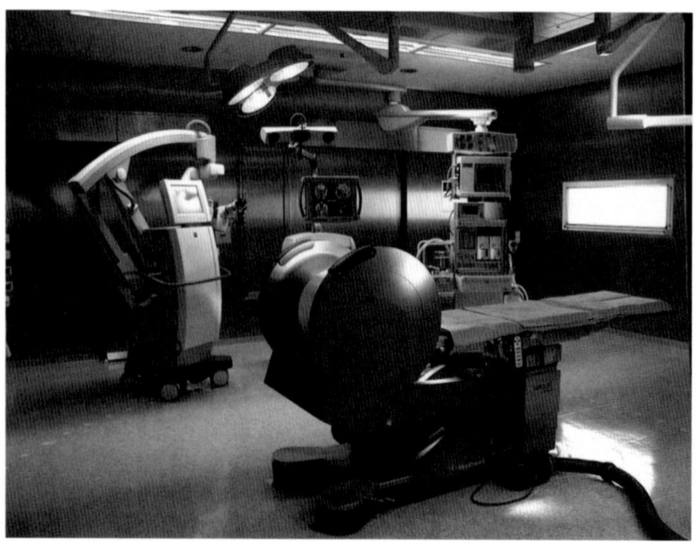

Fig. 2 Medtronic PoleStar N20 0.15 T low field intraoperative MR scanner. The magnetic poles are elevated into the position for scanning the head during surgery (Image courtesy of Medtronic)

operate between the magnets as with the 0.5 T ioMRI system.

Other low field MRI systems that have been used for diagnostic and ioMRI have a vertical gap or biplanar design where the magnet strength is either 0.2 or 0.23 T (Fonar, Melville, NY; Hitachi Medical, Twinsburg, OH). These systems have two horizontal 25–40 cm diameter magnetic poles that allow access to the patient from the side. A modification to this system resulted in a C-arm design (Siemens Medical Systems, Erlangen, Germany; Marconi Medical, Highland Heights, OH) where a column on one side of the magnet supported the upper magnetic pole which allowed for 240° of access to the patient and the ability to biopsy lesions of the neck and high cervical spine. The 40 cm gap between the magnetic poles again delimits the size of the patients that can be treated with these systems. Even though these ioMRI systems seem to be more open than short bore cylindrical scanners, during surgery the head of the patient is as far away from the surgeon as it is with high field systems.

Initially some centers would use these systems for intraoperative imaging by performing the surgery in another room and then transporting the patient to the magnet for imaging. Others would operate immediately adjacent, but outside the 5 Gauss line, and yet others would work within the magnet itself. Of note, while these ioMRI systems seem to be more open than short bore cylindrical scanners, it is important to point out that during surgery on these systems; the head of the patient is actually as far away from the surgeon as it is with high field systems.

All low field systems have reduced temporal resolution, spatial resolution per unit time, and reduced signal-to-noise ratio (SNR) compared to high field ioMRI systems [1]. These imaging constraints mandate an increase in imaging time that is sufficient to achieve image quality that will allow for accurate surgical decision making.

Mid Field ioMRI Systems

The prototype 0.5 T mid field system was the Signa SP "double donut" ioMRI system that was designed specifically for interventional use. With this system, two cylindrical magnets were set up such that an intervening gap was allowed for the surgeon and patient. Each magnet generated an inhomogeneous magnetic field, which because they were inverted relative to each other, created a homogeneous magnetic field of 30 cm diameter. This magnet configuration where the superconducting magnets are separated by a 56 cm gap allows for lateral and vertical access to the imaging isocenter. During procedures, the surgeon stands in this gap which requires special radiofrequency coils that diminish gradient strength and limit the field of view. The decreased field strength found at isocenter of the gap results in reduced SNR, longer imaging times, reduced spatial resolution, and a limitation of functional and physiological imaging capabilities. The advantage of this ioMRI system, greater access to the patient, ultimately was overshadowed by the reduced image quality generated at isocenter and the more broad acceptance of either moving the patient a short distance in and out of the scanner in a higher field strength scanner or shuttling the scanner in and out of the surgical field, as described below.

High Field ioMRI Systems

High field ioMRI systems have the advantage over low and mid field systems of advanced functionality including fat suppression, perfusion studies, MRA, MRV, MRS, MR thermometry, and fMRI [1, 3]. One of the initial problems identified with operating using mid and high field ioMRI systems was the inability to use standard surgical instrumentation near the magnet. In order to obtain intraoperative images of the surgical site the patient had to be transported into the scanner or the scanner had to be moved to the patient. Our initial ioMRI system (ACS-NT, Philips Medical Systems, Best, Netherlands) required that a modified angiography table serve as the operating table which was rotated to dock with the MRI gantry so that the patient could be rapidly transported into and out of the scanner on a floating table top. Access to the patient was enhanced with this system because of the shore-bore magnet configuration and 100 cm flared openings on both sides of the scanner. The infrequent need to scan the patient during a brain tumor resection supports the performance of surgery outside the 5 Gauss line using conventional surgical instruments. In contrast, brain biopsies were performed within the magnet in order to enable the visualization of the passage of the biopsy needle toward the target in near-real time. A comparable approach to patient access was adapted at other high field ioMRI sites (University of Erlangen, Erlangen, Germany and University of California Los Angeles, Los Angeles, California) where a rotating surgical table could be turned into the axis of a 1.5 T Magnetom Sonata Maestro Class scanner (Siemens Medical Solutions, Erlangen, Germany) [4]. With our updated 1.5 T ioMRI scanner (Intera I/T, Philips Medical Systems, Best, Netherlands), we performed craniotomies for brain tumor resection entirely within the magnetic field using MR-compatible instrumentation and anesthesia equipment.

Another alternative high field ioMRI system design utilizes a mobile 1.5 T magnet with a 92 cm bore diameter (Magnex Scientific, Abingdon, Oxon, UK) that moves on a ceiling-mounted track to a stationary operating table (Fig. 3). This system has the disadvantages that it requires repositioning local radiofrequency shielding each time an intraoperative MRI is performed to maintain high SNR and all ferromagnetic instrumentation must be removed prior to scanning. Initially, this system design did not allow access to the patient during imaging so that minimally invasive procedures such as brain biopsy were not possible. A more recent version of the system where the back end of the scanner is now open allows for access to the patient so MR-guided minimally invasive procedures can be performed in near-real time.

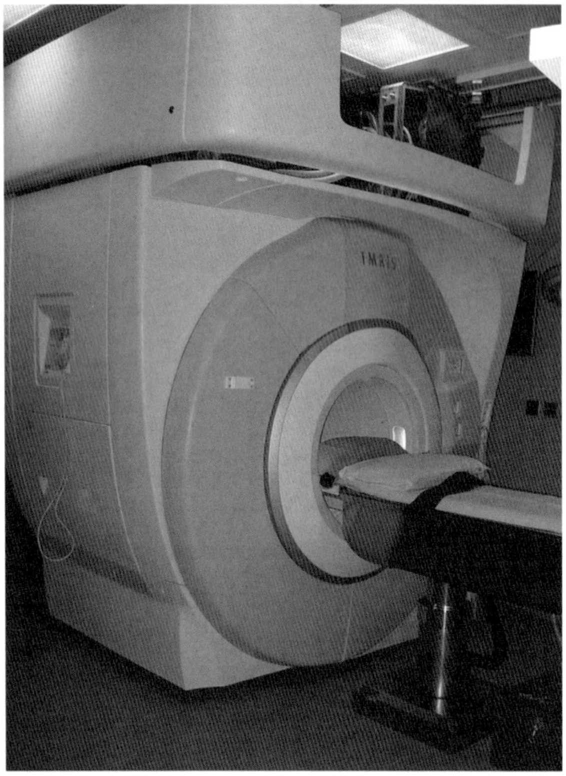

Fig. 3 IMRIS 1.5 T intraoperative magnetic resonance imaging system with the magnet suspended from ceiling rails. In the foreground is the MRI-compatible surgical table

Most recently 3 T MRI scanners have been modified to allow for MR-guided neurosurgical procedures at the back end of the magnet (Intera, Philips Medical Systems, Best, The Netherlands) entirely within the magnetic field due to the greater availability of MR-compatible instruments and equipment (Fig. 4). Both craniotomies and minimally invasive brain biopsies can be performed with minor limitations in patient positioning and a significant improvement in patient flow and throughput due to more rapid acquisition of intraoperative images [5]. All major vendors have now modified diagnostic 3 T MR scanners to allow for MR-guided surgical procedures.

Results

Surgical Indications

The primary indication for 0.15 T ioMRI system is to guide the resection of brain tumors such as gliomas, pituitary tumors, and meningiomas. Another group found that their 0.2 T low field ioMRI system was best suited for the resections of gliomas and pituitary adenomas. Gliomas and pituitary adenomas were found to be those lesions that were also

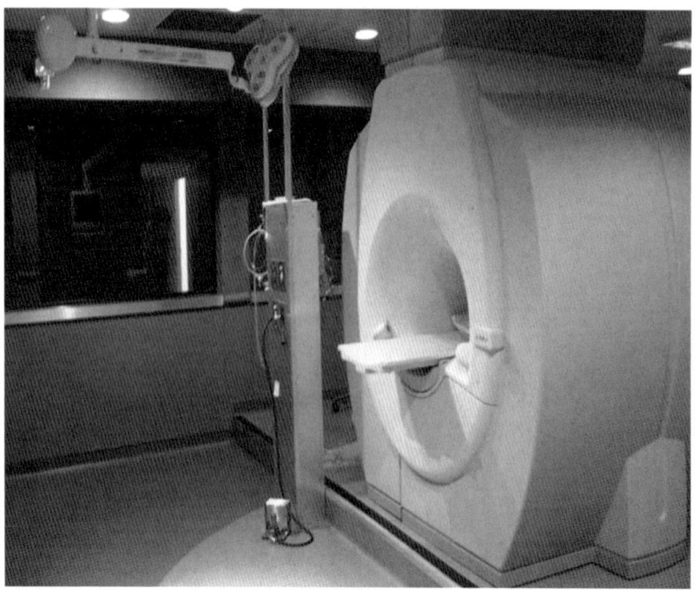

Fig. 4 Philips 3.0 T Intera intraoperative MRI system where surgical procedures are performed at the back end of the scanner with direct neurosurgical access to the patient's head. The patient can be transported rapidly into the scanner for frequent repeat imaging. The column to the left of the back end of the scanner serves as the source for suction and anesthetic gases

most appropriate for 1.5 T MR-guided neurosurgery either with a stationary patient or a stationary magnet.

Brain Shift

As accurate as neuronavigational systems are, they can suffer significant spatial inaccuracy due to the brain shift that occurs once the cranium is opened and CSF is drained upon opening the dura mater. These devices do not allow the neurosurgeon to compensate for brain shift without repeat imaging of the operative site and reregistration of those intraoperative images. The average amount of surface displacement that has been estimated to occur with the resection of a tumor is 1 cm with gravity representing the main force causing brain shift [1]. Peritumoral brain edema secondary to the effects of surgery also distorts the local environment with consequent brain shift. This shift can lead to incomplete tumor resection in the face of the neuronavigation system suggesting complete resection. Alternatively, there is the potential for surgical encroachment on normal brain parenchyma adjacent to the tumor resection cavity, in the face of safe passage suggested by neuronavigation. The percentage of cases where neuronavigation reregistration was felt to be necessary in ioMRI-guided cases due to brain shift was 11–16% [6]. The occurrence of brain shift has been in part responsible for causing unsuspected residual tumor in 2–35% of cases depending on the type of tumor being resected with pituitary adenomas representing the most likely tumor to be incompletely resected.

Brain Biopsy

The initial ioMRI-guided brain biopsies were performed in a freehand manner much like the first computed tomography-guided brain biopsies. Clinicians recognized early on that there was no way to either guide the biopsy needle to the intended target or to stabilize the needle during the acquisition of the tissue samples. The need for a device to stabilize the biopsy needle led to the rapid design and development of such instrumentation (MRI Devices, Waukesha, WI; Snapper-Stereo-Guide, MagneticVision, Zurich, Switzerland; Image-Guided Neurologics, Melbourne, FL). A disposable trajectory guide called the Navigus that was combined with a unique targeting technique known as prospective stereotaxy that allowed for the performance of brain biopsy in near-real time at 1.5 T (Fig. 5). Biopsies are generally performed under general anesthesia at most ioMRI sites for patient comfort because of the length of the procedure and to prevent the inadvertent displacement of the biopsy needle once the target has been reached.

Prospective stereotaxy is a novel biopsy technique that starts at the target and moves away distally toward an alignment stem that acts similarly to a computer joy stick. With this alignment technique three points are aligned: biopsy site (target point), tip of the alignment stem (pivot point), and the cross section of the alignment stem (rotation point). Once all three points are collinear, the passage of the biopsy needle through the guide tube which had held the alignment stem will result in the biopsy needle encountering the target. The entire alignment process takes 2–5 min and following the procedure a series of three scans (half-Fourier acquisition

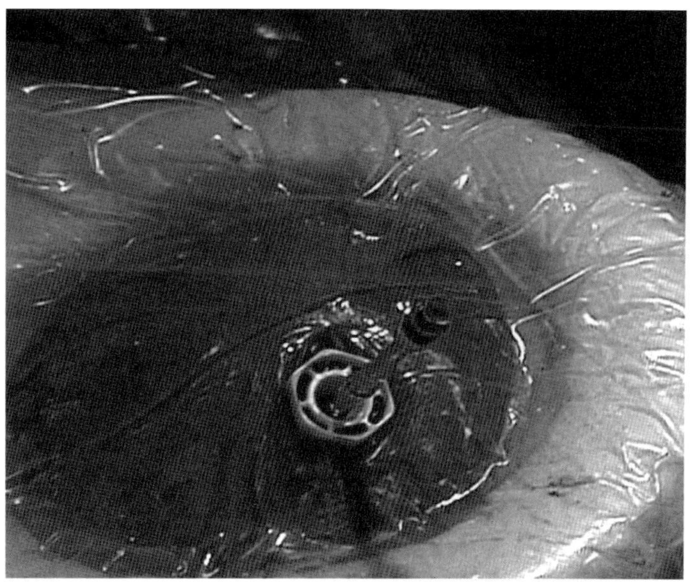

Fig. 5 The skull-mounted Navigus trajectory guide in position for brain biopsy. The alignment stem is inserted into the guide tube and the white plastic locking nut is visible. The procedure is being performed through a gauze wrapped radiofrequency surface coil, which combined with its partner beneath the patient's head, allows for parallel imaging, affording both high signal-to-noise ratio and improved imaging efficiency

single-shot turbo spin echo (HASTE), turbo fluid-attenuated inversion recovery (FLAIR), and gradient echo (GE)-T2*) are reviewed to exclude the presence of intraoperative hemorrhage before the conversion of intracellular oxyhemoglobin to deoxyhemoglobin (Fig. 6). More recently, susceptibility-weighted imaging has supplanted the imaging protocols due to its increased sensitivity to hemorrhage that is still largely in the intracellular oxyhemoglobin phase and only slightly in the intracellular deoxyhemoglobin phase.

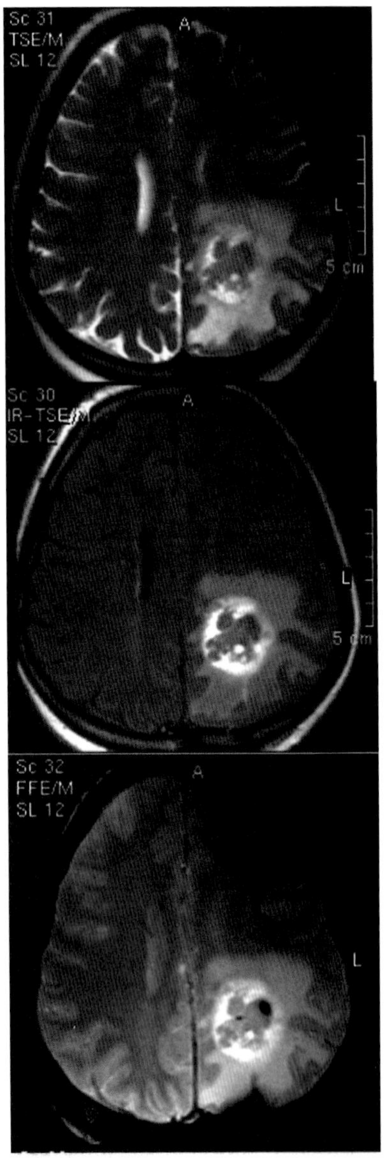

Fig. 6 Following the brain biopsy, a series of three axial scans (half-Fourier acquisition single-shot turbo spin echo (HASTE) (*top*), turbo fluid-attenuated inversion recovery (FLAIR) (*middle*), and gradient echo (GE)-T2* (*bottom*)) are reviewed to exclude the presence of intraoperative hemorrhage before the conversion of intracellular oxyhemoglobin to deoxyhemoglobin has occurred. An area of signal loss in the same location on all three scans would indicate the presence of air

In order to enhance the diagnostic yield of brain biopsy, we have combined intraoperative guidance with MRS, initially with single-voxel spectroscopy (SVS) and subsequently with turbo spectroscopic imaging (TSI). Single voxel spectroscopy targets a region of interest in the brain and compares it to the similar location in the opposite cerebral hemisphere and TSI is performed on a single axial slice where specific brain metabolites (phosphocholine, creatine, *N*-acetyl aspartate (NAA), and lactate/lipid) are measured [2]. Regions of elevated phosphocholine on SVS and TSI, in the presence of diminished NAA, suggest increased cellular density due to rapid membrane turnover that is consistent with tumor tissue and *N*-acetyl aspartate which is a neuronal marker is increased in normal brain [1].

Craniotomy for Tumor Resection

At our site, patients are intubated and receive general anesthesia before they arrive in the ioMRI suite. The head is secured in the operative position in a carbon fiber head holder in order to facilitate repeat intraoperative imaging in the exact orientation that will allow for comparison of scans during surgery. The craniotomy site is localized over the tumor using MRI-visible markers before the hair is clipped and the skin prepped. For nonenhancing brain tumors, HASTE and turbo FLAIR imaging sequences are acquired for intraoperative scan comparison; for enhancing tumors, the administration of intravenous contrast is withheld until the majority of the tumor has been removed to prevent the imbibition of contrast into the edematous peritumoral brain where the blood–brain barrier has been disrupted. The interpretation of intraoperative images can be difficult even with the repeat administration of the intravenous contrast because of its continued diffusion around the resection cavity that occurs related to surgical trauma from the use of electrocautery and the ultrasonic aspirator.

Typically, tumor resections require three imaging sets during the surgery. The first set is acquired prior to the opening of the cranium (Fig. 7) before brain shift has occurred. After the tumor has been either partially (Fig. 8) or completely resected (Fig. 9) in the estimation of the surgeon, a second, and truly intraoperative set of images is acquired. Finally, after the craniotomy has been closed, a third set is obtained, in order to evaluate the surgical site for intraoperative hemorrhage. In addition, at any point during the surgery, where there could be a question concerning brain physiology or the extent of resection imaging can be repeated with a 5 min delay in order to maintain the sterility of the operative field and to allow for removal of all non-MR-compatible instrumentation before transport into the scanner. Imaging of the operative site in any orientation is possible to enable the surgeon to visualize those areas of the brain that may

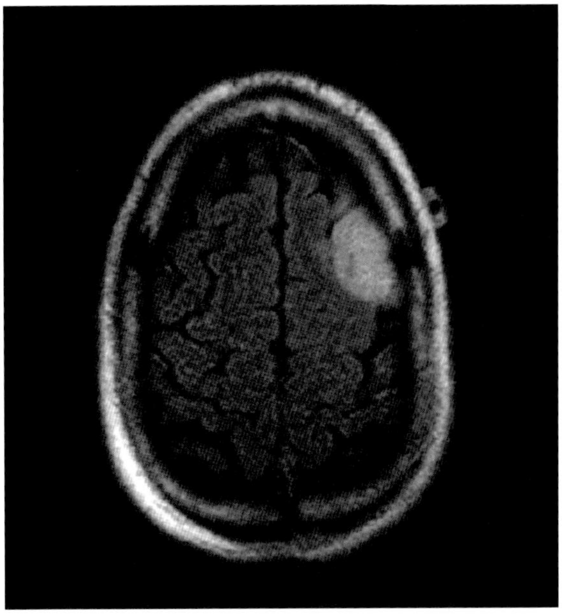

Fig. 7 Preoperative axial turbo fluid-attenuated inversion recovery (FLAIR) MRI scan demonstrating an area of increased signal in the left frontal lobe directly below the coronal suture consistent with a low grade glioma. There is an MRI-visible marker attached to the scalp in order to localize the craniotomy flap preoperatively and delimit the size of the cranial opening and operative field

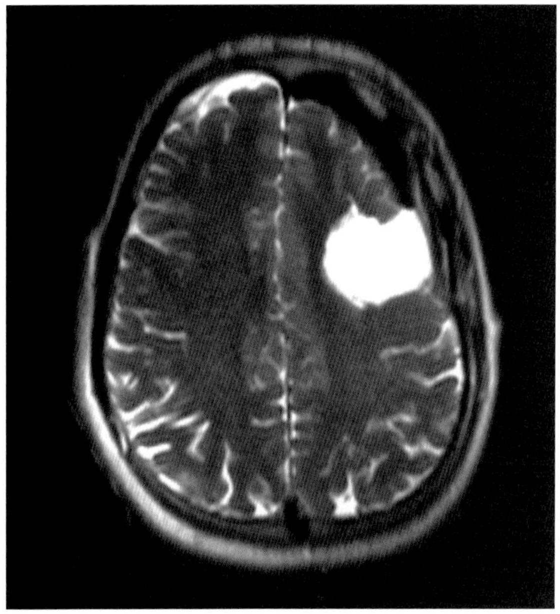

Fig. 9 Postoperative axial half-Fourier acquisition single-shot turbo spin echo (HASTE) scan demonstrating the completion of the tumor resection. The entire tumor footprint has been removed radiographically and the resection cavity has been filled with cerebrospinal fluid. There is pneumocephalus still present over the left frontal lobe and the craniotomy has been closed

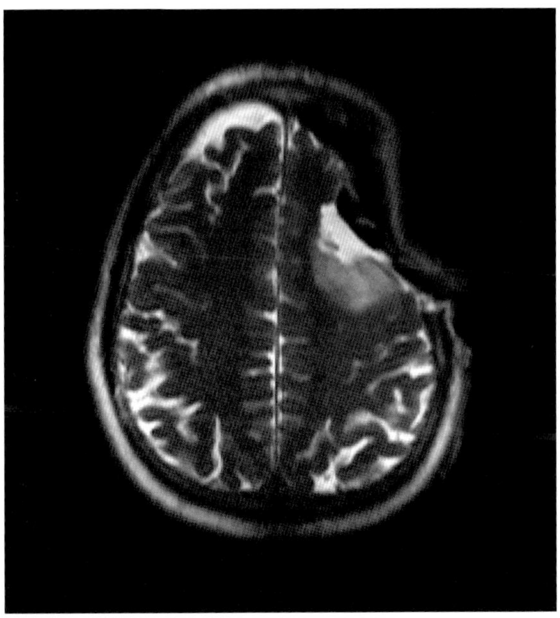

Fig. 8 Oligodendroglioma. Intraoperative axial half-Fourier acquisition single-shot turbo spin echo (HASTE) scan demonstrating the extent of the tumor resection and the proximity of the residual disease to the central sulcus and motor cortex. Note the degree of brain shift of the left frontal lobe that is present. This tumor was found on pathological examination to be an oligodendroglioma

contain residual tumor that is not easily seen because of the collapse or "shift" of the brain into or away from the resection cavity (Fig. 10).

After baseline imaging is obtained, at the 1.5 T site, the patient is moved outside the magnetic field to the location where ferromagnetic instruments can be used without risk of projectile injury. Resection of the tumor is carried out in the standard neurosurgical fashion until the surgeon feels it appropriate to assess the completeness of the surgery. Some groups have combined ioMRI-guided brain tumor resections with neuronavigation to improve the safety of the surgery and to increase the overall extent of the tumor resection [4, 6]. During surgery the imaging data set that is performed to assess the extent of the tumor resection is reregistered into the neuronavigational system to further guide the resection of any residual neoplastic disease. Because of the additional time associated with combining neuronavigation with ioMRI-guided surgery, other sites, like ours, have taken a more simplistic approach for detecting residual tumor after the initial attempt at removing the tumor footprint. Prior to obtaining intraoperative images to examine the surgical site for residual disease, we place MRI-visible markers in the resection cavity adjacent to tissue that is suspected to represent tumor. These markers are made of titanium and are in the shape of rods, struts, or burr hole covers (Fig. 11). Bone wax has also been placed is a resection cavity to monitor for residual disease because of its excellent visualization characteristics on MRI (Fig. 12).

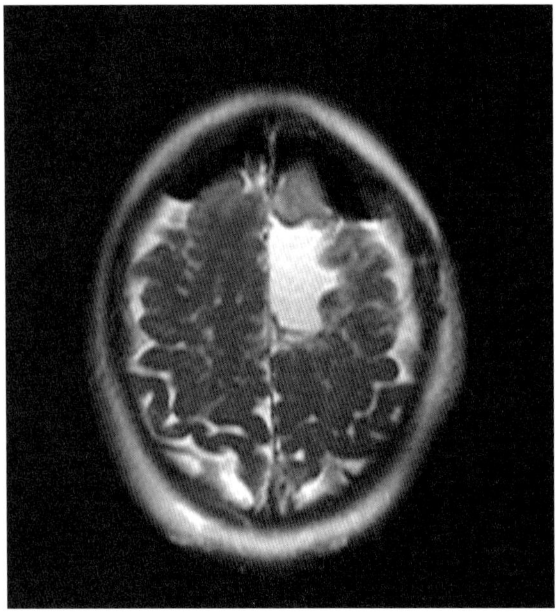

Fig. 10 Postoperative axial half-Fourier acquisition single-shot turbo spin echo (HASTE) scan after the left frontal tumor has been resected and the craniotomy has been closed. The resection cavity is filled with cerebrospinal fluid and there is pneumocephalus over both frontal lobes demonstrating the degree of "brain shift" that can occur within the cranium during surgery despite the tumor being unilateral

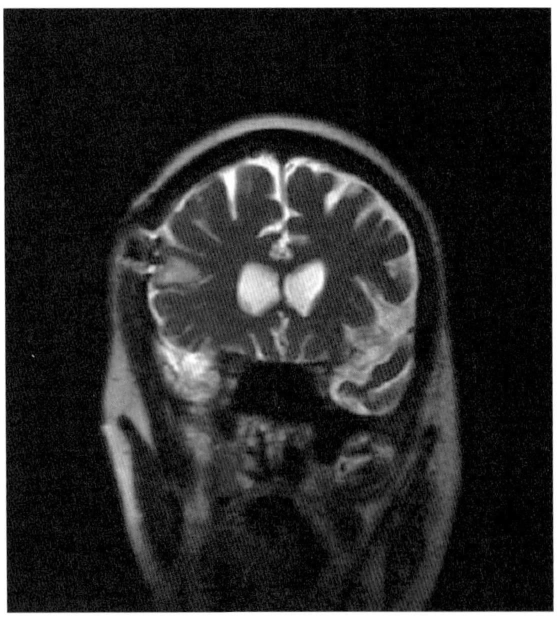

Fig. 11 Intraoperative coronal half-Fourier acquisition single-shot turbo spin echo (HASTE) scan where a titanium burr hole cover has been placed on the right frontal brain surface to localize an area of increased signal in a single gyrus. The cortical surface appeared normal under direct visualization. The gyrus was resected and was found to represent an area of cortical dysplasia that was causing seizures

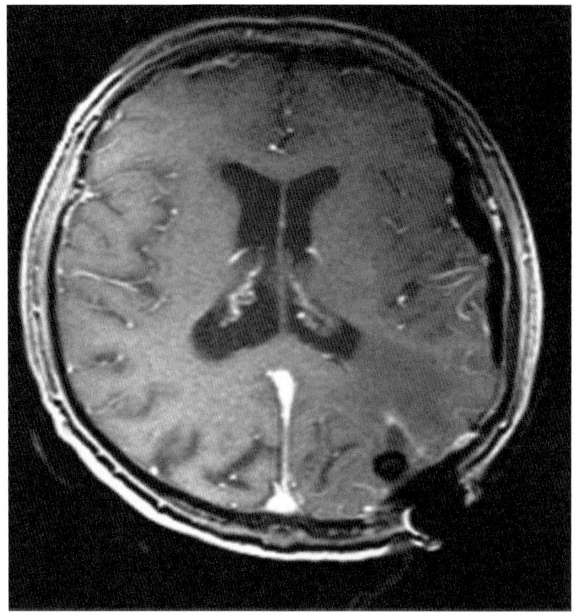

Fig. 12 Axial T1-weighted contrast enhanced MRI demonstrating the complete resection of an enhancing left occipital brain metastasis. The area of signal loss in the resection cavity represents bone wax that was placed adjacent to an area that was felt to be suspicious for residual disease by the surgeon. Notice the degree of "brain shift" over the left cerebral hemisphere that is the result of cerebrospinal fluid loss after the dura mater has been opened

The presence of residual disease near an intraoperative titanium marker will guide the surgeon to that location in order to extend the tumor resection. Once the tumor footprint has been removed the three previously described "hemorrhage" scans are obtained before leaving the ioMRI suite. For tumors adjacent to blood vessels, DWI can be performed at the time of the hemorrhage scans to exclude the presence of ischemia or infarction suggestive of a vascular injury. After imaging is complete, the patient is transported to the recovery room for extubation. In general, each image set requires 10–15 min to obtain and they are rarely repeated within 1 h of the prior imaging. Initially, intraoperative imaging extended the duration of a tumor resection by one-third compared to cases performed in the main operating room, although this time has decreased significantly with increasing experience using this technology.

Functional-MRI-Guided Tumor Resection

To enhance the overall safety of ioMRI-guided brain tumor resection, we have combined fMRI-guidance to the preoperative surgical planning for tumors located near areas of eloquent cortical function. Eloquent cortex represents cortical tissue whereby injury or damage will result in a neurological deficit. Brain activation areas that we have been able to accurately define and avoid during surgery are those for motor function, working memory, and language (Fig. 13). Motor cortex activation will result from finger tapping, tongue tapping on the roof of the mouth, and toe wiggling. Language location is mapped by having patients think of the names of animals starting with the beginning of the alphabet ("silent" speech). Short- and long-term recall using list retention is used to localize memory function to the medial temporal lobe of the dominant cerebral hemisphere. The imaging protocol for fMRI is a single-shot echo planar imaging (EPI) scan. Those areas of blood oxygen level-dependent (BOLD) activation are calculated and then superimposed on high quality anatomic images that can be displayed on liquid crystal display panels in the ioMRI surgical suite for the surgeon to review immediately prior to craniotomy. To assure that the task is being properly performed, a superimposed waveform demonstrates those periods where brain activation is occurring. Acquiring and processing brain activation studies will add approximately 15 min to a surgical procedure provided that they are obtained immediately before the administration of general anesthesia. Some patients will have their fMRI performed several days before the planned surgical procedure if additional surgical planning is felt to be necessary. In our experience, fMRI-guidance for tumor resection has been so safe, reliable, and accurate that we have not combined it with either awake craniotomy or cortical stimulation. For large tumors located adjacent to areas for language activation, the combination of awake craniotomy using total intravenous anesthesia and preoperative fMRI language localization has resulted in the safe and successful resection of lesions that previously would have been biopsied only. Even though most fMRI-guided tumor resections have been performed on high field systems, one group has demonstrated in normal volunteers that brain activation studies are possible on a 0.15 T system [7].

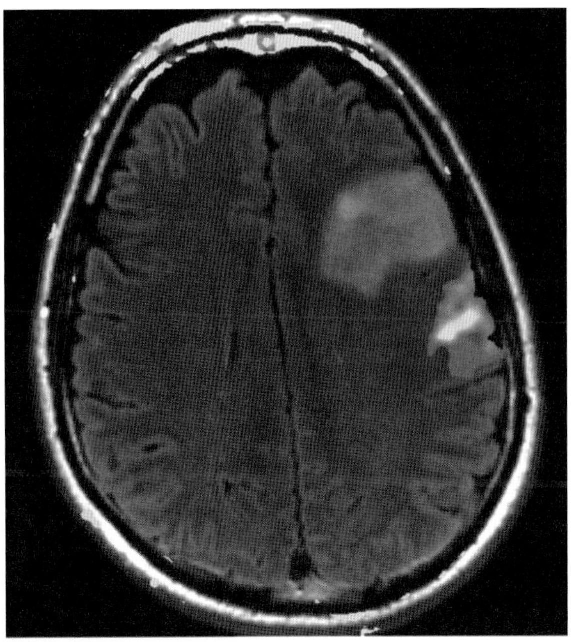

Fig. 13 Axial turbo fluid attenuated inversion recovery (FLAIR) scan demonstrating the area of superimposed brain activation immediately posterior to the area of increased signal that was found to be a low grade oligodendroglioma on pathological examination. The task being performed on the blood oxygen level dependent (BOLD) study was tongue tapping

Diffusion and Perfusion Imaging-Guided Tumor Resection

Using the diffusion energy (Brownian motion) of water molecules, the white matter tracts that pass through the brain can be mapped with diffusion tensor imaging (DTI). This technique was first used to avoid the optic radiations in a child with a low grade glioma where their inadvertent injury would result in a visual field deficit [8]. When comparing the preoperative and intraoperative DTI tractography in glioma resection surgery, the maximum shifting of the white matter ranged from −8 to +15 mm [9]. White matter tracts shifted outward in 62% of patients and inward in 30% [9]. Intraoperative visualization of the white matter tracts has allowed for the safe resection of gliomas near eloquent cortex [10].

Very recently perfusion MRI has been used to guide the resection of residual high grade glioma tissue during ioMRI-guided surgery. Areas of increased perfusion on ioMRI corresponded to areas of residual tumor tissue on pathological examination confirming the need for additional tissue resection. These areas of increased perfusion were also found to correlate with areas of contrast enhancement when the neuronavigation was updated.

Discussion

Intraoperative MRI-guidance has been felt to improve health outcomes for patients by reducing the repeat tumor resection rate, hospital length of stay, and overall hospital costs [11]. High field ioMRI systems clearly offer some advantages over lower field systems namely the higher functionality that allows for advanced MRI that includes MRA, MRV, MRS, DWI, and perfusion MRI. This advanced functionality has led some investigators to consider whether or not there would be an advantage to ioMRI-guided surgery at 3 T [5]. We initially adapted a diagnostic 3 T scanner (Philips Medical Systems) for intraoperative use (Fig. 4) although other

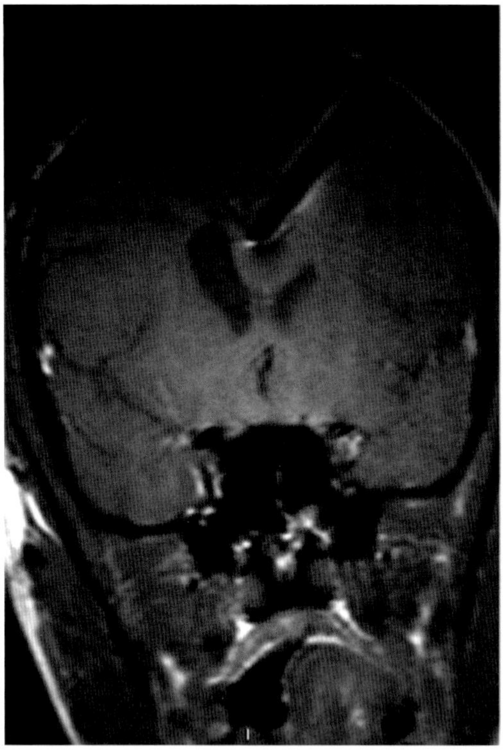

Fig. 14 Coronal T1-weighted contrast-enhanced MRI scan after the MRI-compatible brain biopsy needle has been passed through the Navigus down to the target. The small enhancing focus that was found to be recurrent tumor is obscured by the artifact associated with the biopsy needle in this orientation. Alignment along Bo when possible will delimit the metallic artifact. In this case, as the lesion was along the mesial aspect of the left hemisphere, a long axis approach might have likely injured vascular structures as the needle passed through multiple sulci

vendors followed suit shortly thereafter, such that there are now several 3 T systems modified for surgery. The primary difference between the 1.5 T and the 3 T ioMRI suites is that at the higher field strength everything that enters the room must be MRI-compatible. The only instruments that we have not found a non-ferromagnetic replacement for are the scalpel blade and the suture needles. The scalpel blade that we use has a retractable plastic guard that covers the blade when not in use and the MRI-compatible titanium suture needles are both cost prohibitive and less sharp. To the surgeon, when operating in the 3 T environment, there is virtually no detectable difference as compared to the 1.5 T field strength environment. The advantages that we have seen at 3 T are improved SNR, which provides improved visualization of vascular structures and enhanced performance of MRS and fMRI protocols. There has been no demonstrable increased risk to the patient or staff, while there has been increased efficiency. This improved efficiency, however, may be in part related to the newer configuration whereby the patient table is extended out the far end of the magnet and can be advanced rapidly into the magnet at any time imaging is felt to be necessary. The disadvantages associated with 3 T ioMRI-guided surgery were the limitations associated with not having stainless steel instrumentation with its greater strength over titanium. There is also more pronounced imaging artifact associated with the titanium biopsy needle (Fig. 14). This may also suggest that titanium aneurysm clips will have significant imaging artifact that makes image interpretation difficult and it may not be possible to tell whether there is residual aneurysm neck remaining. There is also a more pronounced artifact when air is in the tumor resection cavity which confounds interpreting the postoperative hemorrhage scans. As at 1.5 T, to minimize such needle related artifact, it is helpful to align the needle whenever possible with the main magnetic field Bo. This works for most intracranial lesions, although is suboptimal for temporal lobe lesions.

After over a decade of experience, intraoperative MRI-guided surgery has finally been embraced by the neurosurgical community as evidenced by five separate systems being operational in one metropolitan area, two at academic centers and three in community hospitals. As to whether there is any advantage to considering magnet strength higher than 3 T is a question for debate. It is more likely that 1.5 T and 3 T ioMRI systems will be combined with state-of-the art computed tomography, angiography, or positron emission tomography equipment or some combination of such.

Conflicts of interest statement We declare that we have no conflict of interest.

References

1. Hall WA, Truwit CL (2008) Intraoperative MR-guided neurosurgery. J Magn Reson Imaging 27:368–375
2. Hall WA, Truwit CL (2005) 1.5 T:spectroscopy-supported brain biopsy. Neurosurg Clin N Am 16:165–172
3. Hall WA, Liu H, Martin AJ, Pozza CH, Maxwell RE, Truwit CL (2000) Safety, efficacy and functionality of high-field strength interventional MR imaging for neurosurgery. Neurosurgery 46:632–641
4. Nimsky C, Ganslandt O, von Keller B, Romstock J, Fahlbusch R (2004) Intraoperative high-field strength MR imaging: implementation and experience in 200 patients. Radiology 233:67–78
5. Truwit CL, Hall WA (2006) Intraoperative magnetic resonance imaging-guided neurosurgery at 3-T. Neurosurgery 58(Suppl 2): ONS338–ONS346
6. Nimsky C, Ganslandt O, Hastreiter P, Fahlbusch R (2001) Intraoperative compensation for brain shift. Surg Neurol 56:357–365
7. Azmi H, Biswal B, Salas S, Schulder M (2007) Functional imaging in a low-field, mobile intraoperative magnetic resonance scanner: expanded paradigms. Neurosurgery 60:143–149
8. Tummala RP, Chu RM, Liu H, Truwit CL, Hall WA (2003) Application of diffusion tensor imaging to magnetic resonance-guided brain tumor resection. Pediatr Neurosurg 39:39–43

9. Nimsky C, Ganslandt O, Hastreiter P, Wang R, Benner T, Sorensen AG, Fahlbusch R (2005) Preoperative and intraoperative diffusion tensor imaging-based fiber tracking in glioma surgery. Neurosurgery 56:130–138
10. Nimsky C, Ganslandt O, Merhof D, Sorensen AG, Fahlbusch R (2006) Intraoperative visualization of the pyramidal tract by diffusion-tensor-imaging based fiber tracking. Neuroimage 30:1219–1229
11. Hall WA, Kowalik K, Liu H, Truwit CL, Kucharczyk J (2003) Costs and benefits of intraoperative MR-guided brain tumor resection. Acta Neurochir Suppl 85:137–142

3 T ioMRI: The Istanbul Experience

M. Necmettin Pamir

Abstract Intraoperative imaging technologies have improved surgical results in glioma and pituitary adenoma surgeries. With improvements and refinements 3 T intraoperative MRI systems offer a potential of further improving these results. Hereby we describe the equipment and technique of a cost-effective shared-resource 3-T Ultra-high field intraoperative Magnetic Resonance Imaging system and report our continuing experience on surgical tumor resection.

A description of the facility design and equipment are given along with examples from our experience on low-grade gliomas and transsphenoidal surgeries. Our facility based on the twin room concept and uses a 3-T Siemens Trio (Siemens, Erlangen, Germany) scanner. The unit consists of adjacent but independent MRI and operative suites, which are connected by a wide door for ioMRI procedure but are used as conventional MRI and operative units. Rigid head fixation during neurosurgery is achieved with a custom designed 5 pin head-rest which also combines a 4+4 channel head coil. Operation is performed using regular non-MRI compatible equipment and the patient is transferred to the MRI during the procedure using a custom designed floating table. Advanced sequences such as diffusion weighted and diffusion tensor imaging, MR angiography, MR venography, MR spectroscopy can be performed with no changes in the setup and result in image quality comparable to outpatient scans.

The intraoperative 3-T ultra high field MRI unit with the twin room concept permits both diagnostic outpatient imaging and image guided surgery in the same setting and is a cost effective solution to afford a highly capable ioMRI system.

Keywords Intraoperative MRI · Low grade glioma · Magnetic resonance imaging · Pituitary adenoma · Ultra-high field MRI

M.N. Pamir
Professor and Chairman, Department of Neurosurgery, Acibadem University, School of Medicine, Inonu Cad, Okur Sok 20, 34742 Kozytagi, Istanbul, Turkey
e-mail: pamirmn@yahoo.com

Introduction

The drive for the development of intraoperative imaging came from the field of neurooncology, due to a need for improving the efficiency of tumor resection. The role of surgery in the treatment of glial tumors is one of the controversial issues in neurosugical practice. Glial tumors grow in an infiltrative fashion which precludes a true oncological-resection of these tumors [1]. However; studies have shown that a more radical resection is associated with longer survival, better quality of life and lower chance of malignant degeneration over time [1–3]. Prospective randomized, multicenter trials have shown that neither radiotherapy nor chemotherapy have a significant effect on patient survival in low-grade gliomas (LGG). Currently the most effective form of treatment for LGG is complete surgical excision [2]. Studies have also indicated that patients do benefit from the extent of this resection with better outcome after more complete resections [1–3].

Another drive for the development of intraoperative MRI systems was their potential use in transsphenoidal surgery. Most studies have indicated that residual adenoma tissue is frequently found after transsphenoidal resections of pituitary adenomas. Intraoperative detection of these residuals carried the prospect of more complete resections.

The Development of ioMRI Technology

The adaptation of an MRI scanner into the operating room is a fairly new concept and therefore the design and technology of the systems have varied considerably. The first intraoperative MRI unit that became operational was installed at Brigham and Women's hospital in Boston in 1994 [4]. The initial design was nicknamed the "double-donut" and was a 0.5-T General Electric magnet (SIGNA SP, General Electric Medical Systems, Milwaukee, WI). In this initial design both the patient and the surgeon were inside the magnet where the surgery was performed using all non-ferromagnetic surgical equipment. Similar low field (0.2–0.5 T) designs worldwide followed this first application including the Erlangen [5] and Toronto Siemens low field systems (Magnetom OPEN; Siemens Medical Systems, Erlangen, Germany) and the Hitachi [6] system (Fonar, Melville, NY; Hitachi Medical, Twinsburg, OH). The short to midterm follow-up results of surgeries performed using low field systems have recently begun to appear in the neurosurgical literature [7, 8]. Analyzing the results for glioma surgery with the initial double donut design from Brigham and Women's hospital, Claus et al. [7] have shown that the odds ratio for recurrence is 1.4, and the odds ratio for death is 4.9 when subtotal vs. total resection using ioMRI was compared.

The adoption of the MRI scanner into the operating room was a significant development in the field of neurooncology, which also sparked the start of a rapid evolution of this technology. The use of high-field MRI equipment in the operating room was the second important development in this field. The image quality and signal-to-noise ratio of the MRI improves with increasing magnet strength and magnetic gradients. Low-field systems suffer from low anatomical resolution, slow speed and the lack of most sophisticated MRI sequences, which are indispensable in today's MRI technology. Application of the 1.5 T technology improved anatomical resolution in imaging; enabled acquisition of good quality T2 weighted images, which are the standard MRI sequence for low grade glioma. Several high-field systems were installed worldwide including the Philips system at University of Minnesota [9], Siemens systems at University of Erlangen [10] and University of California and the IMRIS system at Calgary-Canada [11]. Clinical reports have documented that these systems were capable of increasing the extent of resection [12, 13].

Further evolution in intraoperative MRI technology brought ultra-high field (3 T) scanners into the operating room. This upgrade from 1.5 to 3 T scanners brings further refinements in imaging quality and speed. Few ultra-high field systems have been reported in the literature so far and the technology was pioneered by the 3 T-Philips system at University of Minnesota-USA [9, 14], the 3 T-Siemens at Acibadem University-Turkey [15, 16] and finally the second Philips system at Cliniques Universitaires St-Luc, Université Catholique de Louvain-Belgium [17]. The first clinical series analyzing the results of low grade glioma surgery was reported by our institution and showed an increased gross total resection rate comparable to the results obtained by low- and high- field systems [15]. Probably the most significant gain from installation of the ultra-high field systems was the routine application of very high resolution T2 weighted images as the standard imaging sequence. Other exciting developments also followed: Application of proton MR spectroscopy (MRS) and diffusion weighted imaging (DWI) to differentiate peritumoral T2w MRI changes in normal parenchyma from residual tumor, which can be problematic even in postoperative imaging, was performed without technical difficulties [15]. Diffusion weighted imaging was used to monitor surgically induced ischemia [15]. Previous studies using low field imaging had already shown that complications such as intraoperative bleeding could be demonstrated using ioMRI [18]. With the use of high and ultra-high field ioMRI intraoperative Diffusion Tensor Imaging (DTI) was also performed to demonstrate the corticospinal tract [19, 20]. All of these technologies are still being validated, further investigated and undergoing refinement and their impact on long-term patient outcome and quality of life still needs to be investigated.

While some designs aimed at adopting more sophisticated magnet designs into the operating room, alternative strategies have emerged which aimed at developing low-cost, low-bulk systems, exemplified by the 0.12-T system which had permanent magnets of 40 cm diameter placed 25 cm apart from each other [21]. Use of a 0.15-T version of ultra-low field designs for LGG surgery was reported by Johann Wolfgang von Goethe University in Germany (Polestar N20 system, Medtronic Navigation, Louisville, CO) [8].

Along with this evolution in magnet technology there was also a significant refinement in operating room designs. The initial Signa SP system was designed to be dedicated operative equipment [4]. The design was based on the concept of surgery inside the magnetic field and therefore required the use of non-ferromagnetic equipment, which significantly increased the installation and running costs of such a system. These costs increase further with increasing magnet strength. Financing such a big system is a major burden for most academic or private institutions. An alternative was offered by Siemens [5] and Hitachi [6] low-field systems by designing shared-resource facilities where the MRI gantry and the operating room were separated and the MRI was used both for operative and outpatient purposes. Similar designs were developed for high-field systems [22]. Siemens ioMRI design reverted to single dedicated operating room in the Siemens 1.5-T Brain Suite design [10, 23]. The Siemens system installed at our institution in Istanbul-Turkey used the twin-room philosophy to reduce cost by allocating the equipment to diagnostic outpatient imaging at times when MRI is not needed intraoperatively [15, 16, 24]. A similar design was also adopted by the Philips system installed in Belgium [17].

The Acibadem University ioMRI Facility Design

The Acibadem University-ioMRI suite brings together a Siemens Trio 3 T MRI scanner and a twin-room facility design. This shared resource 3 T-ioMRI setup is not the adoption of an existing facility but a completely novel design. To complete the system several additional pieces of equipment were specially designed which include a 5 pin head-fixation device/4+4 channel head coil combination and a floating-patient transfer table. The unit became operational in June 2004 and after initial optimization of the setup the first ioMRI procedure was performed in November 2004. Within the first 3 years of use a wide array of neurosurgical procedures were successfully performed in the 3 T-ioMRI environment. During this first 3 years a total of 19,217 diagnostic scans were performed using the same MRI equipment. Most commonly performed operations at our institution were tumor resections and transsphenoidal explorations. Other procedures such as brain biopsies, deep brain stimulations, aneurysm and epilepsy surgery were also performed.

The advantages of the shared-resource Siemens Trio 3 T system at Acibadem University are several fold (1) This is an ultra high-field system with very high image quality, advanced imaging capabilities and high speed. (2) The system is based on the twin room concept which, by allocating the system both to intraoperative and outpatient diagnostic use, therefore offering economically very appealing solution for institutions which find it difficult to finance a dedicated operating room MRI equipment. MRI compatible surgical instruments are not required and neurosurgery is performed using regular ferromagnetic equipment, which is another factor that limits the running costs.

Image Quality: Imaging Capabilities

The 3 T MRI (Trio; Siemens, Erlangen, Germany) is a commercially available, fully functional diagnostic scanner that is equipped with strong imaging gradients (40 mT/m, 200 mT/m/ms) and state-of the art pulse sequences. The EPI-capable gradient set and Syngo 2004A software platform permits fMRI studies, perfusion/diffusion weighted imaging and proton spectroscopy. The images were reconstructed and displayed immediately after acquisition in the monitoring room.

Our routine 3 T- ioMRI protocol in both low grade glioma and pituitary adenoma patients is based on triplanar very high resolution T2W images. Such very high resolution images were not possible with lower magnet strengths. These intraoperative images are interpreted by direct comparison corresponding baseline images obtained at the start of the operation. Baseline images increase the accuracy and greatly simplify the interpretation of intraoperative images. Intravenous contrast was not a part of routine baseline images, however it was used in certain high grade glioma or pituitary macroadenoma cases on the on the first-look ioMRI session upon special indication. Diffusion weighted imaging to exclude vascular complications, single voxel Proton MRS to differentiate between residual tumor and edema, MRA and MRV to demonstrate vascular structures were performed as needed. An update of neuronavigation was performed when necessary which took an additional 3.5 min. Results were interpreted together by the radiologist and the neurosurgeon.

Early postoperative MRI has been proven effective in accurately evaluating surgical results in glioma surgery [25]. The image quality provided by the current high-field and ultra-high field ioMRI systems is not any inferior to postoperative MRI studies [14–17, 24, 26]. Therefore, an optimal evaluation of the surgical outcome can be obtained during the procedure and further improvements can be carried out before the procedure ends without increasing morbidity.

Although morphologic ioMR images provide valuable data on the extent of resection, in certain circumstances conventional sequences fall short of differentiating treatment effects from residual tumor [27]. On preoperative MR imaging a significant proportion of the glial tumors present with a T2w hyperintense rim around the tumor mass that is suggestive of peritumoral edema or tumor infiltration. In our experience this area expanded slightly after resection and this unexpected peritumoral intensity change prompted further studies. In such instances we used Proton Magnetic Resonance Spectroscopy (MRS) in combination with diffusion weighted imaging (DWI) to identify the nature of this tissue around the resection cavity [15].

When our facility was designed there was no previous experience with the application of a 3 T magnet to intraoperative imaging and therefore we carried concerns that image distortion and artifact due to increased susceptibility could limit image quality. After optimization of the setup the only limitation was in the application of diffusion tensor imaging [15]. Analysis of this problem indicated to field inhomogenities created by ferromagnetic parts in the head coil. These problems have been solved by modifications in the head coil and DTI images are now flawlessly acquired.

Twin Room/Shared Resource Design

Advanced technology certainly has its price: Ultra-high field systems are more expensive than high and low field equipment. Financing such a big system is a major burden for most academic or private institutions. But the design of our facility greatly reduced this burden by allocating the equipment to diagnostic outpatient imaging at times when MRI is not needed intraoperatively. When the scanner is not used for intraoperative imaging the radiology team performed an average of 25 outpatient MRI sessions per day and more than

19,000 outpatient MRI procedures were performed in the first 3 years of the facilities use [15].

In the Acibadem University ioMRI suite the MRI gantry/control room and the operating theatre are totally independent and for ioMRI sessions the patient is transferred from the operating table into the gantry on a custom designed floating table. This 3 m long transfer takes an average of 1.5 min and the routine imaging paradigm another 6–8 min totaling to 10 min for each ioMRI imaging session. This new design neither causes a significant difference in the daily number of outpatient diagnostic studies nor blocks an operating theater only for ioMRI procedures. Former studies have reported patient transfer as a drawback, but the newly designed operation-transfer table setup has greatly simplified and facilitated the process. During the procedure the sliding surface of the patient table is conveniently moved to the docked transfer table and the patient enters the gantry on this floating transfer table. As the head rest is attached to the sliding surface, the patient position does not change. The transfer process is simple and therefore less prone to technical failure. In shared resource designs the gantry room is used both for operative and outpatient purposes and risk of infection is cited as a potential problem [5, 6]. In the Acibadem University ioMRI system the operating room is pressure regulated, the gantry room is sterile cleaned before each procedure and the wound is sterile draped during each transfer. We have not encountered a single case of infection during the first 6 years of use. No anesthesia related problems or complications were encountered either.

In the shared resource design there is no requirement for MRI compatible operative instruments. Regular ferromagnetic neurosurgical instruments, operative microscopes, navigation setup, diagnostic equipment such as ultrasound, electrophysiological monitoring and anesthesia equipment are routinely used during the operation. Compatibility with regular neurosurgical instruments helps in limiting the running costs. Only exceptions are the MRI compatible head-rest and MRI compatible anesthesia equipment that is used inside the gantry.

Application in Low Grade Glioma Surgery

Several studies have consistently indicated that the extra information provided by the low or high field ioMRI aids in optimizing high and low grade glioma resections [3, 6–8, 12, 13, 15, 22–24, 28–30]. The studies analyzed both low and high grade gliomas and the incidence of residual tumor in these reports ranged from 36 to 94% and further resection resulted in gross total tumor removal in an additional 29–41% of these patients.

Our pre-ioMRI experience indicated on the important role of extensive surgical resection in the treatment of low grade gliomas [31]. The first clinical analysis of low grade glioma patients using ultra-high field ioMRI reported by our institution also concluded that the ioMRI detected residual tumor in approximately half of the patients and this finding prompted further tumor resection. In 40% of the cases these residuals could not be detected by visual inspection or by intraoperative ultrasonography. The use of ioMRI led to an increase in the number of gross total resections by one third, bringing it up to almost 75% (Fig. 1).

Use of the ioMRI was also important for safety of the glioma surgery. Cortical mapping studies in patients with hemispheric gliomas have demonstrated that these infiltrative lesions may contain functionally normal tissue within the tumor substance [26]. Resection of gliomas in functional brain regions caries a risk of injury to neighboring cortical areas and/or subcortical pathways. Precise and accurate information on cortical function (from fMRI) and subcortical connectivity (from DTI) is of great importance for protection of valuable brain tissue and preserving functional integrity. The information helps in both defining resection margins and also surgical planning to choose safe entry routes. Our report on low grade gliomas has indicated that close to two thirds of the cases were located in eloquent areas and preoperative imaging indicated presence of functional tissue inside the tumor tissue in one tenth of cases [15]. Resection of the involved area was not attempted such cases. Also, operative complications such as hematomas, ischemia and infarction were effectively monitored using both anatomical imaging data as well as DWI.

Application in Transsphenoidal Surgery

The use of the intraoperative MRI during transsphenoidal surgery is another major focus of interest in our institution. Our previous experience showed that early postoperative imaging was very important in determining the surgical outcome after transsphenoidal surgery for pituitary adenomas [32]. We have recently analyzed our initial results with ioMRI during transsphenoidal surgery. During the initial 4 years ater the setup of our facility 42 patients underwent transsphenoidal resections for nonsecretory adenomas. 21.4% of these cases were previously operated recurrent cases. Our surgical aim was total surgical excision. In cases with frank cavernous sinus invasion the the surgical aim was excision of the extrcavernous portion followed by radiosurgery for the intracavernous portion. The ioMRI procedure took less than 10 min including the transfer and very high resolution T2w images are obtained without the use of contrast (Fig. 2). Intraoperative MRI findings were

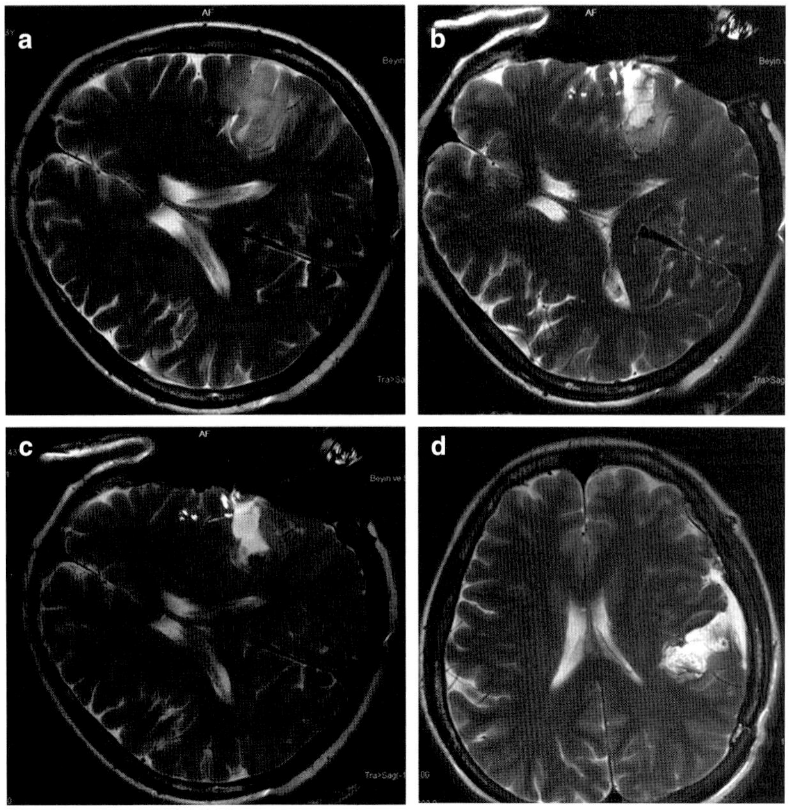

Fig. 1 A left frontal low-grade glioma (**a**) was operated using 3 T-Ultra High Field intraoperative MRI. The first intraoperative scan performed after initial resection and ultrasonography control revealed tumor remnant at the posterior margin of the resection cavity (**b**), which was further resected to yield a gross total resection at the end of the operation (**c**). A follow-up MRI 3 months after surgery confirms gross total resection (**d**)

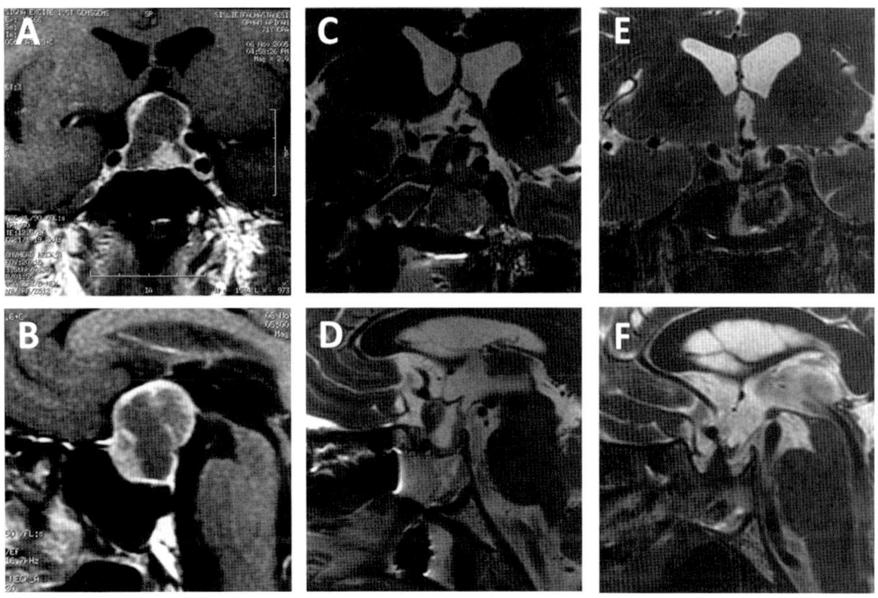

Fig. 2 Pituitary macroadenoma wlth suprasellar extension (as can be seen on coronal (**a**) and sagittal (**b**) contrast enhanced images) was operated using 3 T-ultra high field intraoperative MRI. Intraoperatively acquired coronal (**c**) and sagittal (**d**) high resolution T2 weighted images revealed total resection. Identical coronal (**e**) and sagittal (**f**) T2 weighted images performed at the third month follow-up study confirmed the findings from intraoperative images

confirmed at the first follow-up examination 3 months after surgery. In cases with frank cavernous sinus invasion resection of the extracavernous portion was attempted. A first-look MRI led to further resection in 3 of 13 cases and further tumor resection was achieved in all re-explorations. In cases with no cavernous sinus invasion a total resection was attempted. At the first-look ioMRI total resection was confirmed in 69%. In 6.9% no further resection was attempted. A re-exploration was prompted in 24.1%, based on residual, potentially resectable residual adenoma. In 57% of these, a total resection could be achieved which increased the overall total resection rate to 82.8%. In one patient the intraoperative MRI detected a hematoma in the resection bed, which was managed with immediate evacuation and hemostasis without resultant morbidity.

Conclusions

- This is a novel intraoperative MRI system and combines the shared resource design with an Ultra-high field scanner.
- The shared resource design, and use of normal surgical equipment and instruments makes the design cost effective.
- 3 T-ioMRI was effectively used in neurooncology with the most dramatic results in low grade glioma resections and transsphenoidal surgery
- Advanced imagines sequences such as Proton MR Spectroscopy (MRS), diffusion weighted imaging (DWI) diffusion tensor imaging (DTI) were effectively used intraoperatively. Intraoperative Proton MR Spectroscopy (MRS) was useful in differentiating peritumoral parenchymal changes from residual tumor tissue.

Conflict of Interest Statement We declare that we have no conflict of interest.

References

1. Piepmeier JM (2009) Current concepts in the evaluation and management of WHO grade II gliomas. J Neurooncol 92:253–259
2. Keles GE, Lamborn KR, Berger MS (2001) Low-grade hemispheric gliomas in adults: a critical review of extent of resection as a factor influencing outcome. J Neurosurg 95:735–745
3. Sanai N, Berger MS (2008) Glioma extent of resection and its impact on patient outcome. Neurosurgery 62:753–764, Discussion 264–266
4. Schwartz RB, Hsu L, Wong TZ, Kacher DF, Zamani AA, Black PM, Alexander ER, Stieg PE, Moriarty TM, Martin CA, Kikinis R, Jolesz FA (1999) Intraoperative MR imaging guidance for intracranial neurosurgery: experience with the first 200 cases. Radiology 211:477–488
5. Steinmeier R, Fahlbusch R, Ganslandt O, Nimsky C, Buchfelder M, Kaus M, Heigl T, Lenz G, Kuth R, Huk W (1998) Intraoperative magnetic resonance imaging with the magnetom open scanner: concepts, neurosurgical indications, and procedures: a preliminary report. Neurosurgery 43:739–747, discussion 747–748
6. Bohinski RJ, Kokkino AK, Warnick RE, Gaskill-Shipley MF, Kormos DW, Lukin RR, Tew JMJ (2001) Glioma resection in a shared-resource magnetic resonance operating room after optimal image-guided frameless stereotactic resection. Neurosurgery 48:731–742, discussion 742–744
7. Claus EB, Horlacher A, Hsu L, Schwartz RB, Dello-Iacono D, Talos F, Jolesz FA, Black PM (2005) Survival rates in patients with low-grade glioma after intraoperative magnetic resonance image guidance. Cancer 103:1227–1233
8. Senft C, Seifert V, Hermann E, Franz K, Gasser T (2008) Usefulness of intraoperative ultra low-field magnetic resonance imaging in glioma surgery. Neurosurgery 63:257–266, discussion 266–267
9. Hall WA, Liu H, Martin AJ, Pozza CH, Maxwell RE, Truwit CL (2000) Safety, efficacy, and functionality of high-field strength interventional magnetic resonance imaging for neurosurgery. Neurosurgery 46:632–641, discussion 641–642
10. Nimsky C, Ganslandt O, Fahlbusch R (2005) Comparing 0.2 tesla with 1.5 tesla intraoperative magnetic resonance imaging analysis of setup, workflow, and efficiency. Acad Radiol 12:1065–1079
11. Kaibara T, Saunders JK, Sutherland GR (1999) Utility of a moveable 1.5 Tesla intraoperative MR imaging system. Can J Neurol Sci 26:313–316
12. Hatiboglu MA, Weinberg JS, Suki D, Rao G, Prabhu SS, Shah K, Jackson E, Sawaya R (2009) Impact of intraoperative high-field magnetic resonance imaging guidance on glioma surgery: a prospective volumetric analysis. Neurosurgery 64:1073–1081, discussion 1081
13. Nimsky C, Fujita A, Ganslandt O, Von Keller B, Fahlbusch R (2004) Volumetric assessment of glioma removal by intraoperative high-field magnetic resonance imaging. Neurosurgery 55:358–370, discussion 370–371
14. Hall WA, Galicich W, Bergman T, Truwit CL (2006) 3-Tesla intraoperative MR imaging for neurosurgery. J Neurooncol 77:297–303
15. Pamir MN, Ozduman K, Dincer A, Yildiz E, Peker S, Ozek MM (2009) First intraoperative, shared-resource, ultrahigh-field 3-Tesla magnetic resonance imaging system and its application in low-grade glioma resection. J Neurosurg
16. Pamir MN, Peker S, Ozek MM, Dincer A (2006) Intraoperative MR imaging: preliminary results with 3 tesla MR system. Acta Neurochir Suppl 98:97–100
17. Jankovski A, Francotte F, Vaz G, Fomekong E, Duprez T, Van Boven M, Docquier MA, Hermoye L, Cosnard G, Raftopoulos C (2008) Intraoperative magnetic resonance imaging at 3-T using a dual independent operating room-magnetic resonance imaging suite: development, feasibility, safety, and preliminary experience. Neurosurgery 63:412–424, discussion 424–426
18. McClain CD, Soriano SG, Goumnerova LC, Black PM, Rockoff MA (2007) Detection of unanticipated intracranial hemorrhage during intraoperative magnetic resonance image-guided neurosurgery. Report of two cases. J Neurosurg 106:398–400
19. Nimsky C, Ganslandt O, Hastreiter P, Wang R, Benner T, Sorensen AG, Fahlbusch R (2007) Preoperative and intraoperative diffusion tensor imaging-based fiber tracking in glioma surgery. Neurosurgery 61:178–185, discussion 186
20. Nimsky C, Ganslandt O, Merhof D, Sorensen AG, Fahlbusch R (2006) Intraoperative visualization of the pyramidal tract by diffusion-tensor-imaging-based fiber tracking. Neuroimage 30: 1219–1229
21. Hadani M, Spiegelman R, Feldman Z, Berkenstadt H, Ram Z (2001) Novel, compact, intraoperative magnetic resonance imaging-guided system for conventional neurosurgical operating rooms. Neurosurgery 48:799–807, discussion 807–809
22. Ramina R, Coelho Neto M, Giacomelli A, Barros EJ, Vosgerau R, Nascimento A, Coelho G (2009) Optimizing costs of intraoperative magnetic resonance imaging. A series of 29 glioma cases. Acta Neurochir
23. Maesawa S, Fujii M, Nakahara N, Watanabe T, Saito K, Kajita Y, Nagatani T, Wakabayashi T, Yoshida J (2009) Clinical indications for high-field 1.5 T intraoperative magnetic resonance imaging and neuro-navigation for neurosurgical procedures. Review of initial 100 cases. Neurol Med Chir (Tokyo) 49:340–349, discussion 349–350
24. Pamir MN, Ozduman K (2009) 3-T ultrahigh-field intraoperative MRI for low-grade glioma resection. Expert Rev Anticancer Ther 9:1537–1539

25. Ekinci G, Akpinar IN, Baltacioglu F, Erzen C, Kilic T, Elmaci I, Pamir N (2003) Early-postoperative magnetic resonance imaging in glial tumors: prediction of tumor regrowth and recurrence. Eur J Radiol 45:99–107
26. Truwit CL, Hall WA (2006) Intraoperative magnetic resonance imaging-guided neurosurgery at 3-T. Neurosurgery 58:ONS-338–ONS45, discussion ONS-345–ONS-346
27. McBride DQ, Miller BL, Nikas DL, Buchthal S, Chang L, Chiang F, Booth RA (1995) Analysis of brain tumors using 1H magnetic resonance spectroscopy. Surg Neurol 44:137–144
28. Duprez TP, Jankovski A, Grandin C, Hermoye L, Cosnard G, Raftopoulos C (2008) Intraoperative 3T MR imaging for spinal cord tumor resection: feasibility, timing, and image quality using a “twin” MR-operating room suite. Am J Neuroradiol 29: 1991–1994
29. Nimsky C, Ganslandt O, Buchfelder M, Fahlbusch R (2006) Intraoperative visualization for resection of gliomas: the role of functional neuronavigation and intraoperative 1.5 T MRI. Neurol Res 28:482–487
30. Ntoukas V, Krishnan R, Seifert V (2008) The new generation polestar n20 for conventional neurosurgical operating rooms: a preliminary report. Neurosurgery 62:82–89, discussion 89–90
31. Kilic T, Ozduman K, Elmaci I, Sav A, Necmettin Pamir M (2002) Effect of surgery on tumor progression and malignant degeneration in hemispheric diffuse low-grade astrocytomas. J Clin Neurosci 9:549–552
32. Kilic T, Ekinci G, Seker A, Elmaci I, Erzen C, Pamir MN (2001) Determining optimal MRI follow-up after transsphenoidal surgery for pituitary adenoma: scan at 24 hours postsurgery provides reliable information. Acta Neurochir 143:1103–1126

Intra-operative 3.0 T Magnetic Resonance Imaging Using a Dual-Independent Room: Long-Term Evaluation of Time-Cost, Problems, and Learning-Curve Effect

X. Pablos Martin, G. Vaz, E. Fomekong, G. Cosnard, and C. Raftopoulos

Abstract We present a short and comprehensive report of our 39-month experience using a 3.0 T intra-operative magnetic resonance imaging (ioMRI) neurosurgical-MR twin room, including a description of the problems encountered and the associated time-delays. Forty-seven problems were experienced during the 189 ioMRI procedures (two ioMRI were performed in five of the 184 surgical procedures) performed in the 39-month period, including a blocked transfer table, failure of anesthetic monitoring material, and specific MRI-related problems, such as head and coil positioning difficulties, artefacts, coil malfunctions and other technical difficulties. None of these problems prevented the ioMRI procedure from taking place or affected image interpretation, but they sometimes caused a significant delay. Fifteen (32%) of these problems occurred during the initial learning curve period. The mean duration of the ioMRI procedure was 75 min, which decreased slightly with experience, although an average waiting-for-access time of 24 min could not be avoided. These results illustrate that although performing ioMRI at 3.0 T with the dual room is a challenging procedure, it remains safe and feasible and associated with only minor dysfunctions while offering optimal image quality and standard surgical conditions.

Keywords Intra-operative magnetic resonance imaging · Neuroimaging · Neurosurgery

X. Pablos Martin, G. Vaz, E. Fomekong, and C. Raftopoulos (✉)
Department of Neurosurgery, Cliniques Universitaires St-Luc, Université Catholique de Louvain, Avenue Hippocrate, 10, Brussels 1200, Belgium

G. Cosnard
Department of Radiology, Cliniques Universitaires St-Luc,Université Catholique de Louvain, Brussels Belgium

Introduction

The first system to use intra-operative Magnetic Resonance Imaging (ioMRI) for neurosurgical procedures was built in the Brigham and Women's Hospital in Boston in 1994 [1]. Since then, a wide range of ioMRI models has been developed, each with its own advantages and limitations (see [2] for a review). Regardless of the type of ioMRI system used, operating room time has been shown to be increased [3–12] (but see [13]). The additional time needed to perform an ioMRI procedure is closely related to the configuration of the specific ioMRI system, and to the occurrence of technical difficulties. Based on our 39-month experience with the ioMRI dual-independent room suite built in our academic hospital [14], we present the first detailed report of the time-cost associated with ioMRI and the technical difficulties encountered. This report provides useful information to anyone interested in advanced ioMRI development.

Materials and Methods

Between February 2006, when the first ultra high-field ioMRI was performed at our institution, and May 2009, 180 patients underwent 184 surgical procedures using the 3.0 T. ioMRI complex (Table 1; five patients had two ioMRI so that 189 ioMRI were performed). The mean age of these patients at the time of surgery was 44 years, ranging from 1.6 to 81 years. The cohort consisted of 88 female patients (mean age 43 years, range 1.6 to 80 years) and 92 male patients (mean age 45 years, range 2 to 81 years). Among the 184 surgical procedures, 153 were a first operation and 31 were repeated surgery for tumor progression. Histopathological examination and clinical evaluation revealed that the lesions were glioma ($n=64$, WHO grade I: $n=11$; grade II: 9; grade III: 15; and grade IV: 29), pituitary adenoma ($n=48$), meningioma ($n=14$), metastasis ($n=14$),

DOI 10.1007/978-3-211-99651-5_21,

Table 1 Characteristics of patients who underwent ioMRI between Feb 2006 and May 2009

Tumors and other pathology	Patients, *n* (%)	Sex F/M	Age (min–max)	Primary/recurrent	Surgery
Primary					
Glioma	64 (46)	29/35	47 (1.6–81)	59/9	68[a]
WHO grade I[b]	11 (6)	4/7	27 (2–68)	11/0	11
WHO grade II[c]	9 (5)	7/2	40 (25–67)	9/0	9
WHO grade III	15 (8)	7/8	38 (26–49)	14/4	18
WHO grade IV	29 (16)	11/18	62 (35–81)	25/5	30
Pituitary adenoma[d]	48 (27)	19/29	48 (15–77)	39/9	48
Meningioma	14 (8)	11/3	59 (35–80)	12/2	14
Schwannoma	3 (2)	1/2	68 (60–75)	3/0	3
Metastasis	14 (8)	9/5	54 (25–78)	10/4	14
Cavernoma	3 (2)	3/0	38 (30–44)	1/2	3
Medically refractory epilepsy					
Without lesion	13 (7)	7/6	15 (3–29)	13/0	13
With lesion[e]	7 (4)	3/4	15 (4–37)	5/2	7
Other[f]	14 (8)	6/8	31 (2–63)	11/3	14
Total	180	88/92	44 (2–81)	153/31	184

[a]Including 4 surgical procedures for tumor progression (3, 6, 15 and 17 months)
[b]Patient #145: LG glioma or DNET, Patient#147 glioma vs. dysplasia
[c]Including three gangliogliomas
[d]For six patients, normal tissue was found on histological examination
[e]Lesions were: Tubers, dysembryoplastic neuroepithelial tumor ($n=2$), neuronal dysplasia, pilomyxoid astrocytoma, glioneuronal malformation, and astroblastoma GII
[f]Colloid cyst, choroid plexus papilloma, hemangioblastoma ($n=3$), liponeurocytoma, medulloblastoma ($n=4$), chordoma, hemangioma, cranophayngioma, and epidermoid cyst

medulloblastoma ($n=4$), schwannoma ($n=3$), cavernoma ($n=3$), hemangioblastoma ($n=3$), colloid cyst, choroid plexus papilloma, liponeurocytoma, chordoma, hemangioma, cranopharyngioma, and epidermoid cyst ($n=1$ each). In 20 other patients, a deconnection and/or resection procedure was performed for treatment of medically refractory epilepsy (MRE); of these 20 patients, 13 had cryptogenic epilepsy and for seven patients, histological analysis revealed a dysembryoplastic neuroepithelial tumor (DNET, $n=2$), Bourneville's tubers, neuronal dysplasia, pilomyxoid astrocytoma, astroblastoma (WHO grade II), and glioneuronal malformation ($n=1$ each).

The design of the ioMRI suite, including imaging capabilities, architectural setup and surgical equipment, has been described in detail elsewhere [14].

For every procedure, data were collected prospectively concerning the time needed to complete the different ioMRI steps, and problems that occurred during the process, and any consequences of such problems. The data were then integrated into a spread sheet program for further analysis. To evaluate any possible learning-curve effect, the 189 ioMRI procedures were grouped; groups of equal numbers of procedures rather than of equal periods of time were formed since the learning experience may be related more to the number of procedures performed than to the period of time.

Results

There were no adverse events related to ferromagnetic instrumentation in the MRI room during the study period, and no patient or staff member experienced an injury or was placed at risk because of the projectile effect. There were no accidents related to patient transfer between the operating room (OR) and the MRI room.

Table 2 summarizes the problems that were encountered while using the ioMRI. Each problem was immediately resolved in collaboration with technical and radiological staff. None of these problems led to cancellation of the procedure or inability to interpret the MRI.

The most frequent problem was a blocked transfer table ($n=13$), which occurred mostly during the first 7 months of the study period, with a frequency of one in six ioMRI procedures. Technical inspection of the table revealed an internal software fault that was easily resolved. This problem did not recur over the subsequent 5 months and then reappeared, occurring about once in every 21 ioMRI procedures (1/4.33 months). The problem was generally related to an internal software issue that was solved by restarting the system. The actual delay caused by the blocked transfer table was reported in only two cases, as 10 and 17 min. In the other cases, the difference between the actual transfer duration and the average normal transfer duration was estimated as 15 min.

Table 2 Problems associated with the ioMRI system and their evolution over time

ioMRI[a]	Period (month)	Wait for access to ioMRI: Cases no. (%)	Av. time (min)	Other problems: Blocked transfer table	Anesthetist-related problems[b]	MRI-related problems: Unplugged coil and coil position	Missing or non-functional coil	Head position	Other[c]
21	3 (Feb–May 06)	18 (86)	17	3	0	2	0	2	1
21	4 (May–Sept 06)	20 (95)	20	4	2	0	0	0	1
21	5 (Sept 06–Jan 07)	21 (100)	25	0	0	1	0	0	1
21	5 (Jan–Jun 07)	20 (95)	21	1	1	0	1	1	0
21	4 (Jun–Oct 07)	21 (100)	30	1	1	0	0	1	2
21	5 (Oct 07–Mar 08)	20 (95)	27	1	1	0	1	0	1
21	4 (Mar–Jul 08)	13 (62)	19	1	1	1	0	2	1
21	4 (Jul–Nov 08)	16 (76)	27	1	1	1	0	1	0
21	6 (Nov 08–May 09)	18 (86)	28	1	0	0	5	0	1
189	40 (Feb 06–May 09)	167 (88)	24	13	7	5	7	7	8

[a]The 189 ioMRI (two in five patients) were clustered in nine consecutive groups
[b]Anesthetist-related problems included: respirator ($n=2$), SPO_2, monitoring material problem ($n=3$), unknown
[c]Other MRI-related problems included: Metal artifact ($n=2$); air artefact, neuronavigation registration problem; MRI software bug; air equilibration problem; non-MRI-adapted tube; second contrast injection and new MRI

MRI-related technical problems included an unplugged or malpositioned coil ($n=5$), a missing or non-functional coil in the MRI room ($n=7$), problems with positioning the head in the MRI scanner (difficulty placing the isocenter, $n=7$), metal artifacts because of a surgical metal star holder or head clamp ($n=1$ each), air artifacts, registration problems, MRI software bugs, air equilibration problems, a non-MRI-adapted tube, and insufficient contrast agent ($n=1$ each). The artifacts occurring as a result of head position (when repositioning was deemed unnecessary), metal or pneumencephaly did not prevent interpretation of the MRI.

There were two unplugged or malpositioned coil problems in the first three months, but only three in the subsequent 36 months. This problem was solved by re-plugging or repositioning the coil and usually caused a significant delay of about 15 min (5–38 min).

The problem of a missing coil or one that could not be used for technical reasons was solved by using another coil. In one case (patient #170), a body coil was used and, although decreasing the signal-to-noise ratio, this allowed satisfactory MR imaging. These problems occurred mostly in the last 6 months with five incidents (1/4.2 ioMRI) and special attention is being paid to try and prevent this problem. The other MRI related problems occurred evenly though the 39-month period.

There were also delays related to anesthetic issues ($n=7$), with a mean duration of 13 min (2–20 min). These problems included difficulties with monitoring material ($n=3$), the respirator ($n=2$), SPO_2, and one unknown ($n=1$ each), and occurred with a relatively stable frequency of one case every 5.71 months. Each anesthetic problem was successfully handled and there were no related adverse events.

Waiting for access to the MRI room. Because the MRI equipment is also used for routine diagnostic and research activity, neurosurgeons always warn the MRI staff about 1 h in advance that the MRI room should be converted for surgical conditions. Nevertheless, in 167 (88%) cases there was a delay in gaining access to the MRI room, this proportion ranging from 62% to 100% depending on the time period (Fig. 1). The average waiting time was 24 min (range 0–90 min).

Table 3 summarizes the time required to perform the different steps of the ioMRI procedure. Transfer of the patient to the MRI room took a mean of 11 min (range 2–40 min: patient #139, blocked transfer table needing system restart). The transfer time decreased, from a mean of 14 min in the first group of 21 procedures to 8 min in the last cluster, paralleling the incidence of problems with the transfer table. The scanning procedure itself required a mean of 31 min (11–76 min) and the transfer back to the OR took a mean of 8 min (range 2–40 min: patient #27, problem with transfer table). Hence, the ioMRI procedure, including both transfers, was completed in a mean time of 51 min (46–57 min) across the whole study period; this time decreased from 55 min in the first half of the study period (105 procedures, 21 months) to 47 min in the second half (84 procedures, 19 months). Finally, the whole process, including waiting time for access, took a mean time of 75 min (27–140 min), which decreased slightly from 77 min during the first half of the study period (105 procedures, 21 months), to 70.5 min in the second half (84 procedures, 19 months).

Discussion

Our data show that performing ioMRI at 3.0 T is a challenging procedure but remains feasible and safe. To our knowledge, no untoward events related to the magnetic field strength have ever been reported in the literature. Our experience shows

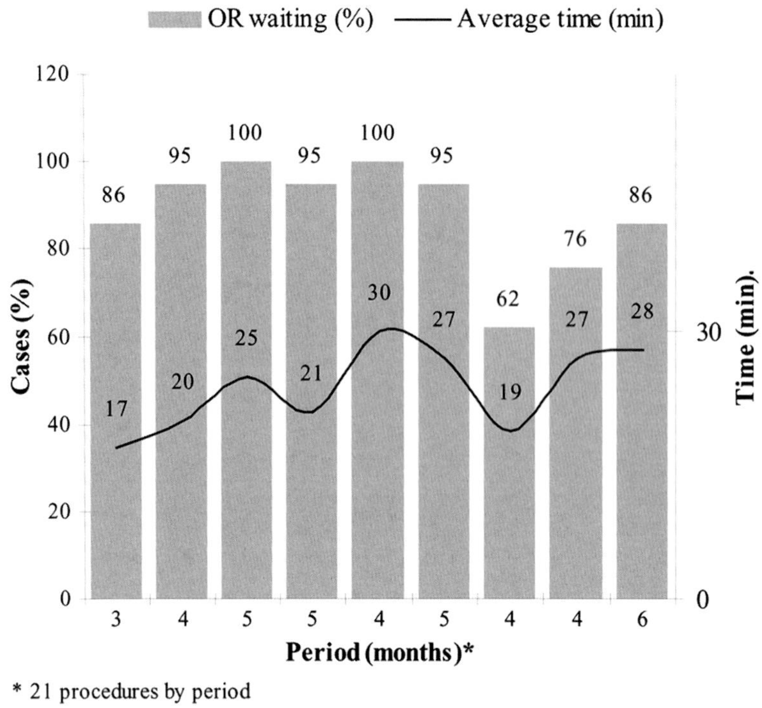

Fig. 1 Percentage of cases when OR had to wait for access to ioMRI and average waiting time in function of team experience

Table 3 Average times in minutes (min–max) for the different steps of the ioMRI process and their evolution over time

ioMRI	Period (month)	OR wait for MR	Transfer to MR	MRI duration	Transfer to OR	Total ioMRI
21	3 (Feb–May 06)	17 (0–75)	14 (7–22)	28 (17–68)	9 (3–21)	72 (37–138)
21	4 (May–Sept 06)	20 (0–44)	13 (7–35)	31 (17–60)	8 (2–40)	74 (53–120)
21	5 (Sept 06–Jan 07)	25 (5–75)	10 (4–15)	35 (16–55)	8 (3–15)	79 (45–135)
21	5 (Jan–Jun 07)	21 (0–65)	11 (5–16)	37 (22–76)	8 (2–18)	78 (42–140)
21	4 (Jun–Oct 07)	30 (10–60)	12 (5–25)	35 (11–70)	9 (3–25)	84 (55–124)
21	5 (Oct 07–Mar 08)	27 (0–55)	10 (5–15)	29 (17–60)	7 (2–25)	73 (35–130)
21	4 (Mar–Jul 08)	19 (0–85)	11 (5–40)	29 (15–55)	8 (3–10)	67 (27–123)
21	4 (Jul–Nov 08)	27 (0–90)	10 (3–30)	31 (15–52)	7 (2–25)	76 (36–138)
21	6 (Nov 08–May 09)	28 (0–60)	8 (2–10)	29 (15–55)	9 (2–23)	74 (34–120)
189	40 (Feb 06–May 09)	24 (0–90)	11 (2–40)	31 (11–76)	8 (2–40)	75 (27–140)

ioMRI intraoperative MRI (189 ioMRI with two in five surgical procedures), *OR* operating room

that even at ultrahigh fields, careful training can insure the ioMRI procedure is safe.

Every planned ioMRI procedure was completed successfully, enabling useful diagnostic information to be obtained. Technical problems occurred more frequently soon after the unit was inaugurated, with 15 technical problems during the first 7 months of activity (32% of the 47 technical problems experienced in more than 3 years). After this period, problems occurred occasionally, except for the non-functional coil problems which occurred mainly in the last 6 months of the study period. In these cases, the coil had to be changed, which did not prevent the ioMRI procedure being performed or limit interpretation of the images, but led to small delays. Our experience (Fig. 2) supports the notion that a learning curve is observed in the initial period, after which specific technical requirements and equipment problems become more common [15–17].

The nature of the technical problems reported here appears very similar to those observed in other series. Artefacts on the MR images, because of ferromagnetic components or pneumencephaly [5, 8, 9, 17–21], did not prevent interpretation. Anesthetic equipment failure [12], difficulty positioning the head in the scanner [15, 22, 23], coil position [10, 20], non-functional coils [17, 24], and internal MRI system failure [15, 17, 19, 21] are difficulties that have been observed irrespective of the ioMRI system used. The number of technical problems reported here may seem somewhat higher than those reported in literature, but in all cases the problems were immediately resolved so that all procedures were performed successfully. These problems should, therefore, be considered as minor issues and confirm the reliability and feasibility of performing ioMRI at 3.0 T.

Transport of the patients in our series required on average 11 min to go and 8 min to return, with a range of 2–40 min

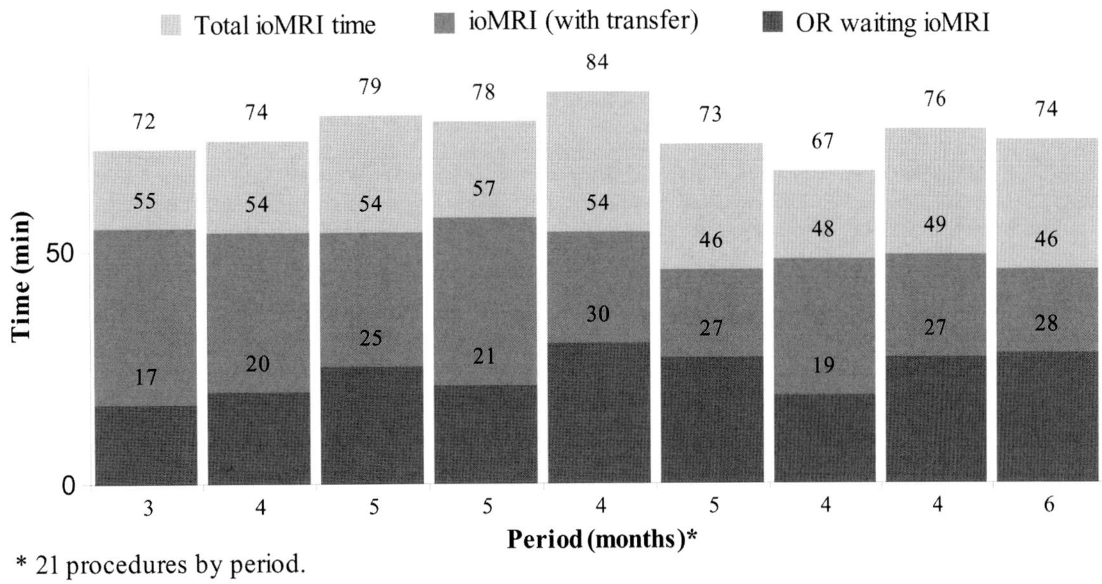

Fig. 2 Average times for ioMRI procedures in function of team experience

for both. These durations are in accordance with other series where an independent surgical room was used [16, 19, 25, 26], although some authors have reported a transfer time of not longer than 3 min [23, 27, 28]. The average additional time required to complete the whole ioMRI procedure was 75 (27–140) min in our series. This duration is closely related to the ioMRI infrastructure and to the numbers and types of scanning sequences performed (e.g., whether or not an intravenous contrast agent is used). ioMRI has been associated with an increased duration of surgery of 1–4 h [3–12], but this could be decreased to 10–35 min [23, 27–30] with some compromises in surgical conditions and imaging protocol.

Another potential source of delay is the time needed to access the ioMRI room, which has not, to our knowledge, been reported in other publications on this subject. Despite an effort to schedule the time when the MRI scanner would be needed, a large number of procedures (88%) were still delayed by having to wait for access to the MRI room. The average waiting time overall was 24 (0–90) min.

The dual independent twin room 3.0 T. ioMRI system offers several advantages as it provides MR images with quality as good as a diagnostic scanner; it does not interfere with the regular operating room in terms of surgical access, patient positioning and instrumentation; it includes an accurate navigation tool; and it enables alternative use of the magnet so that, when not needed by the neurosurgeon, it can be used for routine diagnostic and research activity. Disadvantages include the need to move the patient during craniotomy and sometimes a wait for access to the MRI room. Nevertheless, our large experience over more than 3 years confirms that ioMRI at 3.0 T is a safe and feasible technique with only minor problems.

Conflict of interest statement We declare that we have no conflict of interest.

References

1. Black P, Moriarty T, Alexander E III et al (1997) Development and implementation of intraoperative magnetic resonance imaging and its neurosurgical applications. Neurosurgery 41:831–845
2. Albayrak B, Samdani AF, Black PM (2004) Intra-operative magnetic resonance imaging in neurosurgery. Acta Neurochir 146: 543–557
3. Archer DP, McTaggart-Cowan RA, Falkenstein RJ et al (2001) Intraoperative mobile magnetic resonance imaging for craniotomy lengthens the procedure but does not increase morbidity. Can J Anaesth 49:420–426
4. Black P, Alexander E III, Martin C et al (1999) Craniotomy for tumor treatment in an intraoperative magnetic resonance imaging unit. Neurosurgery 45:423–433
5. Knauth M, Wirtz CR, Tronnier VM et al (1999) Intraoperative MR imaging increases the extent of tumor resection in patients with high-grade gliomas. AJNR Am J Neuroradiol 20:1642–1646
6. Kremer P, Tronnier V, Steiner HH et al (2006) Intraoperative MRI for interventional neurosurgical procedures and tumor resection control in children. Childs Nerv Syst 22:674–678
7. Schulder M (2008) Intracranial surgery with a compact, low-field-strength magnetic resonance imager. Top Magn Reson Imaging 19 (4):179–189
8. Schulder M, Carmel PW (2003) Intraoperative magnetic resonance imaging: impact on brain tumor surgery. Cancer Control 10: 115–124
9. Schulder M, Liang D, Carmel PW (2001) Cranial surgery navigation aided by a compact intraoperative magnetic resonance imager. J Neurosurg 94:936–945
10. Schulder M, Catrambone J, Carmel PW (2005) Intraoperative magnetic resonance imaging at 0.12 T: is it enough? Neurosurg Clin N Am 16:143–154
11. Schulder M, Salas S, Brimacombe M et al (2006) Cranial surgery with an expanded compact intraoperative magnetic resonance imager. Technical note. J Neurosurg 104:611–617

12. Siomin V, Barnett G (1998) Intraoperative imaging in glioblastoma resection. Cancer J 9:91–98
13. Schwartz RB, Hsu L, Wong T et al (1999) Intraoperative MR imaging guidance for intracranial neurosurgery: experience with the first 200 cases. Radiology 211:477–488
14. Jankovski A, Francotte F, Vaz G et al (2008) Intraoperative magnetic resonance imaging at 3-T using a dual independent operating room-magnetic resonance imaging suite: development, feasibility, safety, and preliminary experience. Neurosurgery 63(3):412–424, discussion 424–426
15. Senft C, Seifert V, Hermann E et al (2008) Usefulness of intraoperative ultra low-field magnetic resonance imaging in glioma surgery. Neurosurgery 63(4 Suppl 2):257–266, discussion 266–267
16. Steinmeier R, Fahlbusch R, Ganslandt O et al (1998) Intraoperative magnetic resonance imaging with the magnetom open scanner: concepts, neurosurgical indications, and procedures: a preliminary report. Neurosurgery 43(4):739–747, discussion 747–748
17. Wirtz CR, Knauth M, Staubert A et al (2000) Clinical evaluation and follow-up results for intraoperative magnetic resonance imaging in neurosurgery. Neurosurgery 46(5):1112–1120, discussion 1120–1122
18. Bohinsky RJ, Kokkino AK, Warnick RE et al (2001) Glioma resection in a shared-resource magnetic resonance operating room after optimal imageguided frameless stereotactic resection. Neurosurgery 48:731–742
19. Nimsky C, Ganslandt O, Tomandl B et al (2002) Low-field magnetic resonance imaging for intraoperative use in neurosurgery: a 5-year experience. Eur Radiol 12:2690–2703
20. Schneider JP, Trantakis C, Rubach M et al (2005) Intraoperative MRI to guide the resection of primary supratentorial glioblastoma multiforme – a quantitative radiological analysis. Neuroradiology 47:489–500
21. Wirtz CR, Knauth M, Stamov M et al (2002) Clinical impact of intraoperative magnetic resonance imaging on central nervous system neoplasia. Tech Neurosurg 7:326–331
22. Ntoukas V, Krishnan R, Seifert V (2008) The new generation Polestar N20 for conventional neurosurgical operating rooms: a preliminary report. Neurosurgery 62(3 Suppl 1):82–89
23. Pamir MN, Ozduman K, Dinçer A et al (2009) First intraoperative, shared-resource, ultrahigh-field 3-Tesla magnetic resonance imaging system and its application in low-grade glioma resection. J Neurosurg [Epub ahead of print]
24. Nimsky C, Ganslandt O, von Keller B et al (2004) Intraoperative high-field strength MR imaging: implementation and experience in 200 patients. Radiology 233:67–78
25. Nimsky C, Ganslandt O, Fahlbusch R (2002) From intraoperative patient transport to surgery in the fringe field: intraoperative application of magnetic resonance imaging using a 0.2-Tesla scanner – the Erlangen experience. Tech Neurosurg 7:265–273
26. Nimsky C, Ganslandt O, Gralla J et al (2003) Intraoperative low-field magnetic resonance imaging in pediatric neurosurgery. Pediatr Neurosurg 38:83–89
27. Pamir MN, Peker S, Ozek MM et al (2006) Intraoperative MR imaging: preliminary results with 3 tesla MR system. Acta Neurochir Suppl 98:97–100
28. Ramina R, Coelho Neto M, Giacomelli A et al (2009) Optimizing costs of intraoperative magnetic resonance imaging. A series of 29 glioma cases. Acta Neurochir (Wien) [Epub ahead of print]
29. Iseki H, Muragaki Y, Nakamura R et al (2005) Intelligent operating theater using intraoperative open-MRI. Magn Reson Med Sci 4:129–136
30. Lewin JS, Nour SG, Meyers ML et al (2007) Intraoperative MRI with a rotating, tiltable surgical table: a time use study and clinical results in 122 patients. AJR Am J Roentgenol 189:1096–1110

Multifunctional Surgical Suite (MFSS) with 3.0 T ioMRI: 17 Months of Experience

Vladimír Beneš, David Netuka, Filip Kramář, Svatopluk Ostrý, and Tomáš Belšán

Abstract The 3 T ioMRI in Prague is composed of two independent suites: the operating theatre and the 3 T MR suite, both of which can and do work independently. They are connected by a double door and a special transportation system. The whole operating table is moved on rails to and from the MR gantry. Anaesthesiological equipment is built from paramagnetic material, which is also moved to and from the MR suite. The integral parts of the multifunctional surgical suite (MFSS) are the neuronavigation system, electrophysiological monitoring, surgical microscope with availability of indocyanin green angiography and fluorescence-guided glioma resection technique and endoscopy equipment. The operating theatre is equipped in a normal fashion with the exception of a head holder that is paramagnetic.

MR radiologist and MR assistants are alerted approximately 30 min before the requested intraoperative and outpatient service is interrupted to clean the MR suite. The ioMRI takes 15–20 min and immediately after the door closes the out patient activity is resumed.

Intraoperative MR was performed in 332 surgeries in the first 17 months of operation. The most frequent indications were pituitary adenomas, followed by gliomas. Other indications were less frequent and included meningiomas, cavernomas, aneurysms, epilepsy surgery, intramedullary lesions, non-pituitary sellar lesions, metastases and various other surgeries. In 332 cases no technical or medical complication connected with ioMRI was encountered.

V. Beneš (✉), D. Netuka, F. Kramář, and S. Ostrý
Department of Neurosurgery, Charles University, Central Military Hospital, U vojenské nemocnice 1200, 16902 Prague 6, Czech Republic
e-mail: vladimir.benes@uvn.cz

T. Belšán
Unit of Radiology, Central Military Hospital, Prague, Czech Republic

Keywords Glioma · Intraoperative imaging · Magnetic resonance · Neuronavigation · Pituitary adenoma

Introduction

In the past years the possibility of intraoperative imaging is a fast developing field of neurosurgery [1–6]. Various modalities and systems have been developed. In April 2008, the 3 T intraoperative MR suite was opened at the Central Military Hospital (CMH) in Prague. The system is jointly operated by the Department of Neurosurgery, CMH and Charles University and Department of Radiology, CMH. In the following paragraphs the main features of the MFSS will be described and surgical procedures in which ioMRI has been used will be summarised.

Materials and Methods

Multifunctional Surgical Suite (MFSS) description and workflow (Fig. 1).

The 3 T ioMRI in Prague is composed of two independent suites: the operating theatre and the 3 T MR suite (3.0 T Signa HDx, General Electric). Both can and do work independently. They are connected by a double door and a special transportation system (Maquet Viwas). The whole operating table is moved on the rails to and from the MR gantry. Anesthesiological equipment (anaesthesiological machine Aestiva5/MRI, Datex Ohmeda, vital signs monitor IMM MRI, Datex Ohmeda) is built from paramagnetic material, which can be moved to and from the MR suite. The integral parts of the MFSS are the neuronavigation system (VectorVision Sky, BrainLAB), electrophysiological monitoring (Eclipse, Axon Systems), surgical microscope with availability of indocyanin green angiography and

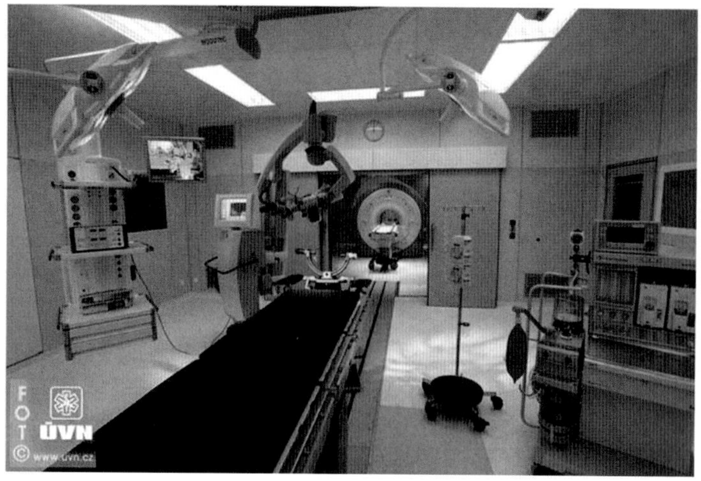

Fig. 1 Operative room with an ioMRI setting

fluorescence-guided glioma resection technique (OPMI Pentero, Zeiss) and endoscopy equipment (both Storz and Wolf endoscope). The operating theatre is equipped in a normal fashion with the exception of a head holder that is paramagnetic (Integra for general electric).

Thirty minutes before the requested intraoperative MR, the radiologists are alerted and out-patient service is interrupted to clean the MR suite. The ioMRI takes 15–20 min and immediately after the door closes the out patient activity is resumed.

Over the past 17 months (April 2008–August 2009), 332 surgeries with single or multiple intraoperative imaging were performed. In the same period the surgical theatre was used for 300 other neurosurgical procedures of all types in which ioMRI was not called into service. Some 15–20 outpatient MR studies are performed daily in the MR suite.

Procedures in Which ioMRI Was Performed

Use of the ioMRI is always determined before surgery. In general, we use ioMRI in all endoscopic endonasal surgeries and in all glioma surgeries. All other indications are individual. Table 1 summarises the types of surgery where ioMRI was performed.

Results

In 332 cases no technical or medical complication connected with ioMRI was encountered. In all cases the quality of imaging was sufficient for the surgeon despite that the quality varied because of technical adjustments, a temporary lack of adequate coils and the learning curve of both neurosurgeons and radiologists.

Table 1 Neurosurgical procedures performed in ioMRI OR in the first 17 months

Pituitary adenoma	122	Hypothalamic hamartoma	3
Glioma	112	Lymfoma	3
Meningioma	23	Carotid endarterectomy	2
Cavernoma	15	Orbital tumor	1
Aneurysm	11	Tuberculoma	1
Other sellar lesions	10	Choroid plexus carcinoma	1
Epileptosurgery	7	Cavernous sinus schwannoma	1
Intramedullary lesions	6	Spinal meningioma	1
Metastases	6	AVM	1
Cyst/Absces	5	Intracerebral hematoma	1

Discussion

The primary use of ioMRI is for all types of glioma, where ioMRI helps in increasing radicality and decreases the risk of surgery. The same is true for pituitary adenomas in which a certain number of surgeries for recurrences can be avoided. These two areas are clear and well documented [7, 8] and the subject of other presentations of our group in this issue.

Immediate Postoperative Imaging

The system very easily allows for immediate postoperative imaging. This imaging is performed immediately after the wound suture and dressing while the patient is still under general anaesthesia. The value of these images is the availability of immediate information. Images provide the neurosurgeon with information about the brain condition and shift after surgery and they improve the decision about postoperative care (e.g., should the patient be ventilated or awakened)? The images also serve as the baseline for subsequent postoperative imaging. An immediate postoperative MR study can also have legal value.

Intraoperative Navigation

Even with the implementation of navigation systems, the surgeon can encounter problems in finding the lesion (e.g., deep-seated small cavernoma). In such a case ioMRI provides an obvious solution. The lesion can easily be re-navigated using the intraoperative images. Navigation and renavigation are also used not only for the lesion remnants but also in biopsies, endoscopic procedures, in multiple cystic lesion targeting, etc.

Intended Partial Resection

In certain cases of very large meningiomas and some other lesions the surgeon plans a partial/subtotal resection for a variety of different reasons, including age or unfavourable general health of a patient and fear of over decompression after the total resection. It is rather difficult to assess the extent of resection in, e.g., a large cribriform plane meningioma. Usually, the surgeon overestimates the extent of resection. It is obvious that the precise extent of surgery required can easily be assessed by ioMRI [9].

Skull Base Tumours

The role of ioMRI is the same as for gliomas and pituitary adenomas, namely enhancing radicality whilst concomitantly decreasing the risks of surgery. However, in these tumours ioMRI can also show the distance to vital structures during piecemeal resection. The shift of the brain structures is easily shown and in skull base tumours intraoperative navigation is always precise and helpful (the skull base structures do not move). ioMRI can be useful in both classical and endoscopic approaches.

Extent of Resection in Epilepsy Surgery

ioMRI can be employed to assess the extent of resection in comparison with preoperative planning [10, 11]. However, because of the intraoperative brain shift, this may be rather difficult and peroperative monitoring is more precise.

Intraoperative Assessment of Acute Ischaemia

DWI images clearly show the extent of ischaemia after, e.g., aneurysm clipping, which would allow for immediate clip replacement. In AVM surgery inadvertent occlusion of the en passage artery can be disclosed.

Biopsies

The exact position of the biopsy needle can be ascertained [12].

Cystic and Multicystic Lesions

The exact and immediate decrease in cyst volume can be shown and subsequent movement and changes of additional cysts in multicystic lesions accurately targeted [13, 14].

Spinal Cord Tumours

The use of ioMRI is the same for spinal cord tumours as for brain gliomas. However, the safe extent of resection is probably more closely monitored by SSEPs and MEPs.

Extradural Spinal Tumours

Control of the extent of resection and resection of any remnants can be enhanced by ioMRI.

Spine Surgery

Mastronardi et al. studied the prognostic relevance of the postoperative evolution of intramedullary spinal cord changes in signal intensity on magnetic resonance imaging after anterior decompression for cervical spondylotic myelopathy [15]. Although we are not convinced whether ioMRI has any real value in this kind of surgery, it should be noted that it might be applied.

All these potential areas have not yet been sufficiently addressed and thus the possible benefits of ioMRI will be

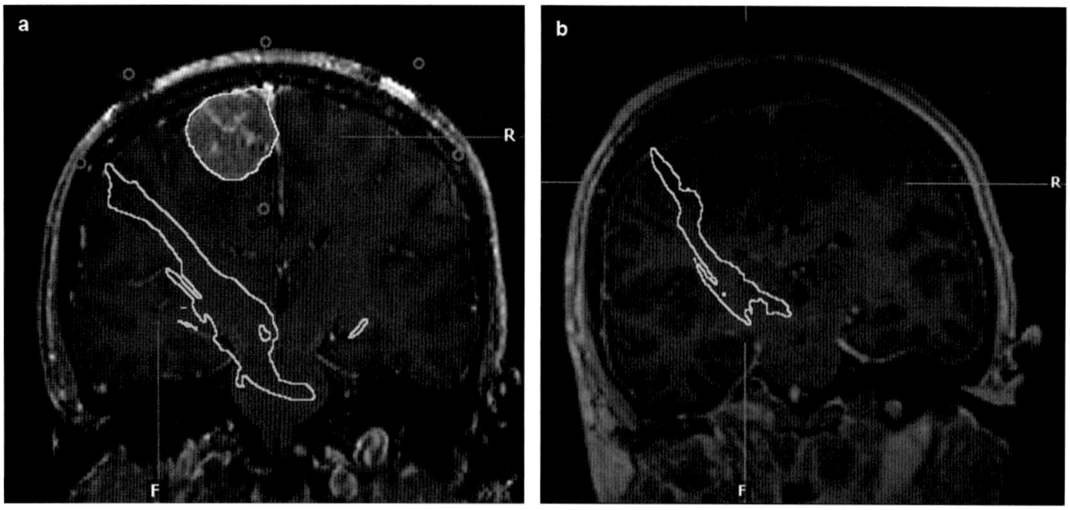

Fig. 2 Preoperative (**a**) and intraoperative (**b**) corticospinal tract tractography in case on convexity meningioma closed to eloquent area

demonstrated more clearly in the future. The use of tractographies during surgery or the integration of functional MR would certainly be of interest. It is probable that software adjustment of functional images to the brain shift shown on peroperative images would facilitate the availability of a sufficient position of eloquent areas on intraoperative images. This multimodal imaging seems to be the most challenging field today (Fig. 2).

We can expect the use of this technology to spread in the near future, similarly to the widespread use of CT in the 1970s, MR in the 1980s and endovascular technologies, radiosurgery and navigation systems in the 1990s. Novel and exciting possibilities of intraoperative imaging can be anticipated.

Conclusions

ioMRI and other types of intraoperative imaging are modern technologies that enable the neurosurgeon to perform precise and safe procedures. Whilst intraoperative imaging is currently used most frequently for gliomas and pituitary adenomas, its potential use in many other areas of neurosurgery will be addressed and studied in future investigations.

Conflict of interest statement We declare that we have no conflict of interest.

References

1. Black PM, Moriarty T, Alexander E 3rd, Stieg P, Woodard EJ, Gleason PL et al (1997) Development and implementation of intraoperative magnetic resonance imaging and its neurosurgical applications. Neurosurgery 41(4):831–842
2. Fahlbusch R, Ganslandt O, Buchfelder M, Schott W, Nimsky C (2001) Intraoperative magnetic resonance imaging during transsphenoidal surgery. J Neurosurg 95(3):381–390
3. Hall WA, Liu H, Martin AJ, Pozza CH, Maxwell RE, Truwit CL (2000) Safety, efficacy, and functionality of high-field strength interventional magnetic resonance imaging for neurosurgery. Neurosurgery 46(3):632–641
4. Jankovski A, Raftopoulos C, Vaz G, Hermoye L, Cosnard G, Francotte F et al (2007) Intra-operative MR at 3T: short report. JBR-BTR 90(4):249–251
5. Steinmeier R, Fahlbusch R, Ganslandt O, Nimsky C, Buchfelder M, Kaus M et al (1998) Intraoperative magnetic resonance imaging with the magnetom open scanner: concepts, neurosurgical indications, and procedures: a preliminary report. Neurosurgery 43(4): 739–747
6. Sutherland GR, Kaibara T, Louw D, Hoult DI, Tomanek B, Saunders J (1999) A mobile high-field magnetic resonance system for neurosurgery. J Neurosurg 91(5):804–813
7. Nimsky C, Ganslandt O, Von Keller B, Romstöck J, Fahlbusch R (2004) Intraoperative high-field-strength MR imaging: implementation and experience in 200 patients. Radiology 233 (1):67–78
8. Nimsky C, von Keller B, Ganslandt O, Fahlbusch R (2006) Intraoperative high-field magnetic resonance imaging in transsphenoidal surgery of hormonally inactive pituitary macroadenomas. Neurosurgery 59(1):105–114
9. Adeolu AA, Sutherland GR (2006) Intraoperative magnetic resonance imaging and meningioma surgery. West Afr J Med 25 (3):174–178
10. Kelly JJ, Hader WJ, Myles ST, Sutherland GR (2005) Epilepsy surgery with intraoperative MRI at 1.5 T. Neurosurg Clin N Am 16 (1):173–183
11. Schwartz TH, Marks D, Pak J, Hill J, Mandelbaum DE, Holodny AI, Schulder M (2002) Standardization of amygdalohippocampectomy with intraoperative magnetic resonance imaging: preliminary experience. Epilepsia 43(4):430–436
12. Vitaz TW, Hushek SG, Shields CB, Moriarty TM (2002) Interventional MRI-guided frameless stereotaxy in pediatric patients. Stereotact Funct Neurosurg 79(3–4):182–190
13. Vitaz TW, Hushek S, Shields CB, Moriarty T (2001) Changes in cyst volume following intraoperative MRI-guided Ommaya reservoir placement for cystic craniopharyngioma. Pediatr Neurosurg 35(5):230–234

14. Walker JB, Harkey HL, Buciuc R (2008) Percutaneous placement of an external drain of the cisterna magna using interventional magnetic resonance imaging in a patient with a persistent cerebrospinal fluid fistula: technical case report. Neurosurgery 63(2): E375
15. Mastronardi L, Elsawaf A, Roperto R, Bozzao A, Caroli M, Ferrante M, Ferrante L (2007) Prognostic relevance of the postoperative evolution of intramedullary spinal cord changes in signal intensity on magnetic resonance imaging after anterior decompression for cervical spondylotic myelopathy. J Neurosurg Spine 7 (6):615–622

Intra-operative MRI at 3.0 Tesla: A Moveable Magnet

Michael J. Lang, Alexander D. Greer, and Garnette R. Sutherland

Abstract This paper presents the development and implementation of an intra-operative magnetic resonance imaging (ioMRI) program using a moveable 3.0 T magnet with a large working aperture.

Methods: A previously established prototype 1.5 T ioMRI program based on a ceiling-mounted moveable magnet was upgraded to 3.0 T. The upgrade included a short, 1.73 m, magnet with a large 70 cm working aperture (IMRIS, Winnipeg, Canada), whole-room radio-frequency shielding, and a fully functional MR-compatible operating room (OR) table. Between January and September 2009, 100 consecutive patients were evaluated at 3.0 T.

Results: The ioMRI upgrade maintained a patient-focused environment. When not needed for surgery, the magnet was moved to an adjacent room. A large aperture and streamlined OR table allowed freedom of patient positioning while maintaining access and visibility. Working at 3.0 T enabled application of advanced imaging sequences to the full spectrum of neurosurgical pathology in the ioMRI environment. The use of ioMRI continues to show unsuspected residual tumor in up to 20% of cases. There were no adverse events or technical system failures.

Conclusion: An ioMRI program based a 3.0 T moveable magnet is feasible. By moving the magnet, the system maintains a patient-focused surgical environment and the ability to share the technology between medical disciplines.

Keywords 3.0-Tesla · Intra-operative imaging · Magnetic resonance imaging · Neurosurgery

Introduction

Intra-operative magnetic resonance imaging (ioMRI) has been used in neurosurgery for over ten years. The technology has varied in respect to magnet design, magnetic field strength, and operating room (OR) configuration [1–5]. Over the past several years, adoption of ioMRI by the neurosurgical community has tended towards higher-field systems. In 1999, results related to the development and integration of an ioMRI system based on a moveable 1.5-tesla (1.5 T) magnet were reported [5, 6]. The system was designed as a patient-focused environment, as, when not needed for surgery, the magnet is moved to an adjacent room. Serendipitously, this configuration was found to facilitate sharing of the technology between surgery and other disciplines, such as diagnostic imaging. The 1.5 T prototype system has since been upgraded to 3.0 T.

Signal-to-noise ratio increases linearly as a function of magnetic field strength [7]. This translates into higher image resolution, decreased acquisition time, enhanced soft-tissue contrast, and improved capability for functional MRI (fMRI), diffusion tensor imaging (DTI), and multi-nuclear MR-spectroscopy [8]. Enhanced image quality, together with advanced software design, has encouraged widespread acceptance of 3.0 T MRI. Several centers have successfully integrated 3.0 T MR systems into various ioMRI configurations (Table 1). Recent advances in 3.0 T technology have resulted in the development of a relatively short magnet with a working aperture of 70 cm, allowing enhanced patient visibility and access, respectively [9]. The present report describes the integration of such a magnet, and its use in 100 consecutive neurosurgical cases.

Materials and Methods

Technology

Magnet and Gradients

The ioMRI system includes a ceiling-mounted moveable 3.0 T magnet (IMRIS, Winnipeg, Canada) capable of transfer into and out of the OR, which measures 1.73 m in length, with

M.J. Lang, A.D. Greer, and G.R. Sutherland (✉)
Department of Clinical Neurosciences, University of Calgary, Calgary, Alberta, Canada
e-mail: garnette@ucalgary.ca

M.N. Pamir et al. (eds.), *Intraoperative Imaging*, Acta Neurochirurgica Supplementum, Vol. 109,
DOI 10.1007/978-3-211-99651-5_23, © Springer-Verlag/Wien 2011

Table 1 Technical specifications of installed 3.0T ioMRI systems

Institution	Scanner	OR configuration	Aperture (cm)	Gradient (mT/m)	Slew Rate (mT/m/ms)
University of Minnesota	Philips	Single-room	60	40	200
Acibadem University	Siemens	Two-room	60	45	200
Université Catholique de Louvain	Philips	Two-room	60	40	120
Barrow Neurological Institute	General Electric	Two-room	60	50	150
University of Calgary	Siemens	Moving magnet	70	45	200

an internal diameter of 90 cm, and a weight of 8,000 kg, compared to the 5,100 kg 1.5 T system. The working aperture is 70 cm with shielded gradients in place. The 5-gauss fringe field measures only 4×3.5 m^2. The system provides a large homogenous field of view measuring $50 \times 50 \times 50$ cm at isocenter, maximum gradient strength of 45 mT/m, and slew rate of 200 mT/m/ms (Table 1).

Operating Table

Success of the ioMRI program at the University of Calgary can, in part, be attributed to a unique MR-compatible OR table [5, 6]. The table includes integrated 3- or 4-pin head-holders and hydraulic motors that allow the full functionality of a standard neurosurgical OR table. Currently in its fifth generation, the table is wider (56 cm), has a thinner vertical profile (14 cm), and now includes table side rails. The table is also able to rotated 90°, increasing the separation from the 5-gauss line, which has allowed the safe introduction of endoscopy and other non-MR-compatible technology into the ioMRI environment.

RF Coils

RF coils are one of the most critical components of an MRI system, owing to their impact on signal-to-noise ratio. Coil design for ioMRI must take into account head fixation compatibility, field sterility, and maintenance of surgical access. The RF system is based on a transmit body coil and a number of different receive coils, depending on the application. The RF train can have up to 102 elements with 32 channels, with software capable of turning elements on or off, depending on the field of interest. This RF technology reduces total acquisition time while maintaining image resolution via the application of parallel imaging techniques.

RF Shielding

In upgrading from 1.5 to 3.0 T, the decision was made to change from local to whole-room copper RF shielding, with attenuation of at least 100 dB. The number of electrical devices in the OR necessitates extensive use of wave guides, filtering, and conversion of electrical signals to fiber optics, where possible. A copper mesh-impregnated glass panel was installed between the MR control-room and the OR, allowing uninterrupted patient visualization during imaging. Wooden doors were constructed for the magnet storage alcove to provide additional safety. The ioMRI suite was fitted with acoustic tiling to minimize emanating noise.

Clinical Material

Prospective study of 100 consecutive patients undergoing 3.0 T ioMRI-assisted neurosurgical procedures was performed from January to September 2009. With the exception of thoraco-lumbar spine and peripheral nerve disease, the patients represent the full spectrum of neurosurgical pathology (Table 2), although the majority underwent treatment for intracranial neoplasia.

Results

Technology

There has not been a single technological system failure in the current series, compared to earlier experience with the 1.5 T prototype, in which 34 out of 986 cases (3.4%) were accompanied by technical failure delaying sequence acquisition (Table 2). The system has been successfully used with patients placed in the supine, prone and lateral positions. In the present series, there has not been a single adverse event. The heaviest patient, who was positioned supine, weighed 111 kg.

A range of imaging sequences, including T_1-weighted, T_2-weighted, FLAIR, DTI and MR-angiography (MRA), were successfully acquired in the intra-operative setting (Fig. 1). The use of a dedicated image processor has greatly improved the speed at which tractography images can be displayed, allowing modification of surgical approach as suggested by white matter anatomy (Fig. 2).

Table 2 Intra-operative MRI cases

Pathologic category	1.5 T (n=986)	3.0 T (n=100)
Tumors		
Glioma	368	39
Meningioma	102	16
Pituitary adenoma	71	9
Metastasis	17	3
Vascular[a]	94	10
Epilepsy	157	7
Spine	38	2
Other[b]	105	14
Technology failure	34	0

[a]AVM, cavernoma, aneurysm, EC-IC bypass, micro-vascular decompression
[b]Ependymoma, choroids plexus carcinoma, neuroblastoma, neurocytoma, schwannoma, craniopharyngioma, lymphoma, radiation necrosis, hydrocephalus

Patients

Patients in this 3.0 T series had a mean age of 43±19 years (range = 13 months–83 years), with seven of the cases in this series performed on pediatric patients, and a male to female ratio of 1.2:1. This compares to a mean age of 42±18 (range = 4 months–83 years) and a male to female ratio of 1.1:1 in 986 patients imaged at 1.5 T. A total of 170 imaging studies were performed on the 100 patients using the 3.0 T ioMRI technology.

For patients undergoing intracranial neoplasm resection, those requiring additional resection following intra-operative imaging are shown in Table 3. Unsuspected residual tumor rates are only reported for the large 1.5 T data set, though residual tumor continues to be observed in up to 20% of cases imaged at 3.0 T. Though not detailed here, ioMRI has demonstrated additional benefits such as accurate craniotomy placement or modified surgical decision-making (Fig. 3). In addition to craniotomy for tumor resection, 3.0 T ioMRI has been applied to uses such as confirmation of spinal decompression during cervical spine procedures and post-operative evaluation of arterial patency following aneurysm clipping.

Discussion

An ioMRI system based on a moveable 3.0 T magnet has been successfully integrated into the operating room while maintaining a patient-centered environment. A highly effective

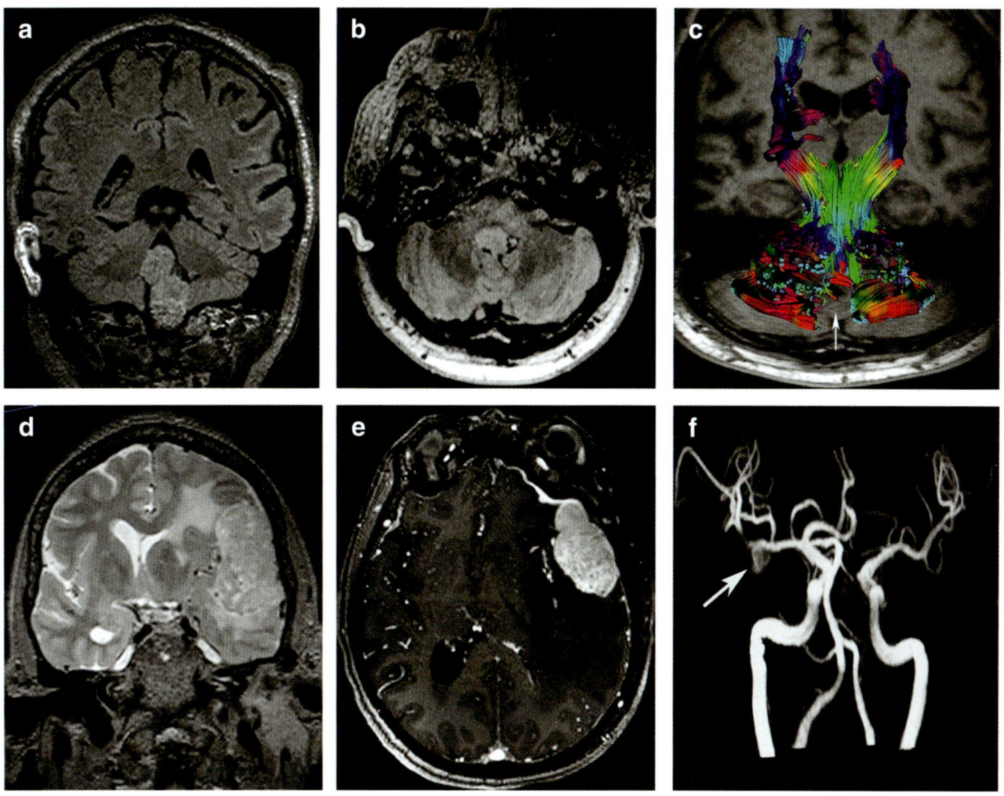

Fig. 1 Imaging quality at 3.0 T: ioMRI images (**a**, coronal FLAIR; **b**, axial FLAIR) obtained from a patient with a 4th ventricle ependymoma. Post-resection images (**c**, DTI imposed on T1 images) with superimposed tractography demonstrate intact cerebellar white-matter anatomy following resection (*arrow*). Images of a sphenoid wing meningioma with dural tail (**d**, T2 coronal; **e**, T1 axial with gadolinium enhancement). MR-Angiography (**f**) demonstrates a small intra-cranial aneurysm (*arrow*)

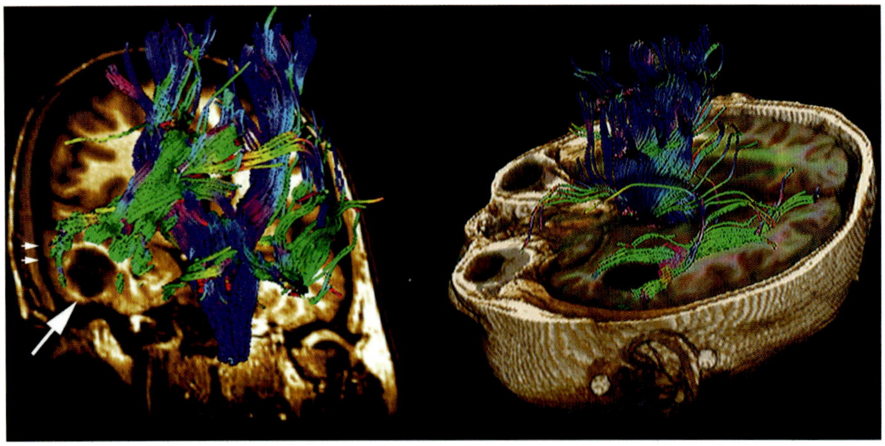

Fig. 2 Effect of pre-operative tractography on surgical planning: Prior to resection of a temporal lobe lesion associated with intractable epilepsy, DTI-based tractography illustrates displaced, yet intact, middle temporal gyrus white-matter tracts (*small arrows*). Absence of functional inferior white-matter tracts (*large arrow*) suggests a sub-temporal surgical approach

Table 3 Impact of ioMRI on intracranial neoplasm resection

Tumor type	Number of cases		Unsuspected residual tumor (%)
	1.5T	3.0T	1.5T[b]
Glioma[a]			
Grade I–II	212	9	27 (13%)
Grade III	89	20	18 (20%)
Grade IV	67	10	15 (22%)
Meningioma	102	16	2 (2%)
Pituitary adenoma	71	9	25 (35%)

[a]World Health Organization classification

[b]Unsuspected tumor data is reported only for experience at 1.5 T due to the small 3.0 T sample size

3.0 T ioMRI program is dependent on the development of multiple, interrelated technologies. Improvements in RF shielding, image processing, and RF coil design have each played a role. However, expanded working aperture and OR table functionality remain key components of a broadly applicable ioMRI system.

The University of Calgary currently possesses the only 3.0 T ioMRI system with a working aperture of 70 cm. An arithmetic increase in working space corresponds to a multiplicative increase in the number of procedures to which ioMRI can be applied. Only with such expanded application will ioMRI be adopted by the neurosurgical community at large. With the availability of a working aperture of at least 70 cm, the ioMRI magnet no longer dictates crucial decisions such as patient positioning and approach. In this way, movable ioMRI technology will empower surgeons to develop novel treatments without impinging upon the current standard of care or exposing patients to undue hazard to obtain imaging. The 70 cm aperture makes all standard patient positions compatible with ioMRI, and expands the use of other surgical adjuncts, such as robotics [10]. While magnets with field strengths higher than 3.0 T have been developed, working aperture size must remain a principal consideration prior to introducing such technology into the OR environment.

In similar fashion, an MR-compatible OR table with full functionality continues to be the focal point of a patient-centered ioMRI system. Paired with a mobile magnet, this system permits the use of standard surgical technique, acquisition of intra-operative imaging, and avoidance of unnecessary and potentially dangerous patient transfer. Notably, as the magnet can be moved out of the operating theatre, the full table functionality is essential for OR use during non-imaging cases.

Three principles must become axiomatic prior to general adoption of ioMRI technology. First, it should be possible to apply ioMRI to the entire spectrum of neurosurgical disease without negatively impacting standard operative technique. Secondly, given the environment of fiscal responsibility, it should be designed to maximize cost-efficiency. Third, the operating room must remain a patient-centered environment. The application of 3.0 T ioMRI to date has upheld these principles to varying degrees. Some investigators employ a research-dedicated design incapable of efficient shared diagnostic usage [11]. A two-room concept, in which patients are transferred from the OR into a separate imaging suite, was created in order to defray cost via shared use, and obviates the need to purchase MR-compatible instruments [12, 13]. Such a layout necessitates transportation of the anesthetized patient out of the OR for imaging, which could place the patient at increased risk. Regardless of OR configuration, all other 3.0 T ioMRI systems currently in place are limited somewhat by a small working aperture. Architectural design and technological development of the ioMRI program at the University of Calgary have sought to systematically address these principles.

Experience with 3.0 T ioMRI in 100 cases has been encouraging as to potential improved patient outcome. It is generally accepted that gross total resection of intracranial neoplasm improves patient survival, and recent studies suggest that high-field ioMRI can increase the rate of gross total

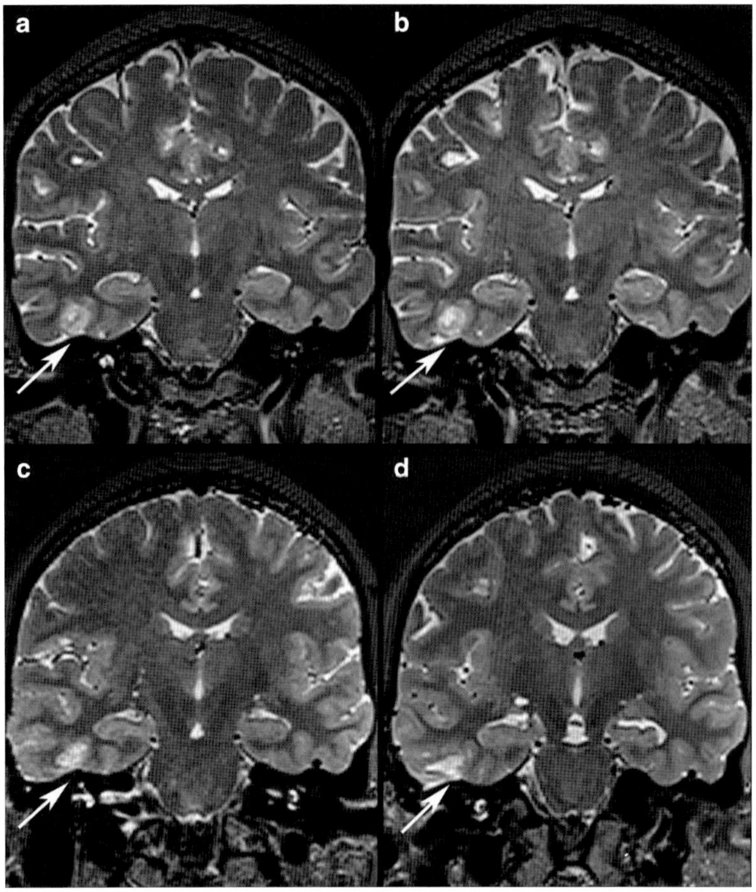

Fig. 3 Changing surgery: Surgical planning (**a** and **b**, coronal T2) ioMRI images obtained from a patient presenting with seizures, associated with a small right temporal lobe lesion (*arrows*). Following resection of the suspected lesion, frozen section showed neurons and glia, consistent with normal brain. Intra-dissection imaging (**c** and **d**, coronal T2) showed complete resection of the lesion, obviating the need for additional biopsy. Subsequent histopathology was consistent with a ganglioglioma

resection [14]. This series demonstrates the utility of intra-operative imaging in neurosurgery, including detection and resection of unsuspected residual lesions. Imaging prior to patient positioning optimizes craniotomy placement and surgical corridor orientation, and provides a unique educational environment for surgical planning. High-resolution DTI-based white-matter tractography has been used extensively in the operating room for surgical planning and intra-operative evaluation of tract preservation [15]. Further research is required to firmly correlate pathologic results with intra-operative imaging.

Continuing development of 3.0 T ioMRI technology portends increasingly comprehensive neurological imaging. Incorporation of fMRI into pre-operative imaging may become a useful tool in the preservation of eloquent cortex [16]. Chemical shift also scales with increased field, which, may make MR-spectroscopy a useful tool for the intra-operative identification of pathologic tissue [7]. MR-angiography may also develop significant intra-operative utility in the setting of vascular disease. However, it has been limited to craniotomy placement (particularly for patients with cavernous angioma or AVM), as image acquisition time complicates aneurysm clip re-application in the event of unintended vascular occlusion. In addition, susceptibility artifact related to titanium clips limits evaluation of the aneurismal neck [17]. Development of MR-invisible clips, based on ceramics, may make such an evaluation possible [18].

Significant challenges remain. Development of MR-compatible anesthesia equipment has advanced significantly, but field exposure continues to inhibit reliable measurement of ST-segment changes within the bore of the magnet. It is for this reason that patients with significant cardiovascular co-morbidity have been excluded from ioMRI-assisted procedures. Some have proposed that barriers, real or perceived, to the ease of ioMRI acquisition limit its practical use. In the current series, workflow disruption has been the largest constraint on the number of studies performed, as surgery is interrupted for up to 30 minutes by the image acquisition procedure. The ability to operate under real-time imaging would allow ioMRI to actively guide surgery, as opposed to confirming the presumed completion of surgical goals.

Ultimately, cost is the true limiting factor in the widespread adoption of 3.0 T ioMRI. Indeed, the cost of high-field ioMRI is routinely cited as the motivation for low-field systems, despite inferior image quality. Were cost not prohibitive, there would be little question as to the superiority of 3.0 T ioMRI. As demonstrated by the case series published to date, 3.0 T ioMRI can be safely integrated into the OR. However, the substantial cost of this technology must first be justified.

It is beyond question that scans obtained at 3.0 T are the highest quality and most widely applicable ioMRI images available today. Integration of this technology will continue to drive innovation in surgical technique and equipment. That said, modern healthcare places increasing emphasis on demonstrable clinical utility prior to the widespread adoption of new technology. Initiation of a randomized controlled trial to assess the impact of this technology on patient outcomes and cost-benefit ratios is desirable and now feasible, given the existing number of higher-field ioMRI units. Importantly, the disruption of traditional surgical workflow caused by intra-operative imaging remains unresolved. Integration of MR-compatible robotics within the magnet bore is, however, an attractive solution to this limitation, and would allow surgery to truly take place within an image.

Conflicts of interest statement Dr. G. Sutherland and A.D. Greer hold shares in IMRIS (Winnipeg, Canada). M.J. Lang declares no conflict of interest.

Acknowledgements This work was supported by grants from Alberta Advanced Education and Technology, Western Economic Diversification, and the Calgary Health Trust.

References

1. Black PM, Moriarty T, Alexander E 3rd, Stieg P, Woodard EJ, Gleason PL, Martin CH, Kikinis R, Schwartz RB, Jolesz FA (1997) Development and implementation of intraoperative magnetic resonance imaging and its neurosurgical applications. Neurosurgery 41:831–842
2. Hadani M, Spiegelman R, Feldman Z, Berkenstadt H, Ram Z (2001) Novel, compact, intraoperative magnetic resonance imaging-guided system for conventional neurosurgical operating rooms. Neurosurgery 48:799–809
3. Martin AJ, Hall WA, Liu H, Pozza CH, Michel E, Casey SO, Maxwell RE, Truwit CL (2000) Brain tumor resection: intraoperative monitoring with high-field-strength MR imaging – initial results. Radiology 215:221–228
4. Nimsky C, Ganslandt O, Tomandl B, Buchfelder M, Fahlbusch R (2002) Low-field magnetic resonance imaging for intraioerative use in neurosurgery: a 5 year experience. Eur Radiol 12:2690–2703
5. Sutherland GR, Kaibara T, Louw D, Hoult DI, Tomanek B, Saunders J (1999) A mobile high-field magnetic resonance system for neurosurgery. J Neurosurg 91:804–813
6. Kaibara T, Saunders JK, Sutherland GR (2000) Advances in mobile intraoperative magnetic resonance imaging. Neurosurgery 47:137–138
7. Lin W, An H, Chen Y, Nicholas P, Zhi GH, Gerig G, Gilmore J, Bullitt E (2003) Practical consideration for 3T imaging. Magn Reson Imaging Clin N Am 11:615–639
8. Tanenbaum LN (2006) Clinical 3T MR imaging: mastering the challenges. Magn Reson Imaging Clin N Am 14:1–15
9. Sadick M, Schock KB, Gretz N, Schoenberg SO, Michaely HJ (2009) Morphologic and dynamic renal imaging with assessment of glomerular filtration rate in a pcy-mouse model using a clinical 3.0 tesla scanner. Invest Radiol 44:469–475
10. Sutherland GR, Latour I, Greer AD, Fielding T, Feil G, Newhook P (2008) An image-guided magnetic resonance-compatible surgical robot: rapid communication. Neurosurgery 62:286–293
11. Truwit CL, Hall WA (2006) Intraoperative magnetic resonance imgaging-guided neurosurgery at 3-T. Neurosurgery 58:ONS-338–ONS-345
12. Jankovski A, Francotte F, Vaz G, Fomekong E, Duprez T, Van Boven M, Docquier MA, Hermoye L, Cosnard G, Raftopoulos C (2008) Intraoperative magnetic resonance imaging at 3-T using a dual independent operating room-magnetic resonance imaging suite: development, feasibility, safety, and preliminary experience. Neurosurgery 63:412–426
13. Pamir MN, Peker S, Özek MM, Dinçer A (2006) Intraoperative MR imaging: preliminary results with 3 tesla MR system. Acta Neurochir 98:97–100
14. Hatiboglu MA, Weinberg JS, Suki D, Rao G, Prabhu SS, Shah K, Jackson E, Sawaya R (2009) Impact of intraoperative high-field magnetic resonance imaging guidance on glioma surgery: a prospective volumetric analysis. Neurosurgery 64:1073–1081
15. Field AS, Alexander AL (2004) Diffusion tensor imaging in cerebral tumor diagnosis and therapy. Top Magn Reson Imag 15:315–324
16. Hall WA, Truwit CL (2006) 3-Tesla functional magnetic resonance imaging-guided tumor resection. Int J Comput Assist Radiol Surg 1:223–230
17. Sutherland GR, Kaibara T, Wallace C, Tomanek B, Richter M (2002) Intraoperative assessment of aneurysm clipping using magnetic resonance angiography and diffusion-weighted imaging: technical case report. Neurosurgery 50:893–897
18. Sutherland GR, Kelly JJ, Boehm DW, Klassen JB (2008) Ceramic aneurysm clips. Neurosurgery 62:ONS400–ONS405

One Year Experience with 3.0 T Intraoperative MRI in Pituitary Surgery

David Netuka, Václav Masopust, Tomáš Belšán, Filip Kramář, and Vladimír Beneš

Abstract A multifunctional surgical suite with intraoperative 3.0 T MRI (ioMRI) has been operating at the Central Military Hospital, Prague since April 2008. Our experiences over the past year and the effect of ioMRI on the extent of pituitary adenoma resection are evaluated.

Eighty-six pituitary adenoma resections were performed in 85 patients with ioMRI in the first year of the ioMRI service. Pituitary adenoma suprasellar extension was present in 60 cases, invasion into cavernous sinus in 49 cases, and retrosellar growth in one case. The surgical goal was set before surgery: either a radical resection (49 cases) or a partial resection (37 cases).

In the group of patients where a decision for a radical resection was taken the results are as follows: ioMRI confirmed radical resection in 69.4% of the cases; ioMRI disclosed unexpected adenoma residuum and further resection led to radical resection in 22.4%.

In the group of patients where a decision for a partial resection was taken, the results are as follows: no further resection was perfomed after ioMRI in 51.3% of the cases and further resection was performed after ioMRI in 48.7% of the cases.

ioMRI seems to be a valuable tool to increase the extent of pituitary adenoma resection.

Keywords Intraoperative imaging · Magnetic resonance · Pituitary adenoma

D. Netuka (✉), V. Masopust, F. Kramář, and V. Beneš
Department of Neurosurgery, Central Military Hospital, Charles University, U vojenské nemocnice 1200, Prague, Czech Republic
e-mail: david.netuka@uvn.cz

T. Belšán
Unit of Radiology, Central Military Hospital, Prague, Czech Republic

Introduction

Intraoperative MRI enables the surgeon to depict the extent of the neurosurgical procedure intraoperatively. This technique has been developed over the past 15 years. Current development goes in two directions. Low-field MRI scanners represent one of the directions [1, 2]. Nowadays, these systems are mobile and less expensive. Moreover, the quality of images obtained by these systems has been improved in the past years. Still, the quality is inferior to preoperative images. The crucial question is whether to use high quality preoperative images and compare them with inferior quality intraoperative images. High-field MRI scanners represent another branch of development [3–5]. These systems are more expensive and less mobile but produce better quality images.

Surgical suite with intraoperative 3.0 T MRI has been operating at the Central Military Hospital, Prague since April 2008. Our experiences over the past year and the effect of ioMRI on the extent of pituitary adenoma resection are evaluated. The operative room and MRI setting are the subject of separate presentation from our group in this issue. Therefore, in this paper we will limit our discussion to our experience and results from endoscopic endonasal procedures.

Materials and Methods

The first endonasal procedure in our ioMRI operative room was performed in April 18, 2008. All procedures were performed using the bilateral endonasal approach. A MRI compatible head holder was applied after induction of anaesthesia. Next, the head of the patient is registered to a frameless navigation system that is used obligatorily. The patient is undraped after tumour resection and transferred to a MRI scanner after tumour resection. New MRI data are

M.N. Pamir et al. (eds.), *Intraoperative Imaging*, Acta Neurochirurgica Supplementum, Vol. 109,
DOI 10.1007/978-3-211-99651-5_24, © Springer-Verlag/Wien 2011

sent to the navigation system and combined with the preoperative navigation data. This enables us to use intraoperative data without any need to re-register the head of the patient. All MRI sequences are analysed for pituitary adenoma remnant or any kind of surgical complication. Then the decision is taken either to continue the surgical resection or to check solely the operative field in order to perform closure of the sella if needed.

Our MRI protocol consists of preoperative 3.0 T MRI scanning followed by ioMRI on the same scanner. Six channel intraoperative coils are used for ioMRI. ioMRI is performed both in T1-weighted images with and without gadolinium and in T2-weighted images. Further, MRI is performed on the first or the second postoperative day. All these images are used to evaluate the extent of surgical resection.

In the first year of ioMRI service 110 endonasal procedures were performed. Non-pituitary adenoma lesions were treated in 15 cases. This group consisted of skull base carcinomas in three cases, surgical revision for cerebrospinal fluid (CSF) leakage (n=3), surgery for spontaneous CSF leakage (n=2), meningioma (n=2), dermoid cyst (n=2), craniopharyngioma (n=1) and revision because of postoperative haematoma (n=1). Altogether, 95 pituitary adenoma cases were treated. No ioMRI was performed in nine cases. The reasons why no ioMRI was performed include CSF leakage after pituitary adenoma resection (n=4), patient with pacemaker (n=1), patient with ferromagnetic material in the skull (n=1), surgery abandoned for medical reasons (n=1), surgery abandoned because of infection of the sphenoid sinus (n=1), or the patient had no insurance coverage (n=1). For the remaining 86 pituitary adenoma surgeries, ioMRI was performed.

The goal of surgery was set before the actual surgery was undertaken: either a radical resection (49 cases) or a partial resection (37 cases). The decision for a partial resection was chosen if there was major cavernous sinus invasion (lateral to internal carotid artery), previous repeated surgeries, previous gamma knife surgery, or parasellar growth. The basic characteristics of patients selected for radical resection are as follows: 48 patients, 49 surgeries, and 21 women, and 27 men (mean age 51.9 years). There were ten microadenomas and 38 macroadenomas in this group. Suprasellar growth of pituitary adenoma was observed in 27 cases and cavernous sinus invasion in 15 cases. The mean vertical diameter of pituitary adenoma was 18.6 mm. Basic characteristics of patients selected for partial resection are as follows: 37 patients, 37 surgeries, and 14 women and 23 men (mean age of 59.1 years). All pituitary adenomas were macroadenomas. Suprasellar growth was present in 33 patients, cavernous sinus invasion in 34 patients, retrosellar growth in one patient and parasellar growth in two patients. The mean vertical diameter was 23.6 mm.

Results

In the group of patients where a decision for a radical resection was taken the results indicated ioMRI confirmed radical resection in 34 cases (69.4%), ioMRI disclosed adenoma residuum in 13 cases (26.5%) and further resection led to radical resection in 11 cases (22.4%).

ioMRI was evaluated as radical resection in two cases (4.1%). However, early postoperative MRI disclosed a small residuum of adenoma. The second surgery was performed in one of these two cases and a residuum of adenoma was resected. ioMRI led to increased radical resection by 22.4% (before ioMRI 69.4%, after ioMRI 91.8%). These results are summarised in Table 1.

In the group of patients where a decision for a partial resection was taken the results showed that no further resection was perfomed after ioMRI in 19 cases (51.3%) and further resection was performed after ioMRI in 18 cases (48.7%) in order to achieve a more extensive but still partial resection (Table 2).

Mortality was 0% in this group of patients while neurological morbidity was 1.1% (one patient suffered unilateral amaurosis; in fact, this patient had temporal field deficit on the same eye preoperatively). CSF leakage requiring redo surgery was present in four cases (4.7%).

ioMRI was perfomed once per surgery in 70 cases, twice in 14 cases and three times in two cases. There was neither technical failure in performing ioMRI nor a patient safety issue.

Discussion

Several papers have focused on ioMRI in sellar region surgery in the past few years. In 1999, Martin et al. published their findings in five patients with pituitary adenoma [6].

Table 1 Results in the group of patients where radical resection was intended

Number of cases	49	100%
ioMRI confirmed radical resection	34	69.4%
Wrong ioMRI evaluation	2	4.1%
ioMRI disclosed adenoma residuum	13	26.5%
Radical resection after ioMRI	11	22.4%

Table 2 Results in the group of patients where partial resection was intended

Number of cases	37	100%
No further resection after ioMRI	19	51.3%
Further resection after ioMRI	18	48.7%

This group used 0.5 T ioMRI. In two cases unexpected pituitary adenoma residuum was disclosed and resected after ioMRI. Seminal papers on this topic are from Erlangen, Germany. Nimsky et al. evaluated the effect of ioMRI in 200 cases [7]. This series consists of both pituitary adenoma and glioma, as well as rare cases where a 1.5 T ioMRI scanner was used. Radical resection was achieved in 56.2% of the piruitary adenoma cases before ioMRI, whereas the proportion of radical resection increased to 87.2% after ioMRI.

The same group evaluated the effect of ioMRI in 33 cases of growth hormone secreting adenomas [8]. ioMRI led to resection of the pituitary adenoma in five cases. Hormone normalization was achieved in three of these cases.

All these papers, including several others [9–11], show the value of ioMRI in pituitary surgery. Our work supports this finding as well.

Conclusions

ioMRI is a valuable tool in pituitary adenoma surgery. The rate of radical resection (radical resection intention group) and more extensive resections (partial resection intention group) are increased. We stress the importace of careful ioMRI evaluation. In our experiences we have not observed any technical ioMRI setting failures or issues involving patient safety. Finally, no increase of morbidity was observed in our series.

Conflict of interest statement We declare that we have no conflict of interest.

References

1. Gerlach R, du Mesnil de Rochemont R, Gasser T, Marquardt G, Reusch J, Imoehl L, Seifert V (2008) Feasibility of Polestar N20, an ultra-low-field intraoperative magnetic resonance imaging system in resection control of pituitary macroadenomas: lessons learned from the first 40 cases. Neurosurgery 63(2):272–284
2. Hadani M, Spiegelman R, Feldman Z, Berkenstadt H, Ram Z (2001) Novel, compact, intraoperative magnetic resonance imaging-guided system for conventional neurosurgical operating rooms. Neurosurgery 48(4):799–807
3. Hall WA, Liu H, Martin AJ, Pozza CH, Maxwell RE, Truwit CL (2000) Safety, efficacy, and functionality of high-field strength interventional magnetic resonance imaging for neurosurgery. Neurosurgery 46(3):632–641
4. Jankovski A, Raftopoulos C, Vaz G, Hermoye L, Cosnard G, Francotte F et al (2007) Intra-operative MR at 3T: short report. JBR-BTR 90(4):249–251
5. Sutherland GR, Kaibara T, Louw D, Hoult DI, Tomanek B, Saunders J (1999) A mobile high-field magnetic resonance system for neurosurgery. J Neurosurg 91(5):804–813
6. Martin CH, Schwartz R, Jolesz F, Black PM (1999) Transsphenoidal resection of pituitary adenomas in an intraoperative MR unit. Pituitary 2(2):155–162
7. Nimsky C, Ganslandt O, Von Keller B, Romstöck J, Fahlbusch R (2004) Intraoperative high-field-strength MR imaging: implementation and experience in 200 patients. Radiology 233(1):67–78
8. Fahlbusch R, Ganslandt O, Buchfelder M, Schott W, Nimsky C (2001) Intraoperative magnetic resonance imaging during transsphenoidal surgery. J Neurosurg 95(3):381–390
9. Jones J, Ruge J (2007) Intraoperative magnetic resonance imaging in pituitary macroadenoma surgery: an assessment of visual outcome. Neurosurg Focus 23(5):E12
10. Nimsky C, von Keller B, Ganslandt O, Fahlbusch R (2006) Intraoperative high-field magnetic resonance imaging in transsphenoidal surgery of hormonally inactive pituitary macroadenomas. Neurosurgery 59(1):105–114
11. Schwartz TH, Stieg PE, Anand VK (2006) Endoscopic transsphenoidal pituitary surgery with intraoperative magnetic resonance imaging. Neurosurgery 58(1 Suppl):ONS44-51

Intraoperative CT and Radiography

Intraoperative Computed Tomography

J.C. Tonn, C. Schichor, O. Schnell, S. Zausinger, E. Uhl, D. Morhard, and M. Reiser

Abstract Intraoperative computed tomography (iCT) has gained increasing impact among modern neurosurgical techniques. Multislice CT with a sliding gantry in the OR provides excellent diagnostic image quality in the visualization of vascular lesions as well as bony structures including skull base and spine. Due to short acquisition times and a high spatial and temporal resolution, various modalities such as iCT-angiography, iCT-cerebral perfusion and the integration of intraoperative navigation with automatic re-registration after scanning can be performed. This allows a variety of applications, e.g. intraoperative angiography, intraoperative cerebral perfusion studies, update of cerebral and spinal navigation, stereotactic procedures as well as resection control in tumour surgery. Its versatility promotes its use in a multidisciplinary setting. Radiation exposure is comparable to standard CT systems outside the OR. For neurosurgical purposes, however, new hardware components (e.g. a radiolucent headholder system) had to be developed. Having a different range of applications compared to intraoperative MRI, it is an attractive modality for intraoperative imaging being comparatively easy to install and cost efficient.

J.C. Tonn (✉)
Neurochirurgische Klinik und Poliklinik, Ludwig-Maximilians-Universität München, Munich, Germany
Neurosurgical Department, Klinikum Grosshadern, Marchioninistr. 15, 81377 Munich, Germany
e-mail: joerg.christian.tonn@med.uni-muenchen.de

C. Schichor, O. Schnell, and S. Zausinger
Neurochirurgische Klinik und Poliklinik, Ludwig-Maximilians-Universität München, Munich, Germany

E. Uhl
Neurochirurgische Klinik, Landeskrankenhaus Klagenfurt, Klagenfurt, Austria

D. Morhard and M. Reiser
Institut für klinische Radiologie, Ludwig-Maximilians-Universität München, Munich, Germany

Keywords Computed tomography (CT) · CT angiography · Intraoperative CT · Intraoperative imaging · Spine surgery

Introduction

The development of neurosurgical techniques and the demand for treating more complex lesions with the aim of continuous reduction of surgery related morbidity has generated an increasing demand for sophisticated intraoperative imaging modalities. Various technologies are available, albeit with different indications. Intraoperative ultrasound has proven to be a rather easy to use, straight forward solution for the intraoperative localisation of deep-seated lesions like cavernomas, metastases or haemorrhages as well as, to a certain extent, for resection control of tumours. Being rather inexpensive with no additional costs of installation, the use of ultrasound is dependent on the personal experience of the user. In addition, despite improved technology, its resolution may be limited depending on the particular type of pathology [1, 2]. For the resection of high grade gliomas, the use of tissue fluorescence after administration of 5-aminolevulinic acid (5-ALA) has been proven to be efficient to delineate tumour margins and residual tumour tissue. The rate of "radicality" in the microsurgical resection of high grade gliomas has been improved significantly hereby. However, this technology is only useful for malignant gliomas, especially glioblastomas; moreover, the drug itself has so far not yet been approved by health care authorities in all parts of the world [3].

Intraoperative imaging using magnetic resonance (MR) scanners, either high field or low field, provide good visualisation of soft tissue abnormalities like gliomas, pituitary adenomas, and other tumours. However, this technology is very expensive and implementation into a pre-existing operating theatre demands a lot of resources. Moreover, the use of intraoperative MRI is limited for cranial applications due to the geometry of the scanner in relation to the table system.

M.N. Pamir et al. (eds.), *Intraoperative Imaging*, Acta Neurochirurgica Supplementum, Vol. 109,
DOI 10.1007/978-3-211-99651-5_25, © Springer-Verlag/Wien 2011

The surgical workflow has to be adapted to the work in a magnetic field with special demands for surgical instruments as well as anaesthesiological monitoring systems [4–6].

Recently, computed tomography (CT) technology has made a tremendous progress. Multislice scanners (e.g. 40-slice scanning systems) provide a very high image spatial resolution with very short imaging acquisition times [7]. Software for image processing has generated tools to provide high quality 3-D CT-angiography, which has been shown to provide images at a quality level superior to MR-angiography. Quantitative perfusion parameters like cerebral blood volume, blood flow and time to peak may be displayed as colour coded maps. By virtue of electronic artefact suppression and use of adequate acquisition parameters, imaging of metallic implants in spine surgery can be achieved and image distorsion can be eliminated to a large extent so that implants are precisely depicted and correction can be performed, if necessary.

For intraoperative applications, CT scanners with a wide bore are superior to those with narrow opening enabling better access to the patient. The longitudinal coverage has also been enhanced so that the whole body of the patient (from head to toe) can be scanned without repositioning. This allows intraoperative CT scanners to be used by many surgical disciplines (e.g. ENT surgeons, vascular surgeons, traumatologists, orthopaedic surgeons) in addition to neurosurgery. Thus, such an installation can be used in a multidisciplinary scenario and thereby enhancing cost effectiveness.

After the development of a setting with a scanner with a sliding gantry on rails and integrating a neuronavigation device for cranial and spinal applications, we analysed the usefulness of this setting for spinal and neurovascular surgery. Moreover, the impact on workflow was examined. Experience has been gained according to the visibility in spinal and vascular surgery as well as work flow analysis, which will be presented here [8, 9].

Methods/Technology

A 40-slice-CT scanner (Somatom Sensation Open Sliding Gantry, Siemens Healthcare, Forchheim, Germany) with a sliding gantry and a diameter of 82 cm mounted on rails within the floor of the OR was installed in a pre-existing operating room. As operating table a carbon table plate, segmented to allow virtually all neurosurgical positionings, was used (Trumpf, Puchheim, Germany). The system was adjusted to a ceiling mounted navigation system (Vector Vision Sky, BrainLab, Feldkirchen, Germany). Invasive head fixation was performed with a radiolucent head clamp (Mayfield radiolucent skull clamp A-2002, Integra, Plainsborough, New Jersey, USA). For application of contrast media in case of CT angiography, a motor injection pump (Stellant MEDRAD Inc., Indianola, Pennsylvania, USA) was employed.

During image acquisition, the gantry moves over the patient without necessity to adjust the position of ventilation systems or catheters for scanning.

CT imaging was performed with a collimation of 40 × 0.6 mm at 120 kV and 140 mAs with a rotation time of 1 s for CTA and 20 × 1.2 mm at 120 kV and 350 mAs for cranial CT. The automated dose modulation software was used. Multiplanar reconstructions (MPR) were calculated with a slice thickness of 1–3 mm in axial, sagittal and coronal planes. Data could be imported into the frameless infrared–based neuronavigation system (Vector Vision Sky). For re-registration, the gantry of the scanner is equipped with fiducials equivalent to the fiducials at the head holder or the spinal fiducial clamp in case of spinal surgery.

Techniques of Intraoperative Computed Tomography Angiography (iCTA) and Perfusion Computed Tomography (PCT)

For the application of contrast agent, the injector is connected to a central line or at least 10 gauge lumen peripheral venous catheter. Monitoring of the whole procedure is secured by direct visual contact through a lead-glass window and indirectly via monitor camera from a neighboring room to get a visual control of all parts of the OR.

For iCTA a CT scout for planning of the scan range of the head and upper neck is acquired first. Then CTA is acquired in caudo-cranial scan direction from C1 to the vertex. A user modified bolus tracking technique (repeated sequential CT scans every 1 s roughly at the level of the carotid bifurcations to monitor the contrast arrival at the cervical arteries, scan is then started manually when contrast enhancement in the arteries is visible) and a weight-adapted contrast agent protocol is used for CTA. This was done to obtain high contrast attenuation values in the cerebral arteries and low contrast enhancement overlay in the veins and sinus.

CTA is then followed by PCT. The scan range is manually selected to avoid beam hardening artifacts starting 1 cm superior to the aneurysm clip and with a distance of at least 1 cm to head clamps. Five second after injection of 50 ml contrast agent (Imeron 300) at 7 ml/s followed by a saline flush of 50 ml at 7 ml/s the PCT starts. Therefore sequential scans with 24 mm slice thickness are acquired every second over a period of 40 s. A standard, vendor given PCT analysis software is used for perfusion analysis. Color-coded parameter-maps of cerebral blood flow (CBF), cerebral blood volume (CBV) and time to peak (TTP) are calculated.

Results

Work Flow

After final positioning of the patient according to the envisioned procedure, a "safety check" was performed. Hereby the gantry is moved over the patient in order to detect any possible collision during the scanning procedure. A special anti-collision system prevents any conflict in case the movement of the gantry is obstructed. All positionings including complex ones like park bench were feasible; the only exception for intraoperative scanning is the semi sitting position.

In case of spinal instrumentation, pre-operative imaging was performed at that time with the data fed into the navigation system in order to allow intraoperative navigation. Hereby, the real position of the spine during surgery is the basis for navigation. This is especially valuable if luxation of the spine has to be reduced in the OR (e.g. in case of cervical instability) since any navigation on the basis of image sets obtained prior to the positioning of the patient on the OR table may be misleading.

The intraoperative examination time for vascular lesions including 3-D CT-angio and a perfusion-CT was 12 min including 3 min for additional draping /undraping of the patient for the scanning procedure, 1:30 min for image acquisition and 3:00 min for reconstruction of the data set. For spinal instrumentation a mean time frame of 9 min was needed for scanning and data acquisition/image evaluation until resumption of surgery.

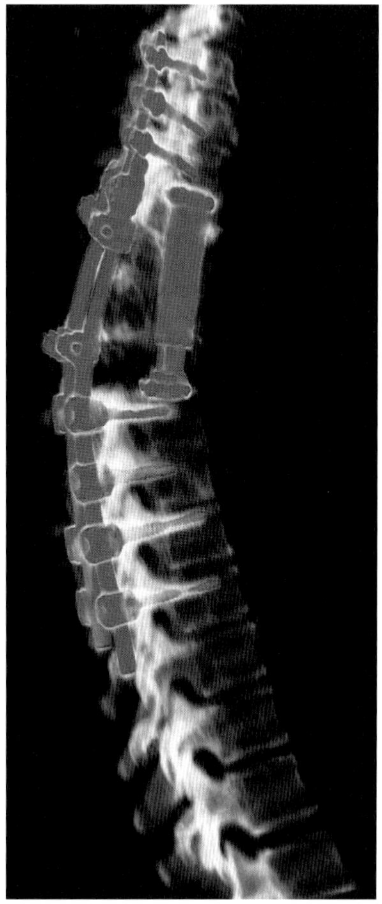

Fig. 1 Reconstructed intraoperative control-CT after cervicothoracic navigated ventrodorsal stabilization C5-Th8 due to metastatic infiltration Th1-4 from mamma-ca, kyphotic instability and compression of the spinal cord

Radiation Exposure

The highest radiation exposure for intraoperative CT-scanning was obtained in CT angiography (including CT perfusion studies). Here, the mean effective dose of CTA and CT perfusion together was 3.69 mSv. This is comparable to 3.6 mSv, which is the value typically required for a 4-vessel catheter angiogram and which does not include a perfusion study [8].

Evaluation of Imaging

With CT guided spinal navigation, a computed spatial accuracy of 0.8 ± 0.1 mm could be achieved. In a first series a total of 414 screws were analysed. Intraoperative CT could detect a minor misplacement (2–4 mm) in 16 screws (3.8% of all screws) and a major misplacement (>4 mm) in four screws (1.0%). All misplaced screws could be re-positioned during the same surgery. Hereby, the necessity for screw revision surgery could be reduced to zero from previously 4.4% in the pre-iCT era (Fig.1). Especially in cervical spine screw placements and in the cranial cervical junction, no major misplacements of screws occurred. There was no increase of infection rate or other procedure related morbidity compared to our pre-iCT series. Duration of surgery in the cranial cervical junction was 127 ± 21 min, thoracic spine stabilisation (eight screws) 170 ± 38 min and for lumbar stabilisation (four screws) 100 ± 24 min, all including the time for imaging [10].

Vascular Neurosurgery

In a pilot series of neurovascular surgery, intraoperative CT angiography and intraoperative CT perfusion were performed. The image quality of CT angiograms was rated excellent by a radiologist (D.M.) in all 13 cases (Fig. 2). CT perfusion imaging was rated excellent or good in 10/11 cases, in one case artefacts resulted in major degradation of the image quality. CT angiography and CT perfusion

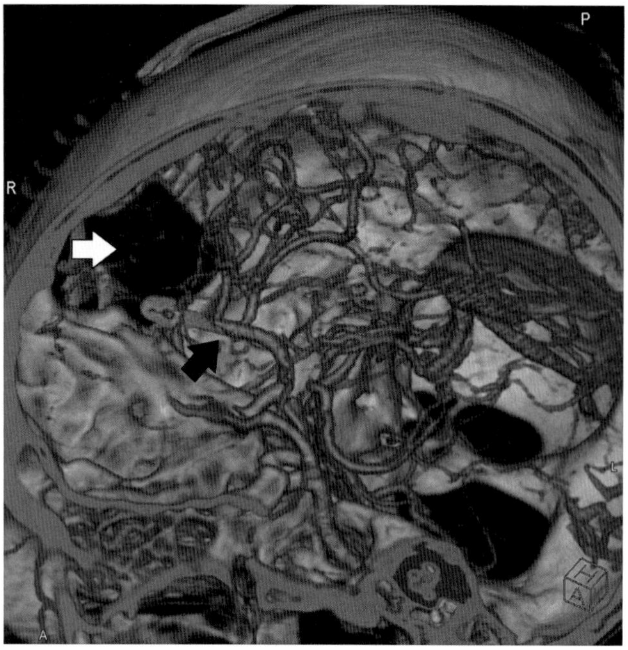

Fig. 2 Intraoperative CTA after clipping of an aneurysm of the *right* medial cerebral artery. View from the *left* side, showing artifact free vascular anatomy of the media bifurcation in the close vicinity of the clip (*Black arrow*). *Right* sided pterional craniotomy (*white arrow*)

changed the surgical strategy in two cases, in which clip repositioning, either due to residual portions of the aneurysm or because of an inadvertent occlusion of a vessel, was corrected. The image quality of iCTA and the intraoperative perfusion map were rated by the surgeon to be adequate for intraoperative decision making [8].

Discussion

The results of our studies indicate that intraoperative CT (iCT) is a promising method enhancing precision of neurosurgery and ameliorating the outcome of patients. State of the art CT technology incorporating multislice (multi detector row) systems (MSCT) allow for very short acquisition times and excellent image quality as well as intuitive multiplanar and 3D representations. Moreover, MSCT enables to perform advanced applications, such as 3-D angiography, cerebral perfusion imaging and the visualization of implants in spinal surgery. In contrast to MR-based intraoperative imaging, there is no need for dedicated surgical instruments. The system can easily be handled with no negative impact on the surgical workflow. Radiation exposure in modern MSCT-systems is acceptable as compared to conventional fluoroscopy. The learning curve for the staff including anaesthesiologists and scrub nurses as well as surgeons was very steep. Even if newly developed radiolucent head clamps with pins made of artificial sapphire were used, artefacts due to the pins may be met. Recently polymeric composite pins proved to be best suited in terms of artefact reduction with grip force comparable to standard titanium pins [11].

In comparison to intraoperative MRI, iCT is definitely superior in intraoperative spinal imaging. Moreover, iCT provides better depiction of bony structures and enables to acquire high quality CT angiography and cerebral perfusion studies. Furthermore, CT is especially useful for the control of catheter placement, e.g. in shunt surgery. MR angiography is severely limited in the depiction of vascular structures adjacent to aneurysm clips, which is clearly a major drawback of MR angiography. As a recent development for vascular imaging, intraoperative fluorescence angiography (ICG) has been shown to be extremely helpful [12]. Whether iCTA and CT perfusion might be complementary is subject of a presently ongoing study. Compared to intraoperative MRI, iCT has a reduced sensitivity in the detection and delineation of low grade gliomas and small pituitary adenomas.

Intraoperative CT imaging is a versatile, cost efficient and easy to handle – easy to install technology, with the potential of a multidisciplinary use especially in spine, skull base and vascular surgery.

Conflict of interest statement We declare that we have no conflict of interest.

References

1. Rasmussen IA Jr, Lindseth F, Rygh OM, Berntsen EM, Selbekk T, Xu J, Nagelhus Hernes TA, Harg E, Håberg A, Unsgaard G (2007) Functional neuronavigation combined with intra-operative 3D ultrasound: initial experiences during surgical resections close to eloquent brain areas and future directions in automatic brain shift compensation of preoperative data. Acta Neurochir (Wien) 149:365–378
2. Roth J, Biyani N, Beni-Adani L, Constantini S (2007) Real-time neuronavigation with high-quality 3D ultrasound SonoWand in pediatric neurosurgery. Pediatr Neurosurg 43:185–191
3. Stummer W, Pichlmeier U, Meinel T, Wiestler OD, Zanella F, Reulen HJ, ALA-Glioma Study Group (2006) Fluorescence-guided surgery with 5-aminolevulinic acid for resection of malignant glioma: a randomised controlled multicentre phase III trial. Lancet Oncol 7:392–401
4. Black PM, Moriarty T, Alexander E 3rd, Stieg P, Woodard EJ, Gleason PL, Martin CH, Kikinis R, Schwartz RB, Jolesz FA (1997) Development and implementation of intraoperative magnetic resonance imaging and its neurosurgical applications. Neurosurgery 41:831–842, discussion 842–845
5. Nimsky C, Ganslandt O, Buchfelder M, Fahlbusch R (2006) Intraoperative visualization for resection of gliomas: the role of functional neuronavigation and intraoperative 1.5 T MRI. Neurol Res 28:482–487
6. Nimsky C, Ganslandt O, Hastreiter P, Wang R, Benner T, Sorensen AG, Fahlbusch R (2005) Preoperative and intraoperative

diffusion tensor imaging-based fiber tracking in glioma surgery. Neurosurgery 56:130–137, discussion 138
7. Hundt W, Rust F, Stäbler A, Wolff H, Suess C, Reiser M (2005) Dose reduction in multislice computed tomography. J Comput Assist Tomogr 29:140–147
8. Schichor C, Rachinger W, Morhard D, Zausinger S, Heigl TJ, Reiser M, Tonn JC (2009) Intraoperative computed tomography angiography with computed tomography perfusion imaging in vascular neurosurgery: feasibility of a new concept. J Neurosurg 112(4):722–728
9. Uhl E, Zausinger S, Morhard D, Heigl T, Scheder B, Rachinger W, Schichor C, Tonn JC (2009) Intraoperative computed tomography with integrated navigation system in a multidisciplinary operating suite. Neurosurgery 64:231–239, discussion 239–240
10. Zausinger S, Scheder B, Uhl E, Heigl T, Morhard D, Tonn JC (2009) Intraoperative computed tomography with integrated navigation system in spinal stabilizations. Spine 34(26):2919–2926
11. Ardeshiri A, Radina C, Edlauer M, Ardeshiri A, Riepertinger A, Nerlich A, Tonn JC, Winkler PA (2009) Evaluation of new radiolucent polymer headholder pins for use in intraoperative computed tomography. J Neurosurg 111(6):1168–1174
12. Raabe A, Nakaji P, Beck J, Kim LJ, Hsu FP, Kamerman JD, Seifert V, Spetzler RF (2005) Prospective evaluation of surgical microscope-integrated intraoperative near-infrared indocyanine green videoangiography during aneurysm surgery. J Neurosurg 103:982–989

Intraoperative CT in Spine Surgery

Wolf-Ingo Steudel, Abdullah Nabhan, and Kaveh Shariat

Abstract *Background*: In spinal instrumentation the misplacement of screws, cages and rods may cause neurovascular complications. Therefore a large variety of methods have been used in recent years to reduce such complications especially by navigation techniques and intraoperative three-dimensional fluoroscopy. The aim of this study is to answer the question: will intraoperative CT improve the efficiency of the treatment as well as the safety for the patient at the spinal instrumentation? Specific questions were: are the implants placed correctly and has decompression been performed sufficiently?

Methods: This is a prospective study in 100 patients mostly with degenerative diseases, tumours and trauma. 80 patients were treated by spinal instrumentation.

A helical CT (Somatom Emotion 2003) was used, which is firmly bound to the OR table by a track system.

Results: 569 implants were used: 159 vertebra body screws and plates, 88 cages, 154 pedicle screws, 73 facet joint screws and 95 rods.

There was malpositioning in seven patients (8.75%). 18 of 154 pedicle screws were misplaced, 2 of 88 cages, and 4 of 73 facet joint screws, for a total of 24 (7.6%).

Conclusions: Intraoperative CT is a useful tool to check the correct position of the implants used, the extent of decompression and the realignment as early as possible. It therefore reduces second operations. A postoperative CT is no longer necessary.

Keywords Intraoperative CT · Intraoperative imaging · Spinal instrumentation

Introduction

Thousands of spine operations are performed every year in Germany with instrumentation. Nowadays, the general standard is to perform intraoperative fluoroscopy as well as a post-operative X-ray control to demonstrate the correct placement of the implants.

Spine surgery, including decompression and stabilization, can be challenging due to the small geometry of important bony structures such as facets and pedicles, anatomical variations (i.e. the course of the vertebral artery within the axis), and the close anatomical relationship of the bone to the spinal cord, roots and vessels [1].

The use of spinal implants may cause neurovascular damage. This despite various intraoperative imaging technique largely depends on the disease as well as on the localization. It seems to be more difficult in the upper cervical, the thoracic spine, the thoracolumbal and lumbosacral region and in patients with idiopathic or degenerative scoliosis [2, 3]. There are various intraoperative methods of spinal image guidance such as preoperative CT-based navigation systems, standard fluoroscopy-based, 3D fluoroscopy and ultrasound methods [4–6]. According to the literature, 3D-fluoroscopy-assisted screw insertion increases the safety of a variety of routine and complex spinal procedures [5, 7]. The authors present a new device for intraoperative imaging in spinal instrumentation, the CT-suite – an operation theatre with a mobile CT. It allows real-time three-dimensional imaging of the whole spine and direct control and visualization of the correct position of the implants, the extent of decompression, especially in patients with degenerative diseases and tumours, and the realignment. In this study we refer exclusively to the correct positioning.

W.-I. Steudel (✉), A. Nabhan, and K. Shariat
Department of Neurosurgery, Universität des Saarlandes, Kirrberger Straße, 66421 Homburg, Saar, Germany
e-mail: ingo.steudel@uniklinikum-saarland.de

DOI 10.1007/978-3-211-99651-5_26,

Patients and Methods

CT-Suite

The CT-suite consists of a mobile CT system (SOMATOM Emotion 2003, Siemens, Erlangen). The system comprises a mobile gantry with a diameter of 70 cm and a scanning length of 153 cm, a mobile carbon OR table (Alphamaquet 1150, Maquet, Rastatt) and a workstation beside the OR with a visual and video connection. There is firm binding of the helical CT to the OR table by a track system in the floor. Slices can be done from 1 to 10 mm. There are different processing options like multiplanar reconstructions and angio sequences with visualization of patient's vessels. An examination of the spine is possible with adequate positioning from the atlanto-occipital junction to the sacrum. The operating table, which includes a special holding device for the head, is a special manufacture made out of carbon fibres (Fig. 1).

Patients

This is a prospective study on 100 patients of different ages and sexes undergoing spine surgery for a variety of indications and therefore using different types of spine fixation devices. The patient was placed in a supine or prone position, depending on the type of surgical procedure. A CT examination was performed after placement of the implants. The patient is always covered by a sterile plastic drape usually used to drape the microscope. The accuracy of the position of the implants was checked according to the classification of Liljenqvist et al. 1997 [8]. Repositioning was immediately done followed by another CT in medial penetration of the pedicles and in complete lateral pedicle screw penetration or in malplacement of a cage.

Results

This is a prospective study of 100 consecutive patients with different pathologies (Table 1). Among them are 20 patients without spinal instrumentation. Only a CT-guided biopsy was done in six patients with spinal tumour and only a decompressive procedure in another four. Only a facet joint infiltration was performed in ten patients with a degenerative radiculopathy.

The Somatotom was easy and safe to handle. Care had to be taken to avoid exposure of the OR team to radiation due to scanning. The team went from the OR into the workstation room during the CT-examination. The intraoperative scanning time amounted to 15–30 min. There was never a problem with sterility. The evaluation of the slices and correct positioning of the implants takes about 5 min. Visualization of the positioning of the implants was good on the images obtained from all patients.

569 different implants were used in 80 patients: 88 cages, 159 vertebra body screws and plates, 154 pedicle screws, 73 faced joint screws and 95 rods (Table 2). The vertebra body screws include four patients with dens screws; the facet joint screws include 8 Magerl screws.

There was an incorrect positioning of the implants in 7 of the 80 patients: The malpositioning occurred in 18 pedicle screws, 4 faced joint screws, twice in vertebra body replacement cages (Table 3).It was observed in two patients with a thoracic tumour, two patients with lumbar degenerative listhesis, two patients with severe spondylodiscitis at the cervical and lumbar region and another patient with a combination of degenerative and idiopathic listhesis.

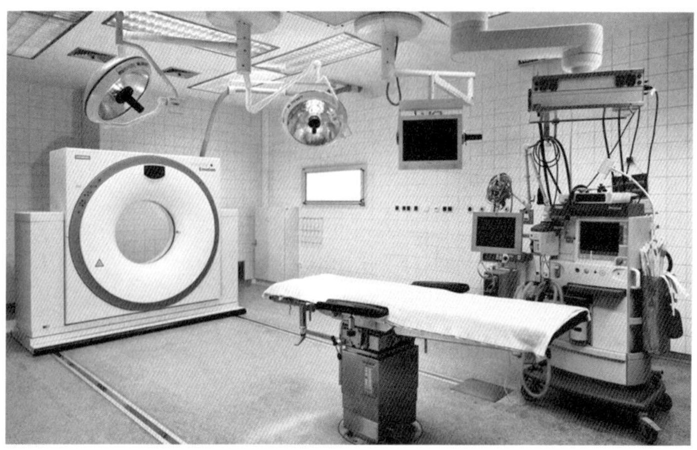

Fig. 1 Technical equipment: The operating room used for surgical procedures in which CT is planned to be used is equipped with a Siemens Somatom Emotion 2003 Helical CT

Table 1 Diagnoses: Characteristics of 100 patients and their surgical procedures

	Number of patients, $N=100$	Age (range)	Sex M	Sex F	Spinal instrumentations, $N=80$	Other procedures
Cervical myelopathy	16	41–86	10	6	16	–
Trauma	15	44–86	9	6	15	–
Radiculopathy	20	30–82	10	11	10	10[a]
Spinal tumor	16	37–80	12	4	6	6[b]
						4[c]
Degenerative lumbar listhesis	16	45–75	8	8	16	–
Congenital lumbar listhesis	7	32–57	3	4	7	–
Spondylodiscitis	4	42–86	3	1	4	–
Malformations	4	19–65	2	2	4	–
Chronic polyarthritis	2	43, 77	–	2	2	–

[a]Facet joint infiltration
[b]Biopsy
[c]Decompression

Table 2 Implants characteristics in 80 patients

Diagnoses	N	Cages	Vertebra body screws, plates	Pedicle screws	Cervical faced joint and transpedicular screws	Rods	Total
Cervical myelopathy	16	29	80	–	22	16	147
Trauma 3 × Kyphoplasty	15	13	12[a]	18	20[b]	12	65
Spinal tumor	6	6	12	14	19	9	60
Degenerative lumbar listhesis	16	19	–	74	–	32	125
Congenital lumbar listhesis	7	7	–	14	–	14	35
Radiculopathy	10	10	46	–	–	–	56
Spondylodiscitis	4	2	2	30	8[b]	8	50
Malformations	4	1	2	4	12[b]	4	23
Chronic Polyarthritis	2	1	5	–	2[b]	–	7
Total	80	88	159	154	73	95	569

[a]Including dens screwing four times
[b]Including 1 case with Magerl screwing C1/C2

Table 3 Evaluations of the positioning of the implants by intra-operative CT

Patients	$N=80$	$N=7$ (8.75%)
Type	Correct positionings	Incorrect
Pedicel screws	154	18
Facet joint screws	73	4
Cages	88	2
Total	315	24 (7.6%)

Discussion

Complication Rate

Various types of spinal operations have relatively different rates of complications, which may include damage to the spinal cord as well as the roots of the nerves, injury to vessels and nearby organs, and hardware failure. Complications occur mostly through malpositioning of the implants. The frequency of complications is given very differently in the literature. The complications depend on the difficulty of the spine operation: firstly on the kind of illness and its seriousness and secondly also on their localisation. There are differences in the region of the occipito-cervical, the thoraco-cervical, the cervical and the lumbo-sacral junction [9]. Furthermore, it has to be considered that the quality of the bone plays an important role as well in spinal instrumentation. A 14–55% misplacement rate for pedicle screws using standard techniques has been reported [10, 11].

Intraoperative Imaging in Spinal Instrumentation

It goes without saying that a wide range of treatments to complement conventional fluoroscopy has been developed over the years to improve and lower the complication rate.

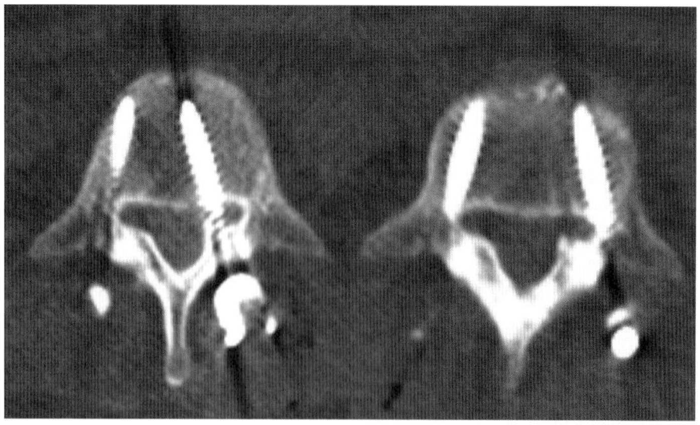

Fig. 2 Intraoperative CT Scan (*left*), orientation misplaced upper right screw. Immediate revision, control CT (*right*)

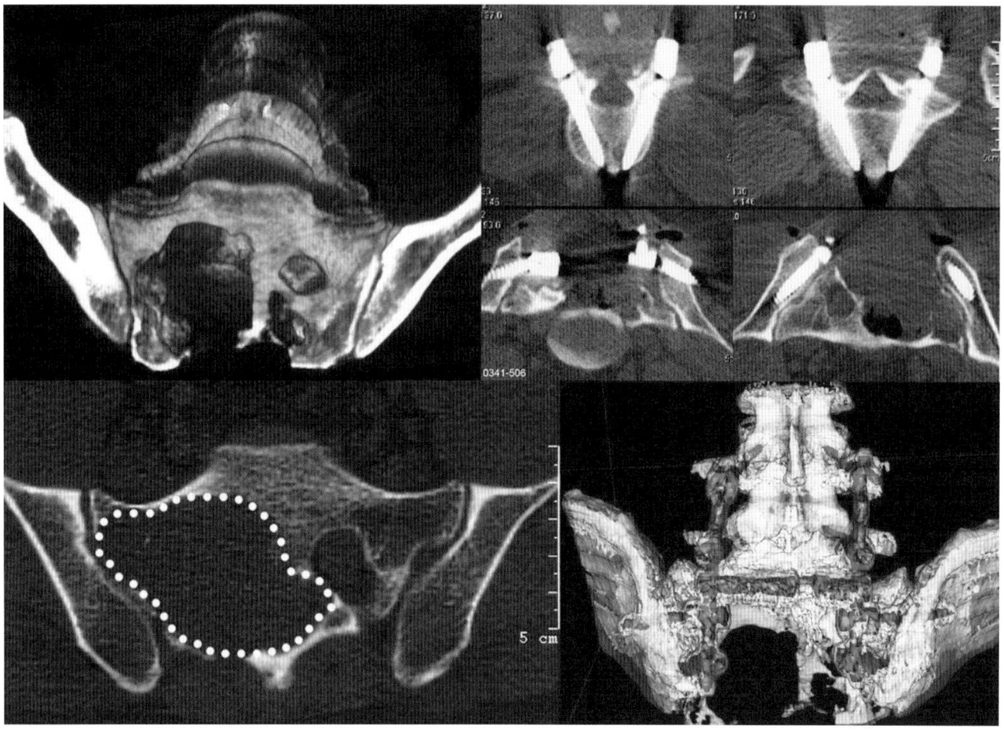

Fig. 3 Intra 3D-CT (*left*) three-dimensional CT (*left*) of a patient harbouring a sacral neurinoma. Tumour removal was done including lumbar-pelvic fixation (*right*). Note the different inclination and orientation of the screws within the spine and the pelvis

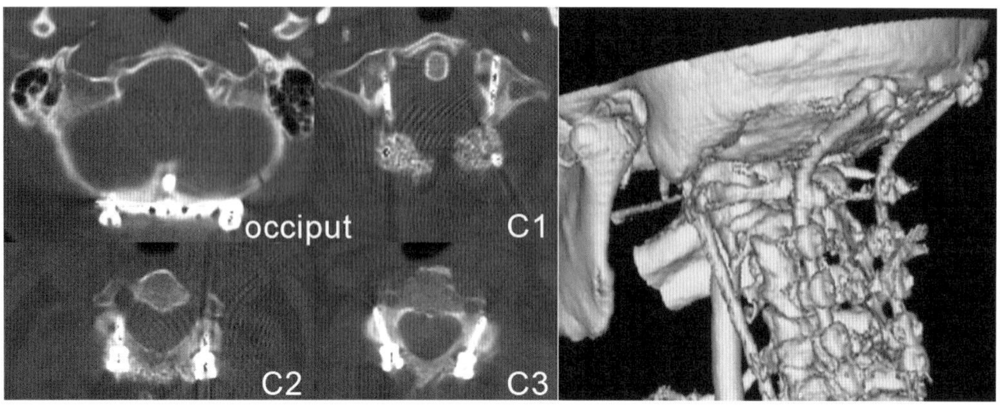

Fig. 4 Intraoperative CT Scan of a patient having received an occipital-cervical fixation down to C3. Note the different orientation of the screws within the occiput. The reconstruction of the position of the implants is on the right

These, such as spinal navigation or 3D fluoroscopy, aim to directly control the implanted material. 3D spinal image guidance significantly reduces the complications and breakage rate and improves safe and accurate placement of spinal instrumentation [11–22]. Using computer-navigated pedicle screw insertion in the lumbar spine, a postoperative CT control no longer seems to be necessary (Bostelmann et al. 2005). Other treatments are ultrasound-methods and neuromonitoring techniques as well as the direct intra-operative control of the anatomic structures of the implants [23]. However, technical problems still exist. It goes without saying that additional treatments are being tested in order to continue to increase the efficiency of the operative treatment. For this, the intraoperative computer tomography is particularly suitable.

Radiation Exposure

Radiation exposure of the surgeon, operating room staff and the patient is a concern when placing instrumentation with the aid of fluoroscopy [24]. This should also be considered in intraoperative CT imaging. But most patients are serially CT scanned after surgery, so in most cases there will be no additional radiation exposure.

Intraoperative CT

Intraoperative CT has the advantage of precisely verifying the position of the implants and the quality of the surgical procedure. In addition, the extent of decompression of the bony structure is nicely visualized. Unlike 3D-fluoroscopy, soft tissue and vessels can be demonstrated during the same examination (Figs. 2–4).

Intraoperative CT has the disadvantage of not being an online control device like spinal navigation. However, in contrast to spinal navigation, which has to be considered to be virtual, intraoperative CT in spinal surgery does verify that the surgical goals have been accomplished. In addition, it is especially useful when implants have to be placed in very different orientations, as for example within the craniocervical, cervicothoracic or spino-pelvic junction.

In addition to the value of this technique for intraoperative imaging, economical advantages should also be mentioned. Surgical revision procedures because of incomplete bony decompression or malpositioning of cages, screws and plates can be avoided. Postoperative CT examinations are no longer necessary to control implant positioning.

Conflict of interest statement We declare that we have no conflict of interest.

References

1. Deinsberger R, Regatschnig R, Ungersböck K (2005) Intraoperative evaluation of bone decompression in anterior cervical spine surgery by three-dimensional fluoroscopy. Eur Spine J 14(7): 671–676
2. Kim YJ, Lenke LG, Cheh G, Rew KD (2005) Evaluation of pedicle screw placement in the deformed spoine using intraoperativ plain radiographs: a comparison with computerized tomography. Spine 30(18):2084–2088
3. Lehmann RA Jr, Sasso RC, Helgeson MD, Dmitriev AE, Gill NW, Rosner MR, Riew KD (2007) Accuracy of intraoperatives plain radiographs to detect violations of intralaminar screws placed into the C2 vertebrae: a reliability study. Spine 32(26):3036–3040
4. Baldauf J, Müller U, Fleck S, Hinz P, Chiriac A, Schroeder HW (2008) The value of intraoperative three dimensional fluoroscopy in anterior decompressive surgery of the cervical spine. Zentralbl Neurochir 69:30–34
5. Holly LT (2006) Image-guided spinal surgery. Int J Med Robot 2 (1):7–15
6. Kantelhardt SR, Bock CH, Larseen J, Bockermann V, Schillinger W, Rohde V, Giese A (2009) Intraosseous ultrasound in the placement of pedicle screws in the lumbar spine. Spine 34(4):400–407
7. Ito Y, Sugimoto Y, Tomioka M, Hasegawa Y, Nakago K, Yagata Y (2008) Clinical accuracy of 3D fluoroscopy-assisted cervical pedicle screw insertion. J Neurosurg Spine 9(5):450–453
8. Liljenqvist UR, Halm HFH, Link T (1997) Pedicle screw instrumentation of the thoracic spine in idiopathic scoliosis. Spine 22 (19):2239–2245
9. Rath SA, Moszko S, Schäffner PM, Cantone G, Braun V, Richter HP, Antoniadis G (2008) Accuracy of pedicle screw insertion in the cervical spine for internal fixation using frameless stereotactic guidance. J Neurosurg Spine 8(3):237–245
10. Kotil K, Bilge T (2007) Accuracy of pedicle and mass screw placement in the spine without using fluoroscopy: a prospective clinical study. Spine 8(4):591–596
11. Nottmeier EW, Seemer W, Young PM (2009) Placement of thoracolumbar pedicle screws using three-dimensional image guidance: experience in a large patient cohort. J Neurosurg Spine 10 (1):33–39
12. Beck M, Moritz K, Gierer P, Gradl G, Harms C, Mittlmeier T (2009) Intraoperative control of pedicle screw position using three-dimensional fluoroscopy. A prospective study in thoracolumbar fractures. Z Orthop Unfall 147(1):37–42
13. Bostelmann R, Benini A (2005) Computer-navigated pedicle screw insertion in the lumbar spine. Oper Orthop Traumatol 17(2): 178–194
14. Darabi K, Reisch R, Müller-Forell W (1998) Intraoperative computed tomography in neurosurgery. In: Lemke HU et al (eds) Computed assisted radiology and surgery. Elsevier Science, New York, pp 605–508
15. Ebmeier K, Giest K, Kalff R (2003) Intraoperative computerized tomography for improved accuracy of spinal navigation in pedicle screw placement of the thoracic spine. Acta Neurochir 85:105–113
16. Haberland N, Ebmeier K, Grunewald JP, Hliscs R, Kalff R (2000) Incorporation of intraoperatives computerized tomography in a newly developed spinal navigation technique. Comput Aided Surg 5(1):18–27

17. Maier B, Zheng G, Ploss C, Zhang X, Welle K, Nolte LP, Marzi I (2007) A CT-free, intra-operative planning and navigation system for mnimally invasive anterior spinal surgera – an accuracy study. Comput Aided Surg 12(4):233–241
18. Nottmeier EW, Foy AB (2008) Placement of C2 laminar screws using three-dimensional fluoroscopy-based image guidance. Eur Spine J 17(4):610–615
19. Ondra SL, Marzouk S, Ganju A, Morrison T, Koski T (2006) Safety and efficacy of C2 pedicle screws placed with anatomic and lateral C-arm guidance. Spine 31(9):263–267
20. Papadopoulos EC, Girardi FP, Sama A, Sandhu HS, Cammisa FP Jr (2005) Accuracy of single-time, multilevel registration in image-guided spinal surgery. Spine J 5(3):263–267
21. Reinhold M, Bach C, Audigé L, Bale R, Attal R, Blauth M, Magerl F (2008) Comparison of two novel fluoroscopy-based stereotactic methods for cervical pedicle screw placement and review of the literature. Eur Spine J 17(4):564–575
22. Yukawa Y, Kato F, Yoshihara H, Yanase M, Ito K (2006) Cervival pedicle screw fixation in 100 cases of unstable cervical injuries: pedicle axis views obtained using fluoroscopy. J Neurosurg Spine 5 (6):488–493
23. Magit DP, Hilibrand AS, Kirk J, Rechtine G, Albert TJ, Vaccaro AR, Simpson AK, Grauer JN (2007) Questionnaire study of neuromonitoring availability and usage for spine surgery. J Spinal Disord Tech 20(4):282–289
24. Nardone E, Chen J, Maggio W, Nauta H (1996) The value of intraoperatives ultrasonography in cervical corpectomy: assessment by postoperative computed tomography. Neurosurgery 39:971–975

O-Arm Guided Balloon Kyphoplasty: Preliminary Experience of 16 Consecutive Patients

Frédéric Schils

Abstract Balloon kyphoplasty is now widely used for the treatment of vertebral compression fractures. Excellent pain relief is achieved with cement injection, but the safety of the procedure relys on excellent radiological exposure. The balloon kyphoplasty technique is usually performed using one or two C-Arm devices to allow correct antero-posterior (AP) and lateral view throughout the surgical procedure. By definition, this minimal invasive spine surgery is associated with radiation exposure for both the patient and the surgeon. In our center, we recently moved from this way of proceeding to the use of an O-Arm image guidance system to perform cement augmentation in vertebral fractures.

To our knowledge, there is no clinical series describing the O-arm use in a balloon kyphoplasty procedure published in the scientific literature. We prospectively evaluate on 16 consecutive patients, the feasibility of the O-Arm guided kyphoplasty procedure with the original, usual tools, and we measured the fluoroscopy time and the X-ray exposure. We didn't experience any device related problem and demonstrated a significant reduction of X-ray exposure and time of fluoroscopy. We believe that using this new intraoperative system, the overall time of surgery and fluoroscopy could still be reduced in a near future.

Keywords Balloon kyphoplasty · Minimal invasive spine surgery · O-arm intraoperative system · Radiation exposure during surgery · Vertebral compression fractures

F. Schils
Department of Neurosurgery, Clinique Saint Joseph, Liège 74, rue de Hesbaye, B-4000 Liège, Belgium
e-mail: frederic.schils@chc.be

Introduction

Vertebral compression fractures represent a major concern amongst elderly patients, frequently leading to pain, disability and quality of life deterioration.

As the population continues to age, the challenge for the treatment of osteoporosis and its complications will become increasingly prevalent [1–3].

Conservative, non-surgical management of vertebral compression fractures is actually challenged by surgical minimally invasive procedures based upon cement augmentation (vertebroplasty and kyphoplasty). These procedures may offer fast and sustained pain reduction, improved function while avoiding the kyphosis progression [4, 5]. Most of the studies in this field were conducted to demonstrate clinical benefit, vertebral deformity correction or risk of cement leakage. To achieve these positive results, the procedure is performed under C-arm radiological exposure in most surgical teams. The C-arm is then manipulated from AP to lateral view several times to provide secure pedicular access and continuous fluoroscopy is required during cement injection. Although an impressive number of papers about kyphoplasty is found in the literature, there is few data about time of fluoroscopy during the surgery or dose of X-ray exposure for the patient and his surgeon [6, 7]. Due to the growing popularity of minimally invasive spinal surgery, efforts to reduce X-ray exposure during the surgical time to the patient and the surgeon may become a critical goal in the future. We believe that new intraoperative tools such as the O-arm system will help us to reach this objective.

Materials and Methods

We started in February 2009 a prospective inclusion of new vertebral compression osteoporotic fractures admitted in our hospital for 3 months.

DOI 10.1007/978-3-211-99651-5_27,

Patients were eligible for enrolment if they experienced one to three acute painful vertebral compression fractures from T5 to L5. Tumors, metastasis and myelomas vertebral fractures were excluded from the study principally due to kyphoplasty reimbursement difficulties in theses indications in Belgium. An hyperintense signal on MRI T2 and/or STIR sequences was required for the definition of recent compression fractures.

Osteopenia evaluation through a bone mineral density dexa scan was systematically used in all of our included patients. Candidates for the study also had to have a minimal back pain score of 5 on a 0–10 visual analog scale (VAS).

Exclusions criteria were chronic fractures, rupture of any kind of the posterior wall of the vertebra, infection conditions and any neurological deficit.

Procedure

Kyphoplasty was performed in all patients with classical instruments: introducers, inflatable bone tamps and polymethylmethacrylate bone cement and delivery devices (manufactured by Medtronic Spine LLC, Sunnyvale, CA, USA), by a bilateral pedicular or extrapedicular approach.

All the procedures were conducted under general endotracheal anaesthesia.

Time of fluoroscopy by procedure and by level were precisely recorded as well as the radiation dose exposure. Overall operation time was also collected for each patient.

Population and O-Arm System

16 consecutive patients with 21 compression osteoporotic fractures were involved in this prospective study and underwent balloon kyphoplasty guided by the O-arm intraoperative system.

O-Arm system is an intraoperative system based on a conventional RX tube and a Flat Panel detector (40 × 30 Varian). The system is used both in 2D mode, as a conventional fluoroscopic system, and in 3D mode. The 3D mode is particularly useful to evaluate cement distribution in the vertebral body immediately after the procedure and to detect any cement leakage, in the vascular system, the spinal canal or the intervertebral disc (Fig. 1).

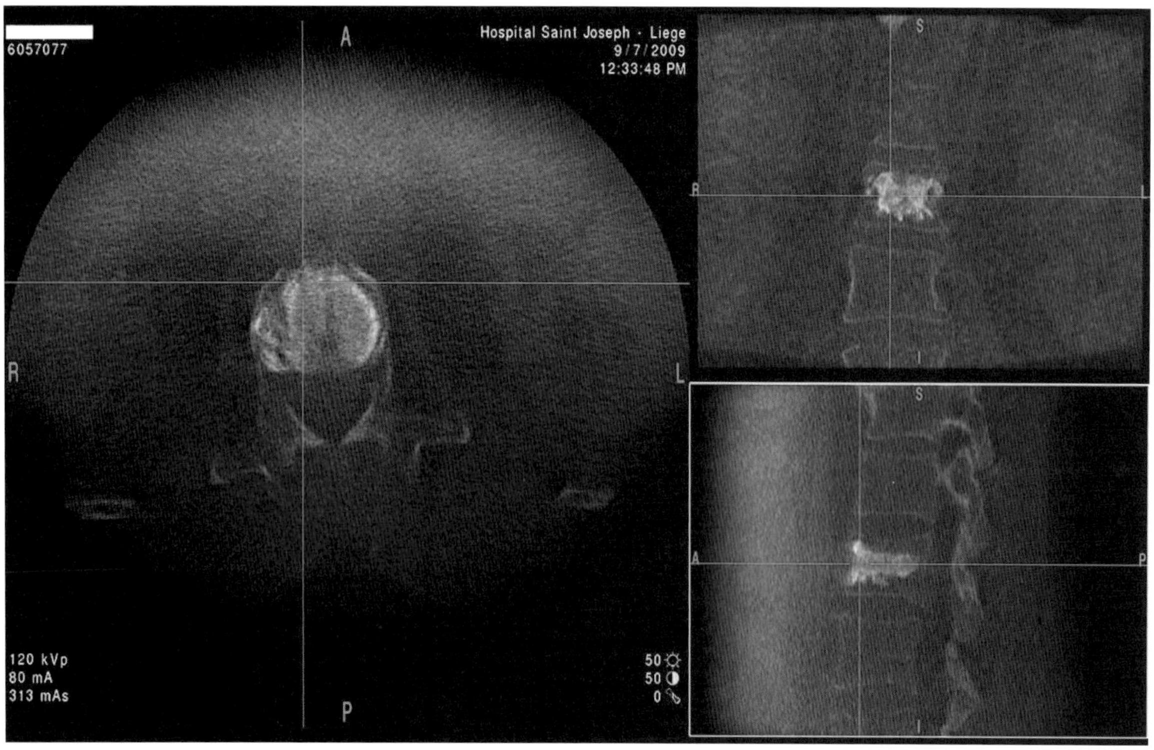

Fig. 1 Illustration of a 3D O-Arm acquisition at the end of the surgical procedure showing, in the three usual planes, the cement distribution in the fractured vertebral body

Results

16 consecutive patients with 21 vertebral compression fractures were evaluated during the three months of the study. Mean patient age was 70 (range 62–88) and male/female ratio was 19%/81%. All the 21 fractured levels were treated (12 patients with one level, three patients with two levels and one patient with three levels). 53% of the levels were lumbar and 47% were thoracic. The mean surgical time (skin to skin) for the procedure was 41 min (range 32–54) with a mean fluoroscopy procedure time of 3.23 min (range 2.68–5.04). The mean fluoroscopy time by level dropped to 2.43 min. Mean irradiation dose by procedure was 247 mGy and mean irradiation dose by level was 192.5 mGy. All patients were addressed for a 3D scan performed at the end of the procedure. No cement leakage was found outside the vertebral body, avoiding any other postoperative radiological control.

Discussion

Several recent studies demonstrated the efficacity of kyphoplasty to provide pain relief, improvement of quality of life, limitation in days of restricted activity and reduction of analgesic use [8–11]. Recent publications also demonstrated the superiority of the kyphoplasty procedure over the non surgical, conservative treatment [5, 12]. Due to these observations, and the growing prevalence of osteoporotic vertebral compression fractures, the number of balloon kyphoplasty procedures increased within the past years [13]. Data concerning physician and patient X-ray exposure during these minimally invasive procedures as well as precise measurement of fluoroscopy time are still lacking.

To perform a kyphoplasty, the surgeon has to achieve perfect visualisation of the pedicles in several planes and has to be aware of possible cement leakage during the filling of the vertebral body. On an another hand, he has to try to reduce as much as possible the X-ray exposure for the patient, the OR staff and of course himself. These two goals may seem to be opposite. Several efforts to reduce the radiation time and dose are made through computer navigation kyphoplasty [14], and preventive protection measures such as protective coats, gloves and glasses. In computer navigation kyphoplasty, an additional incision has to be performed in order to attach the reference clamp, and the cement filling of the vertebral body is still performed under conventional fluoroscopy.

Moreover, navigation represents also an additional recurrent financial cost to the patient, or the hospital, due to numerous disposable single use tools. The O-Arm intraoperative system allows high spatial resolution and may offer several memorized positions (i.e. AP or lateral) reducing the manipulation required with a C-arm use and by the way the amount of unprofitable images and XR doses.

The surgeon may always rely on the same AP and lateral predefined views during the overall procedure which allows for higher security level and perfect visualisation of the vertebral body in any plane at any time. In addition, the immediate 3D acquisition at the end of the procedure is able to detect early, any complication and dispense the need of a radiological postoperative control.

These O-arm kyphoplasty procedures were conducted exactly the same way as C-arm procedures, without any modification of the instruments and without any additional recurrent cost. We observed a mean fluoroscopy time of 3.23 min for a total procedure duration of 41 min. The time of fluoroscopy by level was 2.43 min. These numbers seems to be lower than those classically reported for operative or fluoroscopy time. For example, Izadpanah et al. recently reported an operative time superior to 60 min with computer navigation balloon kyphoplasty [14]. Boszczyk et al. observed a mean fluoroscopy time of 3.8 min for single level cases [7]. We are convinced that, due to a natural learning curve, our values should be lowered in a very near future. New intraoperative devices such as the O-arm may provide the surgeon easy and excellent radiological exposure of bone structures and may help to drastically reduce the X-ray exposure, the time of fluoroscopy and the duration of the overall procedure with a highest degree of security.

Conflict of interest statement We declare that we have no conflict of interest.

References

1. Borgstrom F, Zethraeus N, Johnell O et al (2006) Cost and quality of life associated withe osteoporosis-related fractures in Sweden. Osteoporos Int 17:637–650
2. Johnell O, Kanis JA (2006) An estimate of the worldwide prevalence and disability associated with osteoporotic fractures. Osteoporos Int 17:1726–1733
3. Silverman SL, Minshall ME, Shen W, Harper KD, Xie S (2001) The relationship of health-related quality of life to prevalent and incident vertebral fractures in postmenopausal women with osteoporosis: results from the Multiple Outcomes of Raloxifene Evaluation Study. Arthritis Rheum 44:2611–2619
4. Garfin SR, Buckley RA, Ledlie J (2006) Balloon kyphoplasty for symptomatic vertebral body compression fractures result in rapid, significant, and sustained improvement in back pain, function, and quality of life for elderly patients. Spine 31:2213–2220
5. Grafe IA, Da Fonseca K, Hillmeier J et al (2005) reduction of pain and fracture incidence after kyphoplasty: 1-year outcomes of prospective controlled trial of patients with primary osteoporosis. Osteoporos Int 16:2005–2012
6. Seibert JA (2004) Vertebroplasty and kyphoplasty: Do fluoroscopy operators know about radiation dose, and should they want to know? Radiology 232:633–634

7. Boszcyk B, Bierschneider M, Panzer S et al (2004) Fluoroscopy radiation exposure of the kyphoplasty patient. Eur Spine J 15:347–355
8. Wardlaw D, Cummings S, Van Meirhaeghe J et al (2009) Efficacy and safety of balloon kyphoplasty compared with non-surgical care for vertebral compression fracture (FREE): a randomised controlled trial. Lancet 373:1016–1024
9. Eck J, Nachtigall D, Humphreys S et al (2008) Comparison of vertebroplasty and balloon kyphoplasty for treatment of vertebral compression fractures: a meta-analysis of the literature. The Spine Journal 8:488–497
10. Bouza C, Lopez T, Magro et al (2006) Efficacy and safety of balloon kyphoplasty in the treatment of vertebral compression fractures: a systematic review. Eur Spine J
11. Ledlie J, Renfro M (2006) Kyphoplasty treatment of vertebral fractures: 2-year outcomes show sustained benefits. Spine 31:57–64
12. Komp M, Ruetten S, Godolias G (2004) Minimally invasive therapy for functionally unstable osteoporotic vertebral fracture by means of kyphoplasty: prospective comparative study of 19 surgically and 17 conservatively treated patients. J Miner Stoffwechs 11 (Suppl 1):13–15
13. Tarantino U, Cannata G, Lecce D et al (2007) Incidence of fragility fractures. Aging Clin Exp Res 19 :7–11
14. Izadpanah K, Konrad G, Südkamp P (2009) Computer navigation in balloon kyphoplasty reduces the intraoperative radiation exposure. Spine 34:1325–1329

Intraoperative Ultrasonography

Intra-operative Imaging with 3D Ultrasound in Neurosurgery

Geirmund Unsgård, Ole Solheim, Frank Lindseth, and Tormod Selbekk

Abstract In recent years the quality of ultrasound (US) imaging has improved considerably. The integration of three dimensional (3D) US with neuronavigation technology has created an efficient and inexpensive tool for intra-operative imaging in neurosurgery. Our experience is based on more than 900 operations with the intra-operative 3D ultrasound equipment SonoWand® and some operations with the research equipment Custux X. The technology has been applied to improve surgery of intraparencymal brain tumours, but has also been found to be useful in a vide range of other procedures, such as operations for cavernomas, skull base tumours, medulla lesions, arteriovenous malformations (AVMs) and for endoscopy guidance. Compared to intraoperative magnetic resonance imaging (ioMRI), 3D US technology is advantageous in different ways: It is flexible and can be used in any operation theatre. There is no need for special instruments, and no need for radiologists or technicians. It adds very little extra time to the operation, and the investment-costs are considerably lower than for ioMRI.

Keywords Arteriovenous malformation · Cavernous malformation · Intraoperative imaging · Intraoperative ultrasound · Resection control · Tumor

Introduction

Neuronavigation systems have become standard tools for planning of neurosurgery, but conventional systems have limited value during the operation of brain tissue lesions due to the brain shift. There is an obvious need for intra-operative imaging. One way to solve this is by intra-operative MRI. Another solution is 3D ultrasound. The main advantages with 3D ultrasound compared to ioMRI are considerably lower cost and higher flexibility. The disadvantage is that the surgeon must learn how to use the technology to obtain optimal benefit.

System Description

SonoWand® is an integration of a high-end ultrasound scanner and a navigation system [1]. It can be used as an ordinary real-time 2D ultrasound scanner or solely as a standard neuronavigation system based on pre-operative MRI. It also can import MRI volumes with functional MRI and tractography. However, it is the intra-operative 3D ultrasound capabilities coupled with navigation technology that makes the system unique. Both 3D tissue and 3D angiography (power Doppler) volumes can be acquired by tilting an ultrasound probe over the area of interest. SonoWand® enables simultaneous navigation in both MR and US volumes. The volumes can be displayed either as axial/coronal/sagital slices or as oblique any plane slices, steered by the pointer or different surgical equipment (biopsy forceps, CUSA or endoscope) with a tracking frame attached. Repeated 3D US uptakes during the operation, makes it possible to navigate in an updated map that is very close to the real time.

Brain Shift

In lesions with sharp definition of the lesion border we always found that the 3D ultrasound was correct (<2 mm off) while navigation based on pre-operative MRI was 2–10 mm off from the true position. We also found considerable inaccuracies in cases where there should be no brain shift, for example in skull base tumours, reflecting the problem with accurate registration in spite of using fiducials.

G. Unsgård (✉) and O. Solheim
Department of Neurosurgery, St Olav University Hospital, Trondheim, Norway
The Norwegian University of Science and Technology, Trondheim, Norway
e-mail: geirmund.unsgard@ntnu.no

F. Lindseth and T. Selbekk
The Norwegian University of Science and Technology, SINTEF Health Research, Trondheim, Norway

M.N. Pamir et al. (eds.), *Intraoperative Imaging*, Acta Neurochirurgica Supplementum, Vol. 109,
DOI 10.1007/978-3-211-99651-5_28, © Springer-Verlag/Wien 2011

Image Quality

The brain is very homogenous, thus enabling ultrasound imaging with very few artefacts. Modern high-end scanners with probes that are tuned optimally for brain scanning will therefore depict all types of lesions with very good image quality (Fig. 1). We mostly use a 5 MHz (4–8 MHz) probe, which gives optimal image quality at a distance of 2.5–6 cm from the probe. For superficial imaging a 12 MHz linear probe is optimal. It produces superb image quality from the first mm down to a depth of 4 cm (Fig. 3).

To be able to obtain good images throughout the operation, the patient must be positioned so that the planned access to the lesion becomes vertical. In that way saline will stay in the cavity during image acquisition. Our experience is that when this is considered during the planning, it is almost always possible to obtain a setup where good quality images can be acquired throughout the operation. The only situation where it is not possible to use ultrasound, is when operating in sitting position.

Delineation of Tumours

Before using the 3D US images to guide operations, we felt it was important to do a study to investigate the concurrence between image delineation of the tumours and histopathology. We found that there was a good concurrence between the image interpretation at the biopsy site and the histopathology for biopsies sampled close to the image borders of the tumours [2].

Image Guided Resection

By putting the optical tracking frame on the resection instrument (CUSA) it is possible to continuously follow the position of the CUSA during resection [3]. By looking partly in the microscope and partly on the navigation monitor the surgeon can follow the position of the CUSA tip relative to tumour borders and blood vessels. By making several 3D US

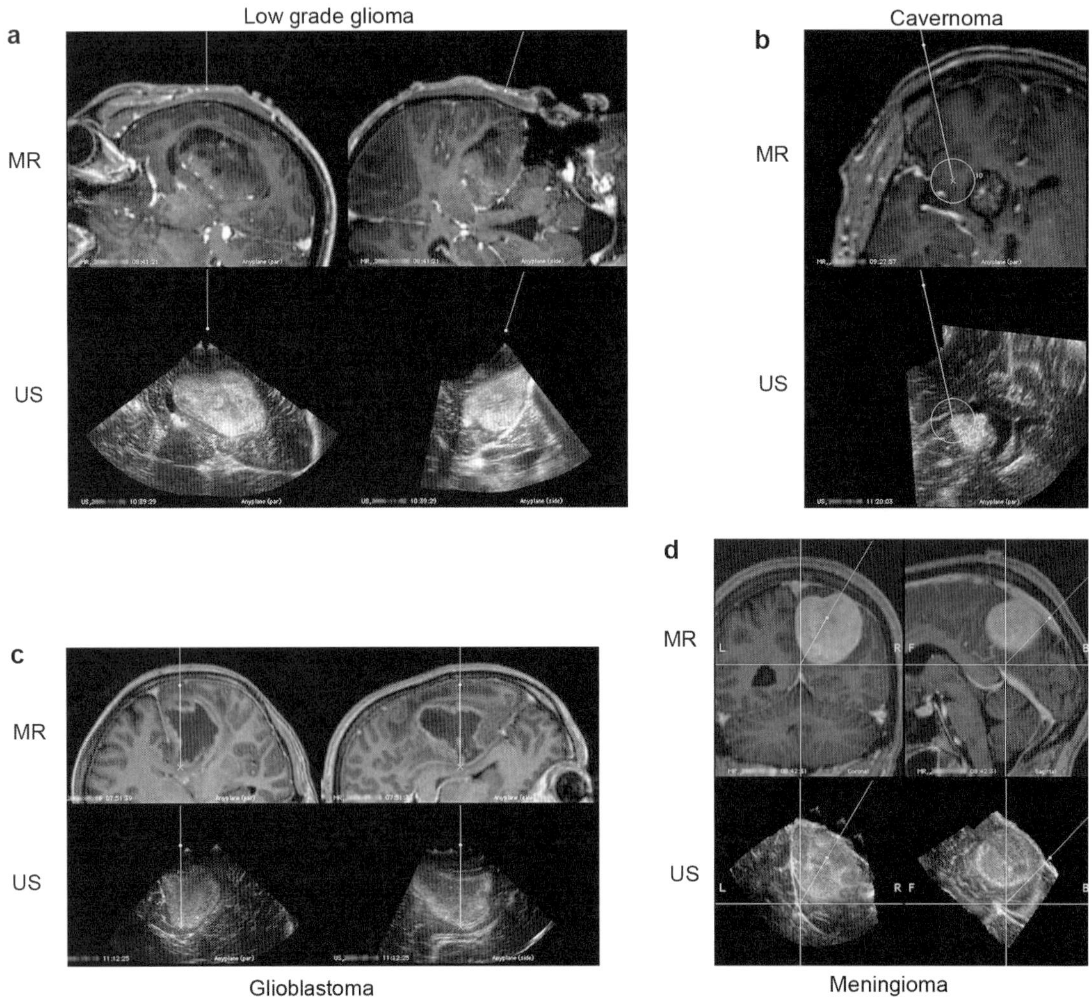

Fig. 1 Simultaneous display of preoperative MR data and intraoperative US data in the SonoWand system, during surgery of a low grade astrocytoma (**a**), cavernoma (**b**), glioblastoma (**c**) and meningioma (**d**)

uptakes throughout the operation the surgeon get a continuous update of his operating site compared to important anatomical structures. This gives the surgeon information in a much more dynamic and precise way than the microscope interface in conventional neuronavigation systems.

Resection Control

We have shown that residual tumour tissue missed during microsurgery can be detected and removed with 3D US [4]. When all suspected tumour volume in the 3D US images has been removed, there is usually no tumour left in the postoperative MRI. It is also our experience that when we stop the resection before the removal of all the high echo volumes on 3D US due to eloquent area, we find tumour suspected areas on postoperative MRI. At the end of the operation there is sometimes artefacts in the wall of the resection cavity (rim-effect). In those cases the images cannot be trusted for the last 1 or 2 mm of resection.

Impact on Surgery

The use of intra-operative 3D US has influenced our operations in different ways:

(a) It is easier to obtain a more radical resection of tumour tissue.
(b) It is much easier to do resections through very small openings in the normal tissue. Thus we are less invasive in the normal tissue with lower patient morbidity.
(c) We can work safer, faster and with more confidence because the position of the resection instrument relative to an updated map of blood vessels, tumour borders and normal tissue is continuously monitored.

Applications Where 2D US Has Improved the Surgical Technique in Transsphenoidal Approaches

A small side-looking high frequency linear array ultrasound probe can be used to ensure orientation in the midline for the transsphenoidal approach, to identify important neurovascular structures to be avoided during surgery and for identification of normal pituitary tissue and residual tumour (Fig. 2), The image resolution is far better than what can be achieved by current clinical MRI technology.

Applications Where 3D US Has Improved the Surgical Technique

Low Grade Gliomas

(a) *Very small low grade tumours.* These low grade tumours would be very difficult to operate without the 3D US technology (Fig. 3).
(b) *Large tumours in eloquent areas.* Preoperative fMRI and tractogrphy imported into the system is useful for the planning of the operation. Intra-operative 3D US combined with the preoperative fMRI and tractogrphy makes it possible to decide the limits of the resection in the 3D US volumes. We found that in cases where the low grade gliomas have "occupied" the expected site of the pyramidal tract without causing neurological deficit, the tract was always pushed away by the tumour. Resection of the tumour visible on 3D US did not create any permanent neurological deficit. Our conclusion is that low grade gliomas in eloquent area depicted by 3D US can be removed without risking permanent neurological deficit.

High Grade Gliomas

3D US is useful to identify and resect all the extensions from the high grade gliomas (Fig. 4). Even resection of high grade gliomas in eloquent areas can be done with very low morbidity and significant improvement of function [5].

Cavernomas

With conventional navigation it is possible to miss small cavernomas due to brain shift and registration error. With 3D US all cavernomas are precisely imaged and localized. Even very small brain stem cavernomas without lesion on the surface are easy to find with 3D US.

Skull Base Tumours

Resection with guided CUSA is useful to minimize the trauma to the normal tissue, especially in meningiomas. After an image guided subcapsular removal, the dissection of the capsule is easier and less traumatic [6]

This navigated subcapsular removal can proceed faster and with more confidence because the surgeon will have 3D update of both the tumour borders and the blood vessels [7], and the surgeon knows exactly the progression of the operation.

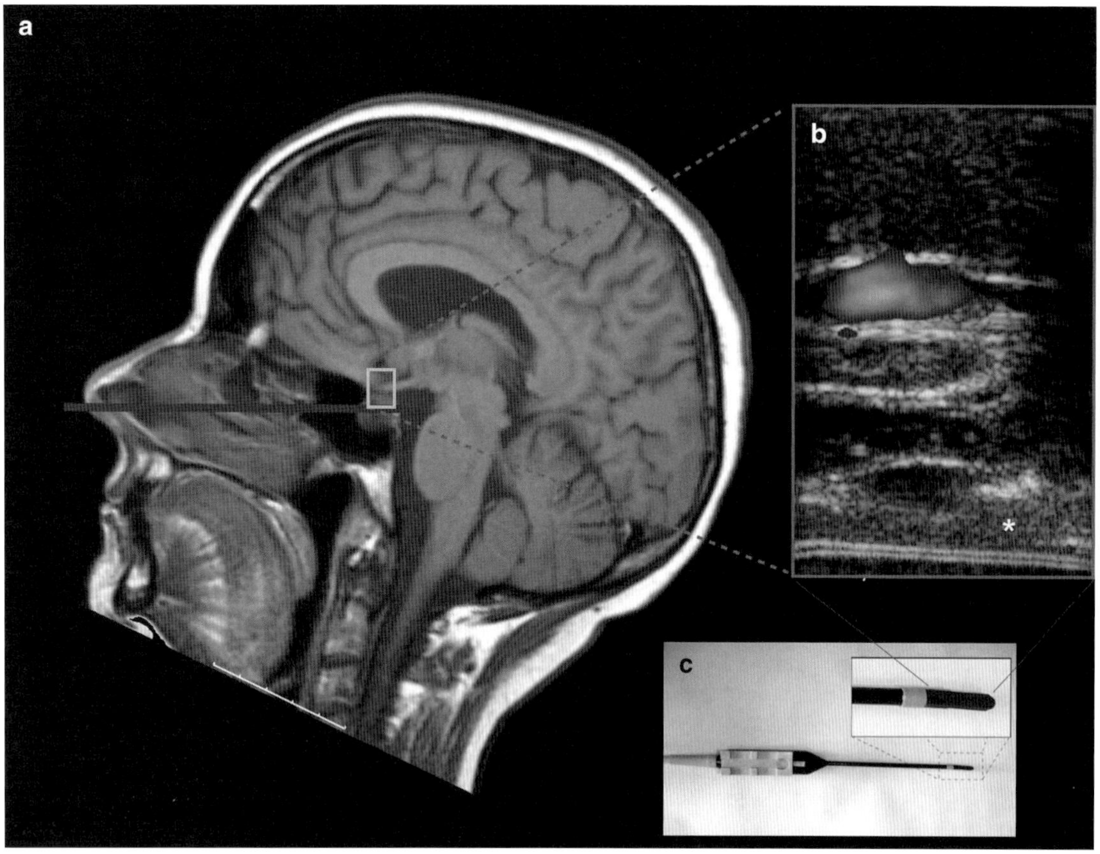

Fig. 2 The use of ultrasound in pituitary surgery, with the probe and dimensions of the image overlaid on a MR image (**a**) and the intraoperative US image showing residual tumour (indicated with *) (**b**), and the US probe with the side firing transducer array (**c**). In the middle of figure **b** is the optic chiasm, and above is the communication artery

Biopsy

It is possible to make 3D US imaging through a15 mm burr holes. Biopsies are sampled either free hand with calibrated biopsy forceps or with a guide.

Ventricle Catheter

3D US imaging of the side ventricle through 15 mm burr hole. Ventricle catheter with the stiff core is fixed to a tracking device, calibrated and then the catheter act as a pointer. The core is removed when the catheter is in the ventricle.

Endoscopy

3D US is useful to guide the endoscope in complex multi-cystic anatomy [8].

Medulla Lesions

3D US has been successfully used for identification and biopsy of lesions in medulla [9], and for syrinxoperations.

AVM

We have used 3D US angiography and stereoscopic display of 3D MR angiography for early identification and clipping of feeders in AVMs [10]. In 25 patients 57 of 70 feeders described in MR angiography could be identified and clipped in the beginning of the operation. This reduced the pressure in the AVM and made it much easier to dissect the AVM from the normal tissue.

Pros and Cons of 3D US

Navigated 3D US (SonoWand®) is not just another navigation system. It is an intraoperative imaging system and a real

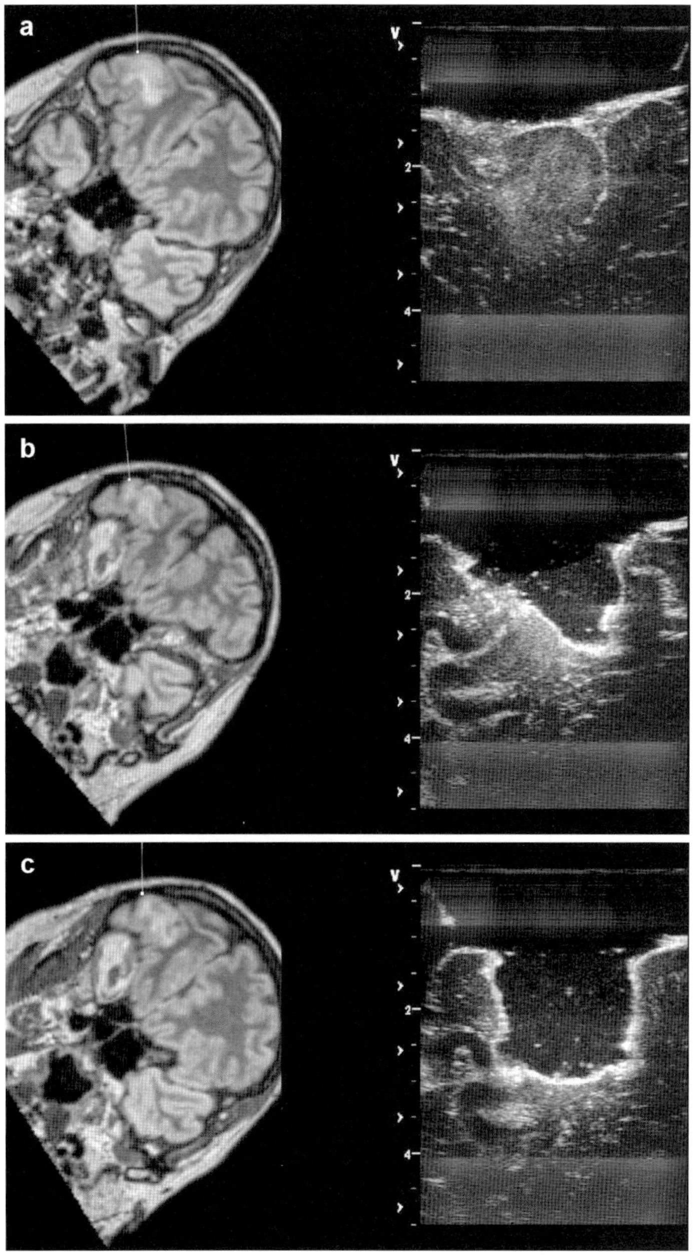

Fig. 3 Preoperative MRI and intraoperative US of a low grade glioma, before (**a**), during (**b**), and at the end of (**c**) resection of the tumour. In figure **b** residual tumour is seen to the left of the cavity

competitor to intraoperative MRI. Even though there has been no randomized study to look at efficiency of 3D US and ioMRI in obtaining radical tumour removal, we have indications to believe that 3D US gives similar intraopertive information as ioMRI. What are the pros and cons when comparing 3D US to ioMRI?

- 3D US is flexible; it can be used in any operation theater
- It is useful for nearly every type of neurosurgical operation
- There is no need for special surgical instruments when using 3D US
- Neither is there any need for extra people (i.e. technicians and radiologists)
- The active use of 3D US claims very little extra time during surgery.
- Investment costs of a SonoWand® system is very low compared to any ioMRI.
- When using 3D US, neurosurgeons have to be more aware of the positioning of the patient.
- Neurosurgeons have to learn to make and interpret US images
- The entire brain cannot be displayed in one 3D US volume, only the region of interest around the surgical approach.

There is a tendency among neurosurgeons to think that US is a too simple technology. They are not aware of the huge

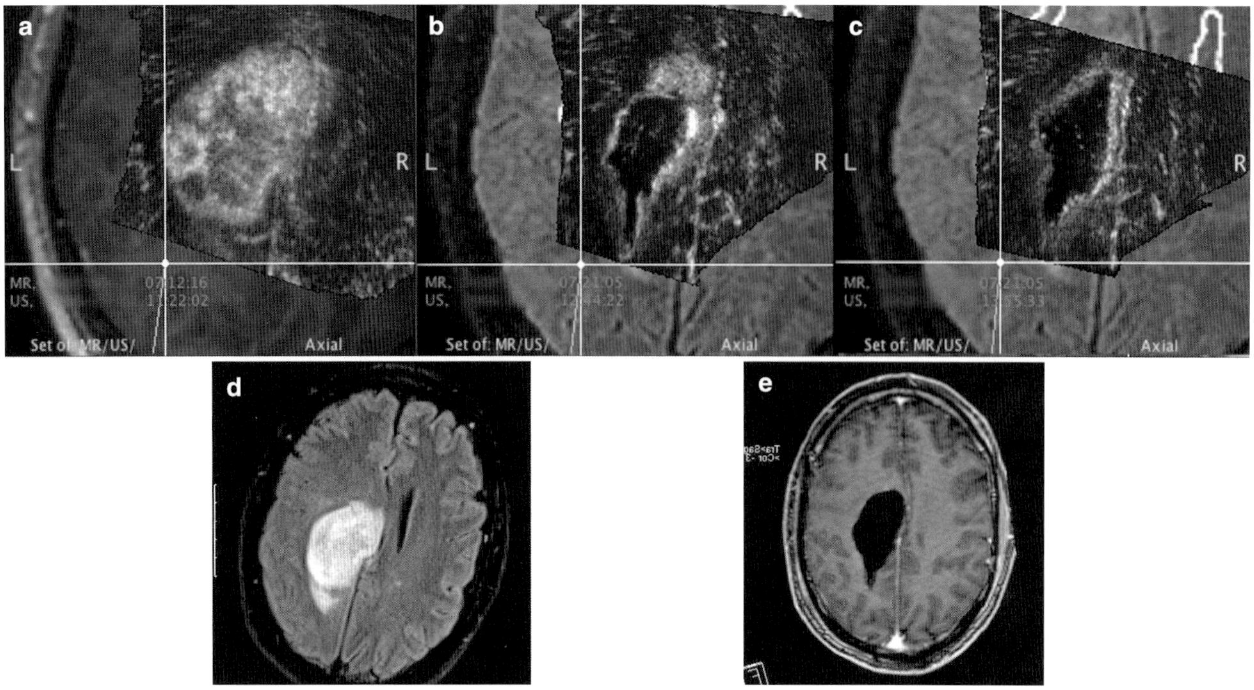

Fig. 4 A high grade glioma. Intraoperative 3D US overlayed the 3D MRI volume, before start of resection (**a**), during resection (**b**) and at the end of resection (**c**). In the lower row is shown preoperative MRI (**d**) and postoperative MRI one day after operation (**e**)

improvement made to US in recent years. Some neurosurgeons are a little afraid of the challenge of learning a new technology. It feels safer to leave the intraoperative imaging to the radiologists. These feelings should not dominate our thinking. Due to the rapidly increasing health care coast we all have an obligation to always go for the most cost-effective equipment.

Conclusion

Intra-operative 3D US is a flexible and inexpensive tool for minimizing the operation injury and increasing the efficiency and confidence of the surgeon during brain and medulla operations. To have optimal benefit from this tool, the surgeon has to learn some principles for the using of this technology in brain operations.

Conflict of interest statement One of the authors (GU) holds 0.5% of the shares in SonoWand.

References

1. Gronningsaeter A, Kleven A, Ommedal S, Aarseth TE, Lie T, Lindseth F, Langø T, Unsgård G (2000) SonoWand, an ultrasound-based neuronavigation system. Neurosurgery 47(6): 1373–1380
2. Unsgaard G, Selbekk T, Müller TB, Ommedal S, Torp HS, Myhr G, Bang J, Nagelhus Hernes TA (2005) Ability of navigated 3D ultrasound to delineate gliomas and metastases – comparison of image interpretations with histopathology. Acta Neurochir 147 (12):1259–1269
3. Unsgaard G, Rygh OM, Selbekk T, Müller TB, Kolstad F, Lindseth F, Hernes TAN (2006) Intra-operative 3D ultrasound in neurosurgery. Acta Neurochir 148(3):235–253
4. Unsgård G, Ommedal S, Muller T, Gronningsaeter A, Hernes TAN (2002) Neuronavigation by intraoperative 3D ultrasound, initial experiences during brain tumor resections. Neurosurgery 50(4): 804–812
5. Gulati S, Berntsen EM, Solheim O, Kvistad KA, Håberg A, Selbekk T, Torp SH, Unsgaard G (2009) Surgical resection of high-grade gliomas in eloquent regions guided by blood oxygenation level dependent functional magnetic resonance imaging, diffusion tensor tractography, and intraoperative navigated 3D ultrasound. Minim Invasive Neurosurg 52(1):17–24
6. Solheim O, Selbekk T, Linseth F, Unsgård G (2009) Navigated resection of giant intracranial meningiomas based on intraoperative 3D ultrasound. Acta Neurochir 151:1143–1151
7. Rygh OM, Selbekk T, Lindseth F, Müller TB, Hernes TAN, Unsgaard G (2006) Intraoperative navigated 3D ultrasound angiography in surgery. Surg Neurol 66:581–592
8. Rygh OM, Cappelen J, Selbekk T, Lindseth F, Hernes TANH, Unsgård G (2006) Endoscopy guided by an intraoperative 3D ultrasound based neuronavigation system. Minim Invasive Neurosurg 49(1):1–9
9. Kolstad F, Rygh OM, Selbekk T, Unsgaard G, Nygaards OP (2006) Three-dimensional ultrasonography navigation in spinal cord tumor surgery. Technical note. J Neurosurg Spine 5(3): 264–270
10. Unsgaard G, Ommedal S, Rygh O, Lindseth F (2005) Operation of arteriovenous malformations assisted by stereoscopic navigation-controlled display of preoperative magnetic resonance angiography and intraoperative ultrasound angiography. Neurosurgery 56(2 Suppl):281–290

Intraoperative 3-Dimensional Ultrasound for Resection Control During Brain Tumour Removal: Preliminary Results of a Prospective Randomized Study

Veit Rohde and Volker A. Coenen

Abstract *Introduction*: The amount of resection is closely related to survival in brain tumours. To enhance resection, especially intraoperative magnetic resonance imaging (MRI) has been applied. The aim of this prospective, randomized study was to test if intraoperative 3-D ultrasound likewise can be used for resection control.

Methods: 16 patients, who underwent surgery for intraaxial tumours in non-eloquent brain areas, were initially included into this prospective study. In two patients, the small size of the craniotomy hindered intraoperative ultrasound imaging. In 14 patients, 3-D ultrasound images were obtained before and after opening of the dura, during tumour removal, prior to evaluation by a blinded investigator for identification of tumour remnants, and after dura closure. Seven patients were randomized to complete tumour removal according to the impression of the surgeon (group 1). Seven patients were randomized to incomplete tumour removal (tumour remnant <1 cm) (group 2); in these patients, the neurosurgeon intentionally left a tumour remnant prior to evaluation by the blinded investigator. The tumour remnant was then removed. It was tested if 3-D ultrasound can correctly identify complete and incomplete tumour resection. All patients underwent early postoperative MRI.

Results: In two patients (one each of the two groups) the image quality was too poor for a meaningful intraoperative evaluation. In the six patients randomized for incomplete tumour removal, 3-D ultrasound correctly identified tumour remnants in four patients (67%). In six patients randomized for complete tumour removal, 3-D ultrasound confirmed complete tumour resection in three patients. In addition, 3-D ultrasound identified correctly one tumour remnant in a patient randomized for complete tumour removal. Thus, the sensitivity for tumour remnant detection increased to 71% (five of seven patients) and that of confirmation of complete tumour removal was 60 % (three of five patients).

Conclusion: The number of investigated patients is still to low to allow definite conclusions. However, the study results suggest, that 3-D ultrasound is especially helpful for detection of overseen brain tumour tissue.

Keywords Glioma · Intraoperative imaging · Intraoperative ultrasound · Resection control

Introduction

Several studies have indicated that time to recurrence in benign tumours and survival in malignant tumours is closely related to the extent of resection [1]. With the aim to enhance the amount of resection, intraoperative magnetic resonance imaging (MRI) and intraoperative computerized tomography (CT) has been introduced into the neurosurgical routine [2–4]. Intraoperative MRI has the major disadvantages of being expensive and requiring special non-ferromagnetic equipment, if the operation is done in the environment of the scanner, or special transport solutions which usually result in a reduced number of intraoperative re-investigations. The image quality of CT is inferior to that of MRI, which even more holds true in the intraoperative situation, and prevented the wide-spread use of intraoperative CT for resection control.

The aim of this preliminary study was elucidate the potential role of intraoperative 3-dimensional ultrasound for intraoperative resection control.

V. Rohde (✉)
Department of Neurosurgery, Georg-August-University Goettingen, Robert-Koch-Strasse 40, 37075 Goettingen, Germany
Department of Neurosurgery, Aachen University of Technology (RWTH), Aachen, Germany
e-mail: veit.rohde@med.uni-goettingen.de

V.A. Coenen
Department of Neurosurgery, Aachen University of Technology (RWTH), Aachen, Germany
Department of Neurosurgery, University of Bonn, Bonn, Germany

Patients and Methods

A total number of 16 patients (nine men, seven women, mean age 44 years) were included in this prospective randomized trial. The patients underwent microsurgery for cerebral metastases ($n=8$), malignant glioma ($n=6$), and benign astrocytoma WHO II ($n=2$); tumours which would not have been completely resectable were excluded. Informed consent was obtained from the patients and approval of the local ethic committee was given. Directly before surgery, imaging studies were performed with a 1.5 T MR scanner. All patients underwent an MRI anatomic navigation sequence preoperatively with fixed skin fiducials. After administration of gadolinium, a T1-weighted 3-D fast field echo sequence was obtained in axial sections for 3-D volume rendering. The data set was transferred to the SonoWand system (Mison AS, Trondheim, Norway), which is an ethernet-linked neuronavigational system with a high-end ultrasound scanner. The system has the capability to trace the navigated ultrasound probe, which allows acquiring 3-D ultrasound volume sets which can be used again for neuronavigational purposes. The system displays preoperative MRI data and the 3-D-ultrasound data simultaneously.

Prior to surgery, the patient was randomized either to complete tumour removal according to the neurosurgeons impression (group 1) or to incomplete tumour removal (group 2); in group 2, the neurosurgeon intentionally left a tumour remnant (<1 cm) prior to intraoperative ultrasound evaluation 4 (see below). Intraoperative 3-dimensional ultrasound images were obtained at five defined surgical steps: 1-after trephination, before dura opening; 2-after dura opening; 3-at least once during tumour removal; 4-prior to evaluation by the blinded investigator (Fig. 1); 5-after dura closure. No information about the course of the operation was given to the investigator, and the video screens displaying the intraoperative microscopic images of the resection cavity were turned off during evaluation. The investigator was allowed to see even repetitively all ultrasound images before making a final decision. It is noteworthy that the intentionally left tumour remnant was removed after the ultrasound evaluation. It was investigated if intraoperative 3-D ultrasound allows differentiating between complete tumour resection and tumour remnants. If the neurosurgeon has had the impression of complete tumour removal but the blinded investigator believed to have identified a tumour remnant on the intraoperative 3-D ultrasound image tissue was harvested for histopathological investigation.

Results

In two patients standard craniotomy was not large enough for obtaining 3-dimensional ultrasound images; sweeping the ultrasound probe was hindered by the craniotomy margins. In additional two patients the image quality was too poor for a meaningful intraoperative evaluation, leaving 12 patients for evaluation. In the six patients randomized for incomplete tumour removal, 3-D ultrasound correctly identified tumour remnants in four patients (67%). In six patients randomized for complete tumour removal, 3-D ultrasound confirmed complete tumour resection in three patients. In this group, 3-D ultrasound identified correctly one tumour remnant which was overseen by the surgeon and which was subsequently removed after histopathological confirmation of tumour tissue. Thus, the sensitivity of 3-D ultrasound for tumour remnant detection increased to 71% (five of seven patients) and the sensitivity for complete tumour removal was 60% (three of five patients). In two patients, tumour remnants were assumed on 3-D ultrasound, but not proven histologically. Overall, the intraoperative situation was correctly predicted by ultrasound in 8 of 12 patients (67%).

Discussion

Increased radicality of tumour resection is closely related to longer survival and longer progression-free survival in malignant brain tumours. The ill-defined border of intraaxial brain tumours often prevents complete resection only with the aid of the operating microscope. Thus, many attempts have been made to improve the amount of resection. Stummer and coworkers convincingly showed that the preoperative intake of 5-aminolevulinic acid and the intratumoural synthesis of fluorescent protoporphyrine IX, which "stains" the tumour, allow reducing the percentage of incompletely resected malignant gliomas significantly [5]. Even more effort was made to bring MRI into the operating room for detection of overseen tumour. Intraoperative MRI has a high sensitivity for detection of tumour remnants, even if extravasation of contrast medium sometimes produces tumour-like artefacts [6]. The high costs of intraoperative MRI and the necessity of using non-ferromagnetic instruments if the operation is done in the environment of the scanner hindered the wide-spread application of intraoperative MRI. A two-room solution with the need of a patient transport system is time-consuming and limits the number of repetitive investigations.

Intraoperative ultrasound has been proposed as a less expensive and repetitively available alternative to MRI. Already in 1989 LeRoux and coworkers showed that the intraoperative ultrasound image correlates well with histopathological findings, and Woydt et al. in 1996 confirmed these results [7, 8]. Both groups used 2-dimensional ultrasound for identifying the tumour borders, and assumed that ultrasound has the potential to enhance the amount of resection. Unsgaard and coworkers, using a 3-dimensional ultrasound in combination with neuronavigation, took tissue samples between 2 and 7 mm from the tumour border as

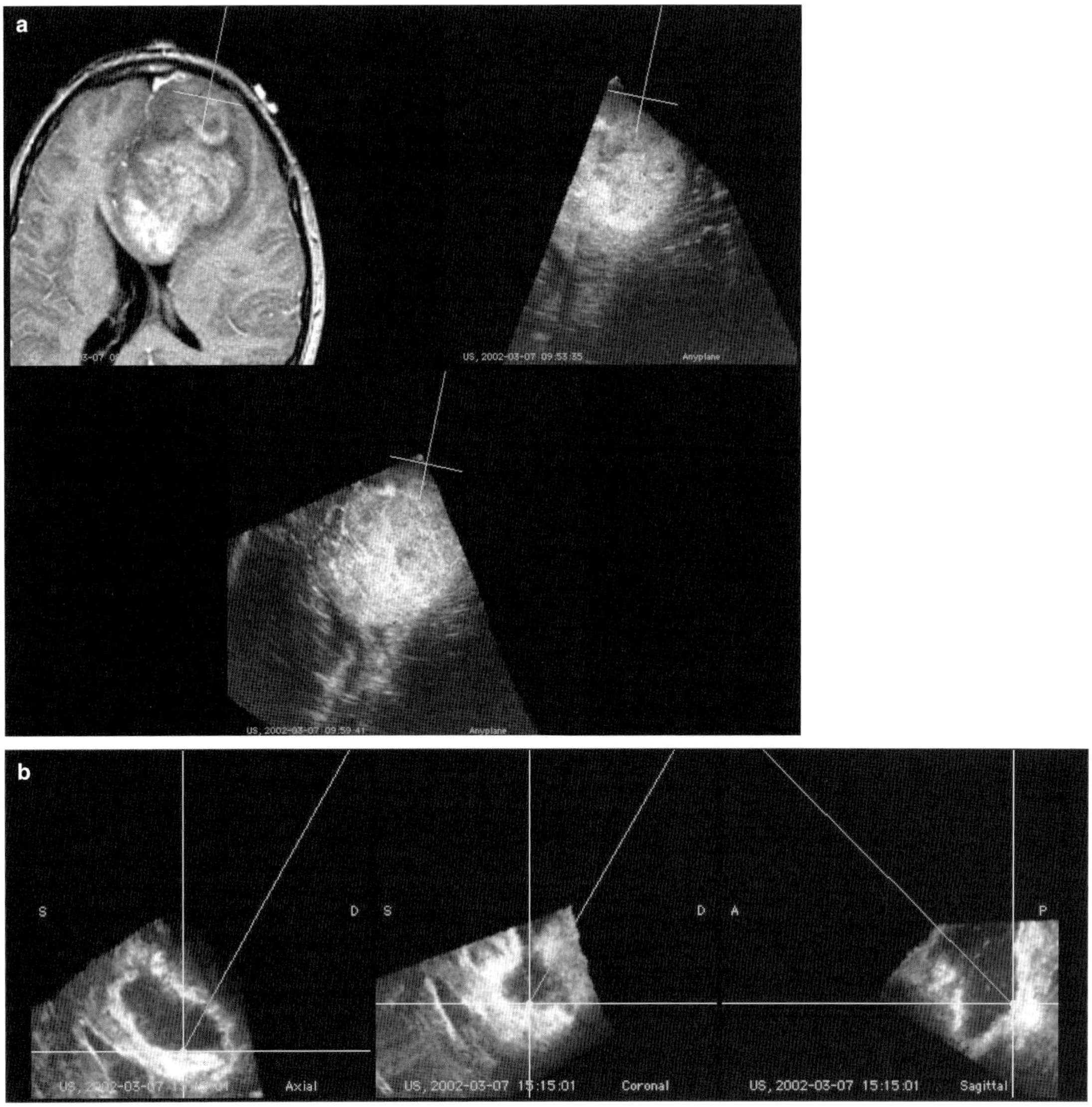

Fig. 1 Intraoperative 3-D ultrasound before (**a**) and after resection (**b**) of a large frontal anaplastic oligodendroglioma

seen on intraoperative 3-dimensional ultrasound images and found a positive correlation of histology and ultrasound imaging in 74% low-grade gliomas, 83% astrocytomas WHO grade III, 77% glioblastomas and 100% metastases [9]. Interestingly, studies focussing on resection control are rare: Lindner et al. used 3-dimensional ultrasound for resection control in 23 patients with metastases, gliomas, cysts, lymphomas and meningiomas. Resection control was possible in 78%, and the intraoperative ultrasound finding correlated with the post-operative MRI in 63.6% of the cases [10]. Gerganov et al. performed a prospective clinical trial and compared the reliability of intraoperative MR imaging and 2-dimensional ultrasound for tumour remnant detection. Tumour remnants were seen in 21 of 26 patients by MR imaging; with ultrasound two tumour remnants detectable by MRI were missed, which indicates that resection control with intraoperative MR imaging might be more effective [11]. Our study is the first prospective randomized study addressing the issue of resection control. As the investigator who has to evaluate the ultrasound images was blinded with respect to tumour remnant or total resection, an overall correct prediction rate of 67% is acceptable, and in line with the few published data [10]. Our study further indicates that the strength of 3-D ultrasound is the identification of tumour remnants; tumour remnants were correctly identified in 71%, which is remarkable because the tumour remnants which have been intentionally left behind were less than 1 cm in diameter. The data of Gerganov et al. suggest that the detection rate would have been higher in cases of larger tumour remnants [11]. The correct identification of complete tumour removal was poorer with 60%; in two of three patients tiny blood clots in the resection cavity were mistaken for tumour remnants. The same phenomenon already has been described [11]. It can be assumed that the predictive value would have been higher if the investigator would have had a close knowledge of the resection cavity or would have performed the operation himself: Suspicious areas of poor delineation between tumour margin and normal brain tissue requiring a closer look up with ultrasound and blood clots which can be mistaken for tumour on ultrasound imaging already would have been known.

The low number of patients in our prospective study limits its value. Nonetheless, our data indicate that 3-dimensional ultrasound has the potential to control resection effectively during brain tumour surgery. The use of contrast-enhancing agents possibly would facilitate identification of overseen tumour further [12].

Conclusion

During brain tumour surgery, 3-dimensional ultrasound can be used for resection control. Intraoperative ultrasound seems to be most valuable for detection of tumour remnants and, thereby, offers the chance to enhance the extent of tumour removal. Proof of already completed total tumour resection by 3-D ultrasound is not as reliable. Normal brain tissue altered by microsurgical resection can be mistaken as tumour. To definitively define the value of 3-dimensional ultrasound for resection control, a larger study is required.

Conflict of interest statement We declare that we have no conflict of interest.

References

1. Lacroix M, Abi-Said D, Fourney DR, Gokaslan ZL, Shi W, DeMonte F, Lang FF, McCutcheon IE, Hassenbusch SJ, Holland E, Hess K, Michael C, Miller D, Sawaya R (2001) A multivariate analysis of 416 patients with glioblastoma multiforme: prognosis, extent of resection, and survival. J Neurosurg 95:190–198
2. Albert FK, Forsting M, Sartor K, Adams HP, Kunze S (1994) Early postoperative magnetic resonance imaging after resection of malignant glioma: objective evaluation of residual tumor and its influence on regrowth and prognosis. Neurosurgery 34:45–61
3. Uhl E, Zausinger S, Morhard D, Heigl T, Scheder B, Rachinger W, Schichor C, Tonn JC (2009) Intraoperative computed tomography with integrated navigation system in a multidisciplinary operating suite. Neurosurgery 64(5 Suppl 2):231–239, discussion 239–240
4. Wirtz CR, Knauth M, Staubert A, Bonsanto MM, Sartor K, Kunze S, Tronnier VM (2000) Clinical evaluation and follow-up results for intraoperative magnetic resonance imaging in neurosurgery. Neurosurgery 46:1112–1122
5. Stummer W, Pichlmeier U, Meinel T, Wiestler OD, Zanella F, Reulen HJ, ALA-Glioma Study Group (2006) Fluorescence-guided surgery with 5-aminolevulinic acid for resection of malignant glioma: a randomised controlled multicentre phase III trial. Lancet Oncol 7:392–401
6. Knauth M, Aras N, Wirtz CR, Dörfler A, Engelhorn T, Sartor K (1999) Surgically induced intracranial contrast enhancement: potential source of diagnostic error in intraoperative MR imaging. AJNR Am J Neuroradiol 20:1547–1553
7. LeRoux PD, Berger MS, Ojemann GA, Wang K, Mack LA (1989) Correlation of intraoperative ultrasound tumour volumes and margins with preoperative computerized tomography scans. An intraoperative method to enhance tumour resections. J Neurosurg 71:691–698
8. Woydt M, Krone A, Becker G, Schmidt K, Roggendorf W, Roosen K (1996) Correlation of intra-operative ultrasound with histopathological findings after tumour resection in supratentorial gliomas. Acta Neurochir 138:1391–1398
9. Unsgaard G, Selbekk T, Brostrup Müller T, Ommedal S, Torp SH, Myhr G, Bang J, Nagelhus Hernes TA (2005) Ability of navigated 3D ultrasound to delineate gliomas and metastases-comparison of image interpretations with histopathology. Acta Neurochir 147:1259–1269
10. Lindner D, Trantakis C, Renner C, Arnold S, Schmitgen A, Schneider J, Meixensberger J (2006) Application of intraoperative 3D ultrasound during navigated tumor resection. Minim Invasive Neurosurg 49:197–202
11. Gerganov VM, Samii A, Akbarian A, Stieglitz L, Samii M, Fahlbusch R (2009) Reliability of intraoperative high-resolution 2D ultrasound as an alternative to high-field strength MR imaging for tumor resection control: a prospective comparative study. J Neurosurg 111:512–519
12. Kanno H, Ozawa Y, Sakata K, Sato H, Tanabe Y, Shimizu N, Yamamoto I (2005) Intraoperative power Doppler ultrasonography with a contrast-enhancing agent for intracranial tumors. J Neurosurg 102:295–301

Advantages and Limitations of Intraoperative 3D Ultrasound in Neurosurgery. Technical note

Oliver Bozinov, Jan-Karl Burkhardt, Claudia Miranda Fischer, Ralf Alfons Kockro, René-Ludwig Bernays, and Helmut Bertalanffy

Abstract Three-dimensional ultrasound (US) technology is supposed to help combat some of the orientation difficulties inherent to two-dimensional US. Contemporary navigation solutions combine reconstructed 3D US images with common navigation images and support orientation. New real-time 3D US (without neuronavigation) is more time effective, but whether it further assists in orientation remains to be determined. An integrated US system (IGSonic, VectorVision[2], BrainLAB, Munich Germany) and a non-integrated system with real-time 3D US (iU22, Philips, Bothell, USA) were recently compared in neurosurgical procedures in our group. The reconstructed navigation view was time-consuming, but images were displayed in familiar planes (e.g., axial, sagittal, coronal). Further potential applications of US angiography and pure US navigation are possible. Real-time 3D images were displayed without the need for an additional acquisition and reconstruction process, but spatial orientation remained challenging in this preliminary testing phase. Reconstructed 3D US navigation appears to be superior with respect to spatial orientation, and the technique can be combined with other imaging data. However, the potential of real-time 3D US imaging is promising.

Keywords Image-guided surgery · Reconstructed 3D ultrasound · Intraoperative sonography · Neuronavigation · Real-time 3D ultrasound · Neurosurgery

Introduction

Recently it has become increasingly attractive to add intraoperative imaging data to the surgical planning/procedure [1], and ultrasound offers an inexpensive and quick alternative to MRI or CT [2–9]. However, neurosurgeons usually have little experience with the interpretation of intraoperative (mainly oblique) US views and have instead been trained to interpret MRI images in the axial, coronal and sagittal display [4, 8, 10, 11]. The growing spread of ultrasound use has been influenced by significant improvements in image quality over the past few years as well as the fact that probes have become small enough to fit into a minimally invasive craniotomy [9, 11, 12]. Our own group has described a two-platform model [13] and a one-platform solution for the combination of MRI neuronavigation and US [11]. This led to increased routine use of this technology by several neurosurgeons previously unfamiliar with US [11, 14]. The recent development of real-time 3D US probes raises the question of whether one modality can replace the other. We present here our initial experience.

O. Bozinov (✉), J.-K. Burkhardt, C.M. Fischer, R.A. Kockro, R.-L. Bernays, and H. Bertalanffy
Department of Neurosurgery, University Hospital, Frauenklinikstrasse 10, 8091 Zürich, Switzerland
e-mail: oliver.bozinov@usz.ch

3D Ultrasound-Assisted Image-Guided Neurosurgery

Technical Aspects

The technical characteristics of the VectorVision[2] (BrainLAB, Heimstetten, Germany) system and the integrated US device (IGSonic) have been reported previously in detail [11]. Briefly, the precalibrated current IGSonic Probe 3000 (4–9 MHz frequency) with multi-focus imaging is connected to the VectorVision navigation station, and the infrared cameras track the reflective marker spheres of a reference clamp attached directly to the probe. No registration of the US probe is necessary when using a one-platform solution. The system provides real-time US information and overlays the ultrasonic images or puts them next to the corresponding classical images of the navigation system. Acquisition of a 3D data set is possible with the most recent version of the system.

M.N. Pamir et al. (eds.), *Intraoperative Imaging*, Acta Neurochirurgica Supplementum, Vol. 109,
DOI 10.1007/978-3-211-99651-5_30, © Springer-Verlag/Wien 2011

3D Ultrasound Acquisition and Display

After craniotomy, the first US investigation is performed once the US probe is automatically registered (approx. 30 s). The draped touch screen allows alteration by the surgeon, who can adjust the parameters for better visualisation and acquire the 3D US dataset. The US probe is moved over the field of interest. Each real-time 2D US image is saved with the specific coordinates recognised by the navigation system through the US reference star. A maximum of 256 slices were collected per dataset, and US data were reconstructed based on spatial resolution. The acquisition time for an entire 256-image set was 1–2 min, and the calculation time was 30–60 s each. Each 3D US dataset can be displayed in the usual planes of neuronavigation (axial, coronal and sagittal) (Fig. 1a, b). If a tumour border has been outlined preoperatively (segmented image) in the MRI or CT dataset, it can be optionally superimposed onto the 3D US image (Fig. 1a, b).

Ultrasound Angiography

As previously reported by our group, intraoperative landmarking of anatomical structures (e.g., vessels or tumour remnants) by US is possible and may be fused to intraoperative 3D US reconstructions [10]. This might provide additional useful intraoperative information for the surgeon in cases of complex glioma or vascular lesion [9, 10, 15, 16]. Three-dimensional acquisition in the Doppler mode stores only colour-coded Doppler information, which in summary will reconstruct a 3D vessel superimposed on the navigation images of choice (Fig. 1b). Eventually, this leads to intraoperative non-invasive angiography. Our system did not provide any surface-rendering program, as CT or MRI angiographies do. Other groups have demonstrated enhanced image qualities by additional surface-rendering [9, 17]. Thus, more promising tools may be available in the near future.

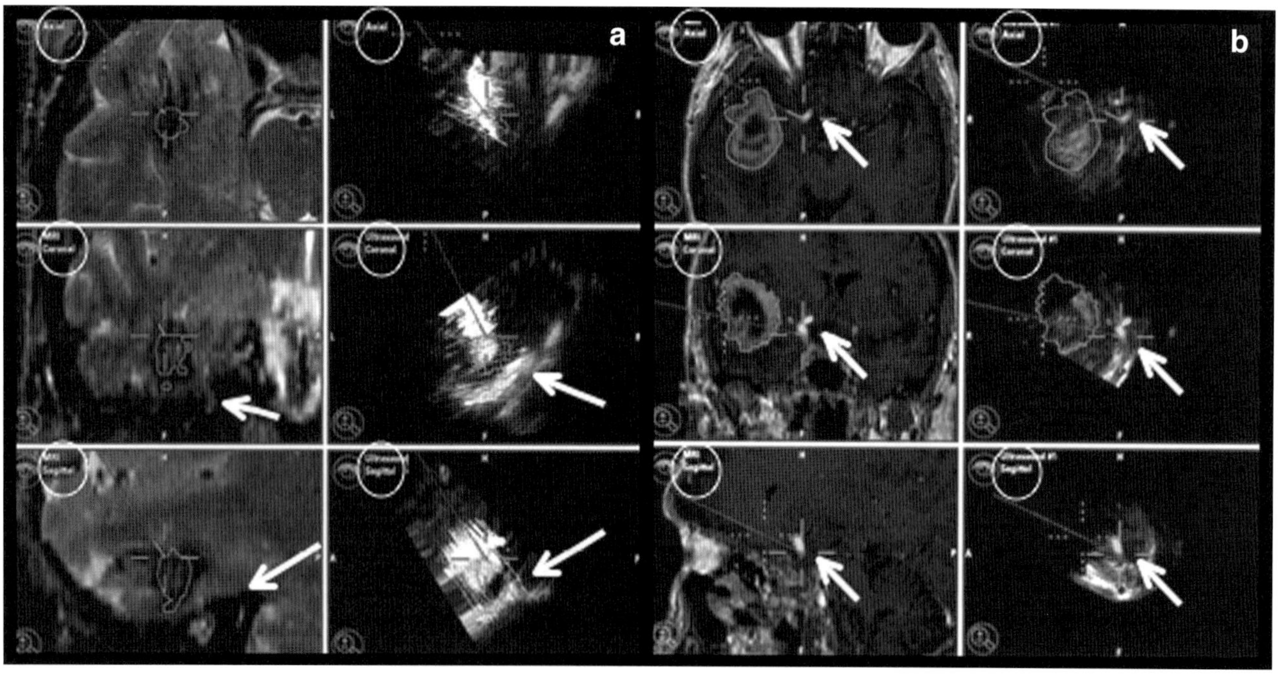

Fig. 1 The *right* side of the *left* navigation screenshot (**a**) of a *right* temporal cavernoma displays all three familiar planes (axial, coronal and sagittal) of the 3D ultrasound reconstruction data corresponding to their preoperative navigated MRI data on the *left* side (highlighted by the *small circles* in all six windows). The *arrows* point to the skull base below the cavernoma (hyperintensive in ultrasound reconstruction). The *right* screenshot (**b**) includes the US angiography of the *right* internal carotid artery and middle cerebral artery (*arrows*) of a *right* temporal glioblastoma case (outlined preoperatively). The navigation images of the preoperative MRI and reconstructed 3D ultrasound acquisition were also placed in (**b**) as described above in (**a**)

Real-Time 3D Ultrasound Imaging

Technical Aspects

The US probe X7-2 (2–7 MHz frequency) used to acquire real-time 3D images (iU22, Philips, Bothell, USA) is predominantly designed for paediatric cardiologists or gynaecologists. The xMATRIX array technology utilises 2,400 fully sampled elements for 360-degree focusing and steering. The array probe enables live xPlane imaging to acquire two full-resolution planes simultaneously from the same heartbeat or region of interest. The system's multi-directional beam steering provides unlimited planes in all directions, and live volume imaging allows the acquisition and rendering of full volume data at true real-time frame rates with unparalleled isovoxel resolution. The settings on the system are not primarily ordered for neurosurgical procedures, according to the company. However, there is increasing corporate interest in further adapting parameters for brain and tumour visualisation, which is crucial for optimal US imaging.

3D Ultrasound Acquisition and Display

An acquisition procedure is not necessary, as the 3D data are immediately available (live). In the "X-Plane" mode, two US images are displayed (Fig. 2c). The left one always shows the 2D US image according to the position of the probe (oblique). The right one displays the corresponding live 2D image according to the chosen degree of turn (from 0° to 360°). For example, if one holds the US probe in an axial position, then a choice of a 90° or 270° turn will illustrate the corresponding coronal (from the lateral approach) or sagittal (from the anterior approach) image of this area of interest (Fig. 2c). The "Live 3D" mode displays all of the US information from the array probe at once in a cone. The width of the cone can be adjusted to the user's needs. The image is displayed online and changes immediately in response to all movements of the probe. In predominant tissue areas (brain and tumour tissue with no cysts or ventricles), visualisation of the field of interest is difficult; it is thus especially complex to demonstrate in a 2D picture (Fig. 3). However, the overall advantage of this mode for

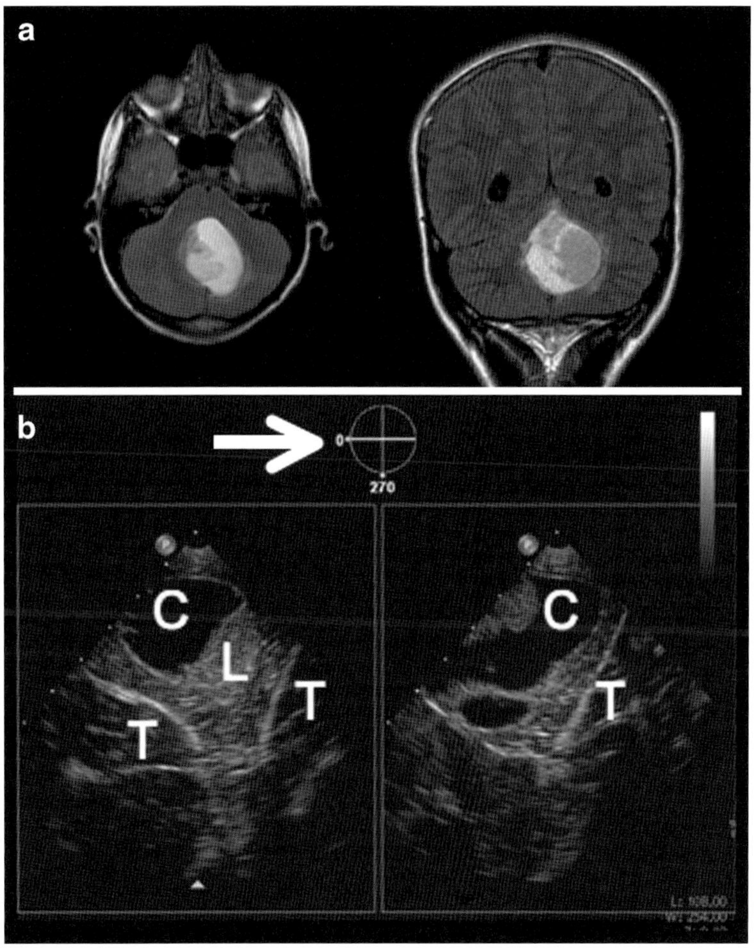

Fig. 2 Images from a 12-year-old male show a cerebellar low-grade astrocytoma with multiple cysts (**a**). The real-time 3D ultrasound images (**b**) display the solid lesion (L), cysts (C) and tentorium (T) in two planes simultaneously. The *arrow* shows the degree of the *right* ultrasound image compared to the oblique *left* side. In this case, the *right* image is a 270° turn of the *left* image (near axial) and should represent a nearly sagittal position. The "X-Plane" mode was used for this image

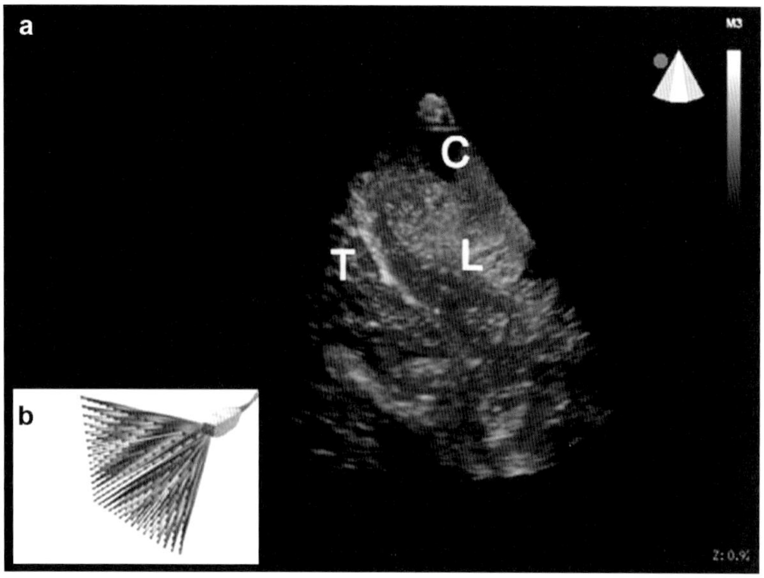

Fig. 3 A cone picture is displayed from the use of the "Live 3D" full volume mode (same case as Fig. 2) with real-time 3D ultrasound (**a**). Basically, all ultrasound data from the array probe are shown in one 3D animation. The width of the cone can be changed according to the user's needs. The orientation is very difficult and anatomical structures not clearly presented. Most of the tissue overshadows the solid lesion (L), cysts (C) and tentorium (T). The small picture from the array probe (**b**) demonstrates the linear ultrasound in a 3D representation (Copyright Philips, Bothell, USA)

neurosurgeons still remains to be discovered. Gynaecologists and pregnant mothers appreciate this "Live 3D" mode, as it is often able to show the surface of the foetus and sometimes even the face. Multiple sets of 3D US images or videos can be stored and reactivated any time during the surgical procedure.

Ultrasound Angiography

The usual Power Doppler and additional modes are available with the real-time 3D US probe, but no advanced reconstruction for angiographies or navigation combination is included.

Comparative Advantages and Disadvantages

Clinical Arrangements

To facilitate optimal US imaging, nearly all patients are positioned during surgery with a nearly vertical craniotomy corridor. In such a position, saline remains in the resection cavity after the dura is opened for ultrasound imaging; the amount of air bubbles can be limited to reduce acoustic shadows [9]. This technique was used to facilitate sonographic resection control with both systems. In all cases, the chosen craniotomy was sufficient for the US probe; our group performed no enlargement of the craniotomy for either US probe. Initial US acquisitions were performed extraduraly. Repeated intraoperative image updating was valuable and easily accomplished, even in inexperienced hands. The best image acquisition was always obtained after filling the cavity with normal saline. After dural closure, images were mostly unacceptable (especially after 3D reconstruction) due to remnant air bubbles. Resection control is therefore recommended intraduraly and directly, either with the navigated 2D mode or real-time 3D probe. The technical installation of both systems for surgery needs no significant aid. However, this is different during surgery. Navigated 3D US can be managed via a draped touchscreen by the surgeon, whereas the real-time US machine has to be managed by an unscrubbed person. It is possible to drape the buttons and a small additional touch screen, but handling the trackball through a drape is impossible.

3D Orientation and Resolution

In all cases, a leading anatomical landmark (falx, tentorium, ventricles, brainstem or skull base) close to the lesions was noted to allow for rapid orientation of the surgeon using the real-time 3D US mode. Anatomical landmarks became unnecessary when reconstructed 3D US images were presented next to their corresponding image slices of the preoperative navigation sets (MR or CT) (Fig. 1a, b). The combination of both 3D data sets (US and MRI) in one picture is also possible, but using the same greyscale for both images makes visualisation difficult. Lindseth et al. [8] introduced multimodal image fusion in US-based neuronavigation by improving the overview and interpretation. These authors integrated preoperative MRI with intraoperative 3D US and added an accuracy study to this combination of two systems. Displaying the 3D data as a specifically oriented image plane was somewhat supportive for the orientation. It was initially challenging to determine the degree that would actually become a true axial, coronal or sagittal slide (Fig. 2). The full real-time 3D US cone image ("Live 3D") provided no additional help regarding orientation (Fig. 3). Unsgaard et al. [9] have published a benchmark review article regarding developments in reconstructed 3D US. They have used the intraoperative imaging system SonoWand (Mison A/S), which is a high-end US platform with a supplementary navigation system [18]. This system has shortened the acquisition time to a very tiny delay of surgery. The resolution of its US probes is also superior to that of the IGSonic probe. The resolution of our real-time 3D probe is very good, but the image pre-settings could be improved.

Comparison via One Lesion Entity (Cavernoma)

Cavernomas provide a favourable group of lesions for US-guided resection [19]. Their significant hyperechogenity (Fig. 1a) is most likely due to the concentrated hemosiderin in and around the lesion, as seen on haemorrhages in US images. After 3D acquisition, neuronavigation was sometimes changed completely to the US mode without using any further preoperative MRI data. Vessels close to the cavernoma (like the often-seen draining vein) can be visualised and landmarked nicely with the Color Doppler mode [10]. Real-time 3D ultrasound was also able to localise and demonstrate such lesions. No disturbing shadows were experienced due to perfect 3D visualisation. However, navigation guidance for further surgery was certainly missing. Navigated 3D acquisition was especially helpful for intraoperative planning of the approach, whereas subsequent postoperative reconstructed 3D resection control was not helpful in our experience. After complete microscopic resection of the cavernoma, the surrounding tissue remained hyperechogenic in 3D US reconstructions and it thus imitated a significant residual lesion or even the condition of no resection at all. We have used real-time 2D US for resection control of cavernomas when using navigated ultrasound. For resection control, real-time 3D US is superior. The images are clearer and immediately available. However, the image quality is not comparable to a high field intraoperative MRI or high frequency multi-focus ultrasound probes, and landmarking of the residual tumour for navigated identification is still not possible.

Standalone Use

One positive aspect of US technologies is their frequently mentioned low cost [9, 11, 12]. Neuronavigation has become a state of the art tool in the last two decades. Even in economically challenging countries, neuronavigation systems are increasingly purchased, however such devices are rarely used in practice because preoperative MRI is often too costly for patients in these countries. Many neurosurgical groups intend to obtain intraoperative imaging technology but often struggle with the enormous costs of intra-operative MRI imaging – and furthermore the running costs should not be forgotten. An integrated US navigation system would offer a cheap intraoperative imaging alternative with familiar orientations (i.e., axial, coronal and sagittal) and basically no running costs. Furthermore, this tool can also be used without any expensive preoperative imaging modality (CT or MRI) and therefore should be very interesting for economically challenging countries as a true alternative to intraoperative MRI or CT. The real-time 3D US system itself (with additional transducers) is certainly a high-end, modern intraoperative imaging device with minimal running costs.

Outlook and Future

Further development of image quality for one-platform solutions would be highly appreciated, but those improvements should not change the convenient manageability, handiness or plug-and-play usage. Most interesting will be further technical developments in real-time 3D US sonography with better image settings, real time segmentation features, higher frequency, multi focus imaging and larger probe arrays. Certainly, more experience with real-time 3D imaging will help as well. Finally, combination with a navigation system could overcome the persistent orientation problem. The surgeon could immediately see the US image in all three familiar dimensions/planes without any time delay due to acquisition or calculation. This would make neurosonography a very strong competitive alternative in intraoperative imaging.

Conclusion

These two presented intraoperative 3D US techniques offer user-friendly and clinically useful imaging modalities and represent further important steps in neurosonography. Orientation in a one-platform solution with neuronavigation remains superior to that in a real-time US system. However, a larger clinical series should look deeper into these preliminary experiences.

Conflict of interest statement We declare that we have no conflict of interest.

Acknowledgment The authors state that both US probes (IGSonic and real-time 3D transducer) have been provided by the companies for research proposes. This is not the case for the navigation system VectorVision or US system IU22, which were bought by the departments. No further financial collaborations, consulting contracts or conflicts of interest exist. The reprint of the image in Fig. 3b has been approved by the company (Copyright Philips, Bothell, USA).

References

1. Bernays RL (2003) Intraoperative imaging in neurosurgery. MRI, CT, ultrasound. Introduction. Acta Neurochir Suppl 85:1–3
2. Bonsanto MM, Staubert A, Wirtz CR, Tronnier V, Kunze S (2001) Initial experience with an ultrasound-integrated single-rack neuronavigation system. Acta Neurochir 143:1127–1132
3. Cannon JW, Stoll JA, Sago IS, Knowles HB, Howe RD, Dupont PE, Marx GR, del Nido PJ (2003) Real-time three-dimensional ultrasound for guiding surgical tasks. Comput Aided Surg 8:82–90
4. Enchev Y, Bozinov O, Miller D, Tirakotai W, Heinze S, Benes L, Bertalanffy H, Sure U (2006) Image-guided ultrasonography for recurrent cystic gliomas. Acta Neurochir 148:1053–1063
5. Jödicke A, Deinsberger W, Erbe H, Kriete A, Böker D-K (1998) Intraoperative three-dimensional ultrasonography: an approach to register brain shift using multidimensional image processing. Minim Invas Neurosurg 41:13–19
6. Jödicke A, Springer T, Böker D-K (2004) Real-time integration of ultrasound into neuronavigation: technical accuracy using a light-emitting-diode-based navigation system. Acta Neurochir 146:1211–1220
7. Lindner D, Trantakis C, Renner C, Arnold S, Schmitgen A, Schneider J, Meixensberger J (2006) Application of intraoperative 3D ultrasound during navigated tumor resection. Minim Invasive Neurosurg 49:197–202
8. Lindseth F, Kaspersen JH, Ommedal S, Lango T, Bang J, Hokland J, Unsgaard G, Hernes TA (2003) Multimodal image fusion in ultrasound-based neuronavigation: improving overview and interpretation by integrating preoperative MRI with intraoperative 3D ultrasound. Comput Aided Surg 8:49–69
9. Unsgaard G, Rygh GM, Selbekk T, Müller TB, Kolstad F, Lindseth F, Nagelhus Hernes TA (2006) Intra-operative 3D ultrasound in neurosurgery. Acta Neurochir 148:235–254
10. Sure U, Benes L, Bozinov O, Woydt M, Tirakotai W, Bertalanffy H (2005) Intraoperative landmarking of vascular anatomy by integration of duplex and Doppler ultrasonography in image guided surgery. Technical note. Surg Neurol 63:133–142
11. Tirakotai W, Miller D, Heinze S, Benes L, Bertalanffy H, Sure U (2006) A novel platform for image-guided ultrasound. Neurosurgery 58:710–718
12. Unsgaard G, Ommedal S, Muller T, Gronningsaeter A, Nagelhus Hernes TA (2002) Neuronavigation by intraoperative three-dimensional ultrasound: initial experience during brain tumor resection. Neurosurgery 50:804–812
13. Sure U, Alberti O, Petermeyer M, Becker R, Bertalanffy H (2000) Advanced image-guided skull base surgey. Surg Neurol 53: 563–572
14. Miller D, Heinze S, Tirakotai W, Bozinov O, Sürücü O, Benes L, Bertalanffy H, Sure U (2007) Is the image guidance of ultrasonography beneficial for neurosurgical routine? Surg Neurol 67: 579–587
15. Sure U, Gatscher S, Alberti O, Witte J, Bertalanffy H (2000) Image-guided duplex and Doppler ultrasound for microsurgery of cerebral AVMs. Zentralbl Neurochir 61(Suppl 1):47–48 (abstract)
16. Woydt M, Horowski A, Krauss J, Krone A, Soerensen N, Roosen K (2002) Three-dimensional intraoperative ultrasound of vascular malformations and supratentorial tumors. J Neuroimaging 12: 28–34
17. Unsgaard G, Ommedal S, Rygh OM, Lindseth F (2007) Operation of arteriovenous malformations assisted by stereoscopic navigation-controlled display of preoperative magnetic resonance angiography and intraoperative ultrasound angiography. Neurosurgery 61(1 Suppl):407–415
18. Gronningsaeter A, Kleven A, Ommedal S, Aarseth TE, Lie T, Lindseth F, Lango T, Unsgard G (2000) SonoWand, an ultrasound-based neuronavigation system. Neurosurgery 47: 1373–1380
19. Winkler D, Lindner D, Strauss G, Richter A, Schober R, Meixensberger J (2006) Surgery of cavernous malformations with and without navigational support–a comparative study. Minim Invasive Neurosurg 49:15–19

Multimodality Integration

Integrated Intra-operative Room Design

Ivan Ng

Abstract The design of intraoperative suites require significant inputs from the neurosurgeons. Prior consideration of specific surgical objectives before investment of capital resources will enable to surgeon to yield maximum value from the project.

We describe the setup of the integrated neurosurgical centre at our institution which comprises of a hybrid high field MRI suite, an OR's consisting of a multi-slice CT scanner and iso-C 3D respectively. The iCT and ioMRI OR's carry ICG angiography capabilities. These ORs are linked to also the Novalis radiosurgery suites and outpatient clinics and offices to facilitate pre-surgical review, planning as well as treatment plans on a common interface via the BRAINSUITE net.

Design considerations include right sit-ing of imaging equipment as well as a focus of ergonomics and design features to maximize workflow. Whenever possible, standard neurosurgical instrumentation is utilized.

With widespread availability of technology, neuroimaging in the operating room may become more prevalent. The surgeon is the lead individual in the team with regards to planning and designing the ORs to accommodate the new imaging equipment.

Keywords Intraoperative imaging · Operating room design

Introduction

For more than a decade, advanced imaging modalities like 3D fluoroscopy [1], computed tomography (CT) [2, 3] and magnetic resonance imaging(MRI) [4–6], catheter [7, 8] and indigo-cyanine green (ICG) angiography [9, 10] have made their way into the operating rooms and considerable experience with a wide array of systems have been accumulated. The move to incorporate various imaging modalities within neurological surgery has been driven by the need to ensure that the desired operative endpoint or objective has been achieved. Examples would be the need to verify optimal clip placement following aneurysm surgery, correct positioning of screws in spinal instrumentation procedures and more recently to ascertain brain tumour- normal brain interface where the margins may not be readily apparent to the visible eye.

The incorporation of these modalities in the operating environment would in some instance require some degree of configuration change of the operating suite as well as workflow modifications to accommodate this change from conventional neurosurgery. This may vary widely; it may require little or no change in operating suite design and construct; e.g. the use of 3D fluoroscopy to one which requires significant planning, pre-design and construction of an operating suite; e.g. the construction of a high field intra-operative MRI facility.

The construction of intra-operative operating rooms (OR's) in our institution for the purposes of neurosurgery was conceptualized to incorporate various forms of neuro-imaging to cover and support the whole spectrum of neurosurgical diseases into a pre-existing operating room complex. In this manuscript, we describe the set-up of the integrated neurosurgical centre focused on its various intra-operative imaging options and objectives of design.

Materials and Methods

The integrated neurosurgical centre at the Singapore General Hospital, Singapore comprised of three intra-operative OR's and a Novalis radiosurgery suite (BrainLAB, Feldkirchen, Germany) which was built on a network platform that was

I. Ng
Departments of Neurosurgery at Singapore General Hospital and the National Neuroscience Institute, Duke-NUS Graduate Medical School, Singapore
e-mail: ivan.ng.h.b@sgh.com.sg

M.N. Pamir et al. (eds.), *Intraoperative Imaging*, Acta Neurochirurgica Supplementum, Vol. 109,
DOI 10.1007/978-3-211-99651-5_31,

designed to enable seamless transfer of imaging information from workstations in the outpatient clinics and individual neurosurgeons' office to the various OR. The design facilitated easy access to the workstations of rendered software to allow for pre-surgical planning in any part of the hospital with wireless access and these data can be stored and transferred to the navigational consoles within individual OR's. These OR suites were specifically organized within the major operating theatre complex and accommodate the building of a brand new operating room with a high field magnetic resonance imaging machine (1.5 T; ioMRI); the remaining two OR's incorporate each an intra-operative imaging modality, namely a 32 slice computed tomography scanner on rails (iCT) and a 3 dimensional fluoroscopy system(i-iso C 3D).respectively in two separate OR's.

Hybrid ioMRI Suite Setup

The ioMRI suite measures 11,225 mm by 7,420 mm (approximately 83 m^2 and was built on space previously used within the major operating complex for post surgical recovery. The control room which includes the server room was an additional 7,865 mm × 3,500 mm. The layout of the operating suite is shown in Fig. 1. The high field 1.5 T MRI(Magnetom Espree, Siemens; Erlangen, Germany) has a 70 cm wide bore open magnet with 30 cm of face space and is 125 cm long and is housed within a pre-fabricated radiofrequency-shielded cabin. The smaller footprint of the magnet allows for greater space conservation and the larger bore allows for surgical procedures in the supine, prone or lateral positions. The operating table (Trumpf, Pucheim, Germany) is fully MRI compatible and in the default position lies within the "sweet spot" of the operating room. It permits rotational movement of the patient enabling the head to be beyond the edge of the 5 Gauss safety line; additionally the layout allows the provision to utilize neurosurgical procedures to be carried out with standard instrumentation. When scanning is planned, the patient is placed in the magnet by rotating the operating table. The patient's head is held in a MRI compatible ceramic head holder which allows 32 coil elements to be seamlessly integrated into one examination and read out into eight independent receiver channels. A ceiling mounted microscope (Pentero, Zeiss, Oberkochen, Germany) with ICG angiography capabilities has a camera for tracking microscope movements is placed at a distance of approximately 1.5 m in the 5-G perimeter (Fig. 2). We use the Automatic Image Registration software & hardware (BrainLAB, Feldkirchen, Germany) which allows for automatic registration of intra-operative images from the ioMRI scanner. The intra-operative images are available for image guided surgery at the navigation system immediately after the scanning process without requiring any manual registration. For this process, a special MR compatible reference structure and a reference star is attached to the upper half of the head coil and the head clamp. We routinely utilize anatomical and functional as well as tractography images for navigation [4, 11–13]. The navigation workstation is placed outside the radiofrequency shielded OR (Fig. 3). Three MRI compatible high resolution flat screen color monitors (57 in.) are available for the purposes of display of navigation guidance, live video streaming of the operating procedure and neuro-images retrieved from the hospital in- house PACS system.

Intra-Operative CT Scan (iCT) OR

The iCT OR was retrofitted into a pre-existing neurosurgical OR and its dimensions are 8,350 mm × 7,000 mm × 3,000 mm [approx. 59 m^2] and incorporates a control room with the dimensions 5,900 mm × 3,150 mm [approx. 19 m^2]. The main components of the OR includes a commercially available 32 multi-slice CT scanner (Somatom Sensation Open Gliding Gantry; Siemens Medical Solutions, Forchheim), CT (32 slice; Siemens, Germany), a motorized radiolucent, flexible rotating table (Trumpf, Pucheim, Germany), and a ceiling mounted frameless infrared-based neuronavigational system (Vector Vision Sky; BrainLab) as in the ioMRI. The setup is represented in Figs. 3 and 4. The operating table allows patient to be positioned in all positions except the sitting position and the CT scanner gantry moves over the patient during scanner by means of rails built on both sides of the operating table (Fig. 3). As in the ioMRI suite, the scanner is controlled by a workstation in a room next to the OR with direct visual contact and video surveillance. This allows for CT image acquisition without radiation exposure to personnel.

Brainsuite Network System

DICOM data generated from the MRI and CT scanner is networked between the BRAINSUITE net (BrainLAB, Feldkirchen, Germany) and the image guided surgery system which allows for automatic registration within the OR suite. The neuronavigation system also functions as a control terminal for BrainSUITE NET allowing for a common simple interface for which to manipulate the data. We deployed a image data management system which allowed for video and still images like the surgical microscope and endoscope as well as the OR light's video camera and room cameras. This features a high end, firewall encapsulation of the complete subnetwork with controlled data link to the MR

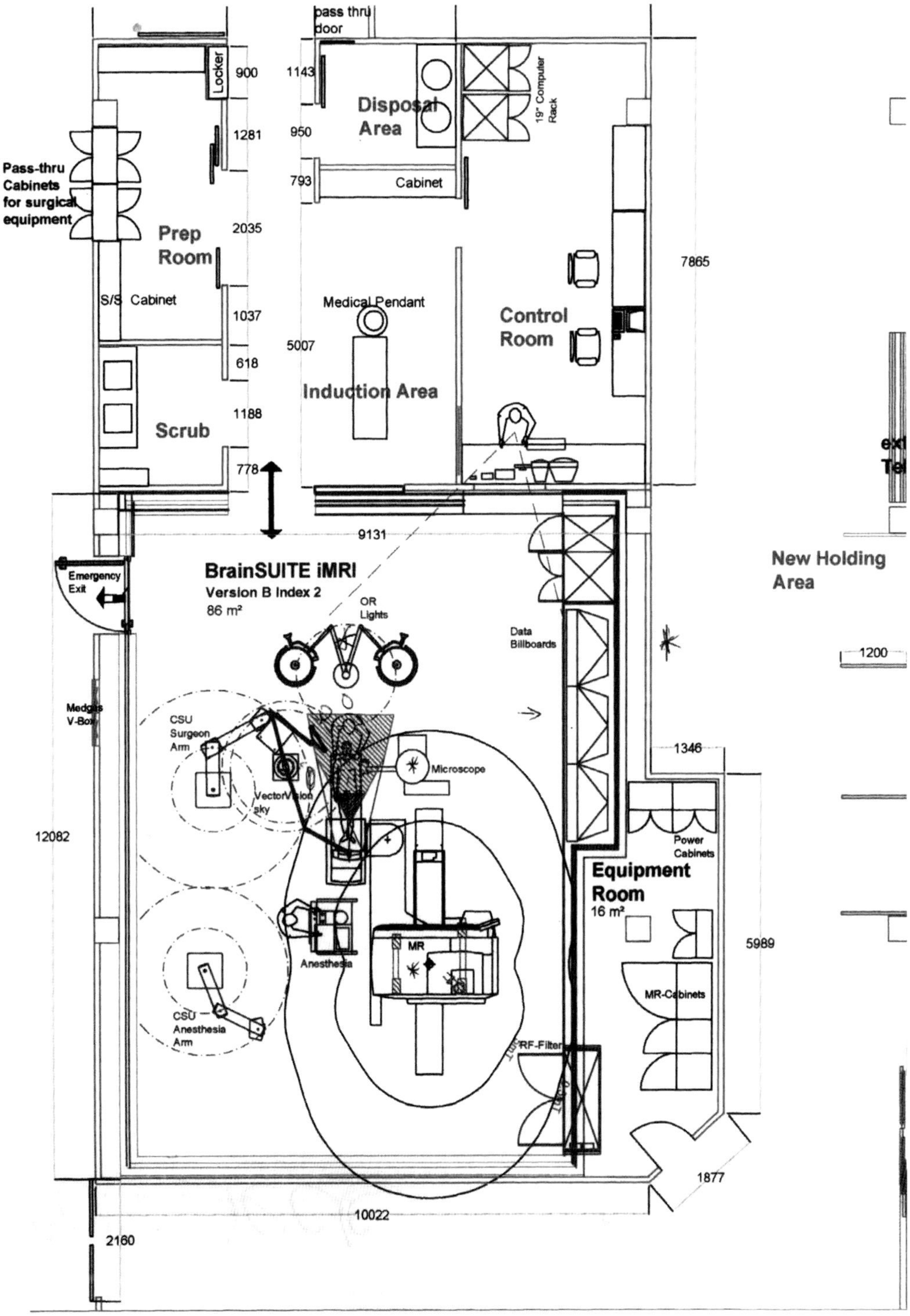

Fig. 1 Schematic overview of the IoMRI suite. The suite consists of the OR proper with its RF cabin; an anaesthetic preparation room, scrub nurse preparation room, dedicated scrubbing area and the control and server room

scanner interface. Configurable connectivity to existing hospital infrastructure like CT, MR. X-ray workstations and PACS for DICOM image data transfer and even the possibility of immediate remote service response was also catered for (Fig. 5).

Results

The casemix for the ioMRI and iCT suites from June 2008 to July 2009 are shown in Table 1 and 2 respectively. Workflow for the surgical team, nursing and anaesthetic team

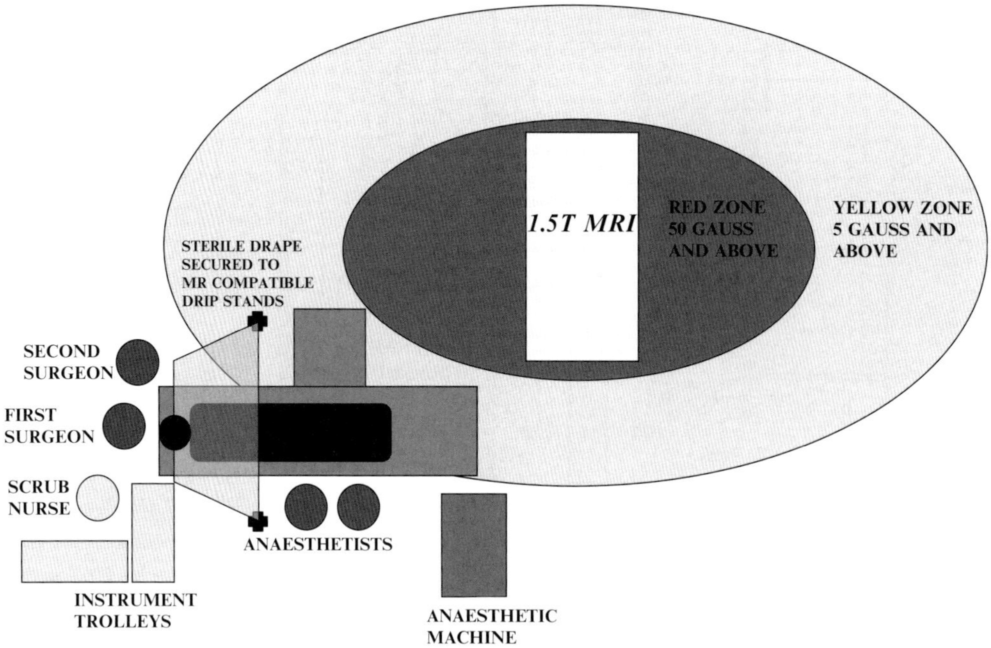

Fig. 2 General surgical layout within the ioMRI OR. Surgery is performed at the area which is beyond the 5G line (*yellow* perimeter). This allows the use of conventional neurosurgical instrumentation. The arrangement allows for our usual OR configuration with regards to position of scrub nurse and assistant

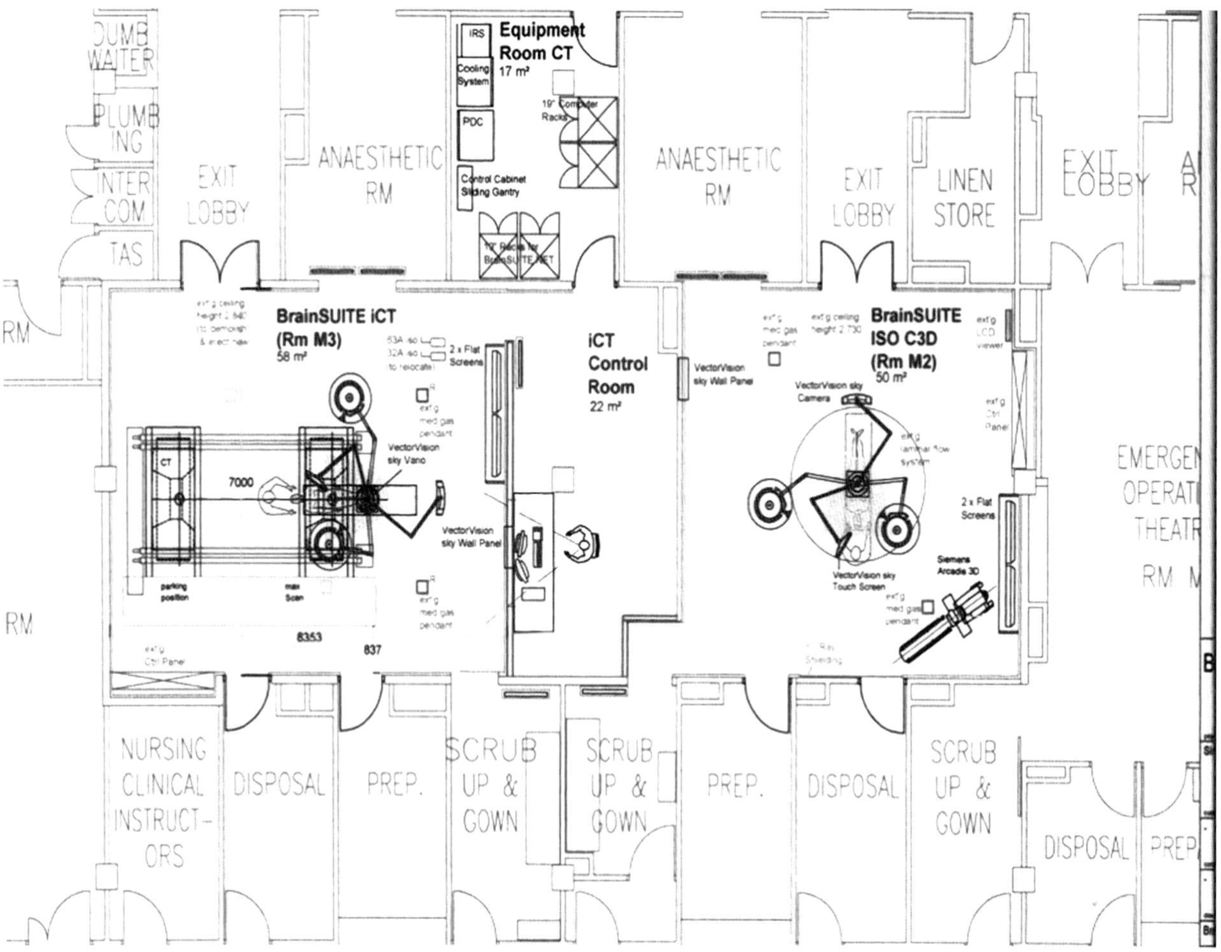

Fig. 3 Schematic overview of iCT and iso C3D suites

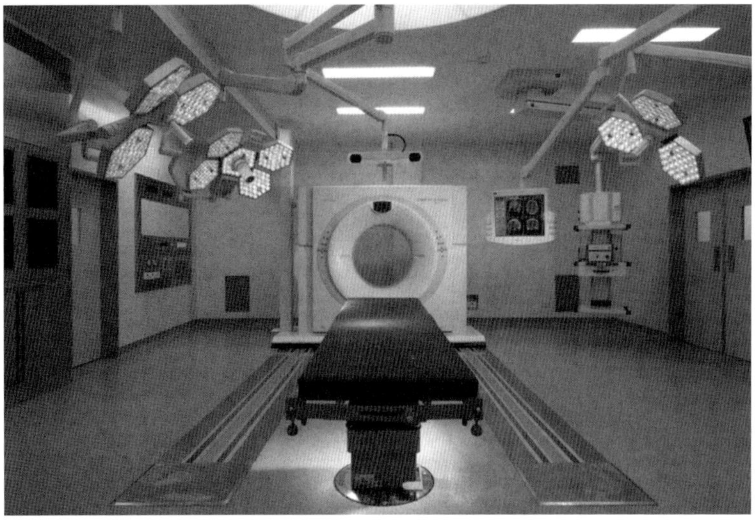

Fig. 4 iCT set-up with a mobile 32 slice CT scanner on rails with the radiolucent operating table at its epicenter

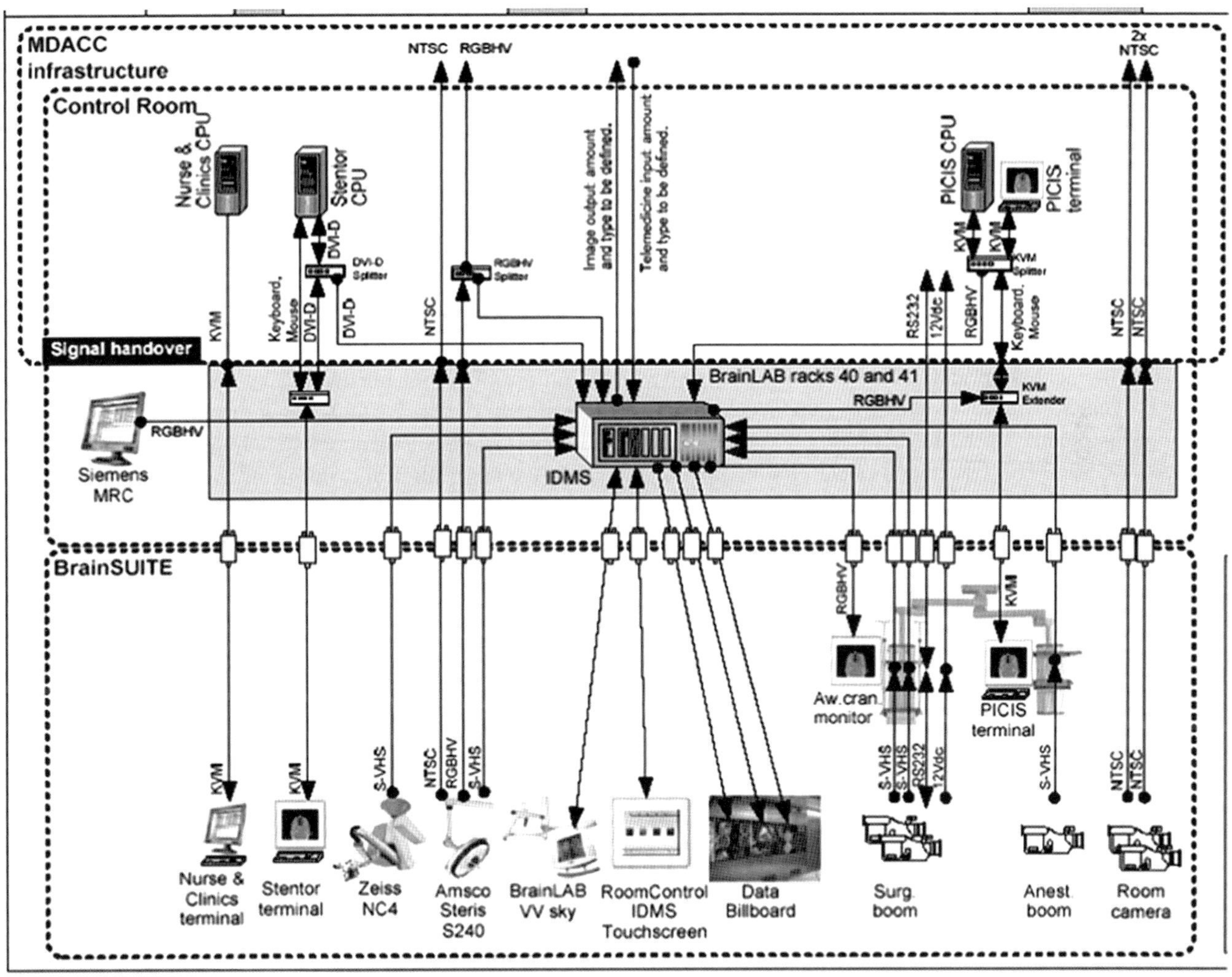

Fig. 5 The BRAINSUITE net setup

Table 1 Casemix of ioMRI from May 2008 to June 2009

	ioMRI
Gliomas	37
Pituitary tumours	55
AVMs	12
Metastasis	11
Biopsy	5
Total	120

Table 2 Case of iCT from May 2008 to June 2009

	iCT
Spinal instrumentation	67
Cranial tumours	131
Stereotaxic biopsy	33
Aneurysms(icg & CTA)	7
AVMs(iCT & CTA)	3
Others (trauma, neuroendoscopy)	140
Total	381

were essentially kept similar with minor modifications. Within the OR, the surgical team and its spatial relationship with the scrub nurse and her instruments were unchanged to maintain efficiency and optimize coordination between the two teams. Standard neurosurgical instruments were used even in the ioMRI OR as the neurosurgical procedure was conducted just beyond the 5 G safety line. To increase patient safety, the anaesthetic team deployment allows for easy access to all vascular access and airway and physiological monitoring and can be continued remotely even during scanning with wireless devices or through cables running through the booms in the roof to the control rooms. All medical equipment are placed on articulated booms to keep heavy and bulky items out of harms way and away from the imaging equipment. In the ioMRI OR, all equipment are secured in place. The OR floor is kept free of clutter as much as possible. All the relevant OR;s utilize a line of sight neuronavigation system with a touchscreen with auto-registration capabilities to minimize time wasted by transferring new data into system and manually re-registering. Duration where navigation is possible during the operation is maximized by having ceiling mounted line of sight navigation systems.

Discussion

Various options for intra-operative modalities have got significant different properties and capabilities to visualize neuroanatomical and potentially neurophysiological entities and the current state of technology has demonstrated value in individual categories of neurosurgical procedures; e.g., the use of the MRI has been shown to potentially benefit transphenoidal resection of pituitary tumours [14] intra-axial tumours particularly gliomas [4, 11–13]; fluoroscopy with or without 3D reconstruction(as been demonstrated to be valuable with spinal instrumentation [10, 15, 16]. We therefore endeavored to build suites that will incorporate imaging modalities which may be best utilized to provide the information necessary to the neurosurgeon for him to make critical decisions and as an adjunct towards the smooth conduct of the operation. In this regard, we surmise that the MRI would be valuable for us in neuro-oncology [4–6, 12], the multi-slice CT scanner would be useful in craniofacial procedures, aneurysms with CT angiography [3], spinal instrumentation and as a peri-operative surveillance tool; the iso C 3D fluoroscopy for spine [10, 15, 16] and ICG angiography incorporated into the operating microscope in both the ioMRI and iCT so that vascular cases may be performed in either OR. With regard to the choice of the MRI, the three choices would be a low field, 1.5 T and 3 T machines to choose from [17–19]. We opted for a 1.5 T MRI for its superior image resolution and its ability to provide in addition to structural anatomical images other sequences such as tractography, diffusion weighted imaging, spectroscopy, MR angiography and venography compared to the low field systems. While there have been some 3 T systems employed in the clinical setting, the advantage at this juncture over the 1.5 T machine for neuro-oncology has not been sufficiently investigated although there may be emerging evidence suggest that the additional information with spectroscopy may further aid glioma resections [17, 19, 20].

The design of these OR's was also predicated on the fact that it would be desirable not to modify too drastically the workflow or arrangements of the respective surgical and anaesthetic teams. We thus sought to ensure design would suit our unique institutional requirements with regards to using the usual surgical instruments as well as relative position of the surgeon and his assistant during the operations well as scrub nurse positions to maintain and maximize surgical efficiency. Optimization of ergonomics and workflow also involved suspending whenever possible all surgical equipment such as the electrocautery machine, suction, craniotomy drills and endoscope trolleys onto booms suspended off the roof so as to minimize clutter on thc floor.

The choice of the imaging system would largely be determined by the institutions' casemix and in most instances, the design and conceptualization would best be served by having surgeons with a vested interest in utilizing the technology leading the project design and implementation. This would ensure that the ORs are built to specifications which would best facilitate and improve on contemporary practice. While turnkey solutions are available commercially, individualized planning is still valuable to maximize efficiency and ensure that the new ORs are appropriately used.

Conclusions

The design and building of hybrid intraoperative OR's despite the increasing availability of turnkey solutions will still need to be led by neurosurgeons with careful thought put towards designing the OR's to suit individual needs within the institution.

Conflict of interest statement We declare that we have no conflict of interest.

References

1. Stubig T, Kendoff D, Citak M, Geerling J, Khalafi A, Krettek C, Hufner T (2009) Comparative study of different intraoperative 3-D image intensifiers in orthopedic trauma care. J Trauma 66:821–830
2. Engle DJ, Lunsford LD (1987) Brain tumor resection guided by intraoperative computed tomography. J Neurooncol 4:361–370
3. Uhl E, Zausinger S, Morhard D, Heigl T, Scheder B, Rachinger W, Schichor C, Tonn JC (2009) Intraoperative computed tomography with integrated navigation system in a multidisciplinary operating suite. Neurosurgery 64:231–239, discussion 239–240
4. Nimsky C, Ganslandt O, Kober H, Buchfelder M, Fahlbusch R (2001) Intraoperative magnetic resonance imaging combined with neuronavigation: a new concept. Neurosurgery 48:1082–1089, discussion 1089–1091
5. Sutherland GR, Kaibara T, Louw D, Hoult DI, Tomanek B, Saunders J (1999) A mobile high-field magnetic resonance system for neurosurgery. J Neurosurg 91:804–813
6. Truwit CL, Hall WA (2006) Intraoperative magnetic resonance imaging-guided neurosurgery at 3-T. Neurosurgery 58:ONS-338–ONS-345, discussion ONS-345–ONS-346
7. Kivisaari RP, Porras M, Ohman J, Siironen J, Ishii K, Hernesniemi J (2004) Routine cerebral angiography after surgery for saccular aneurysms: is it worth it? Neurosurgery 55:1015–1024
8. Tang G, Cawley CM, Dion JE, Barrow DL (2002) Intraoperative angiography during aneurysm surgery: a prospective evaluation of efficacy. J Neurosurg 96:993–999
9. Dashti R, Laakso A, Niemela M, Porras M, Hernesniemi J (2009) Microscope-integrated near-infrared indocyanine green videoangiography during surgery of intracranial aneurysms: the Helsinki experience. Surg Neurol 71:543–550, discussion 550
10. Hott JS, Papadopoulos SM, Theodore N, Dickman CA, Sonntag VK (2004) Intraoperative Iso-C C-arm navigation in cervical spinal surgery: review of the first 52 cases. Spine (Phila Pa 1976) 29:2856–2860
11. Nimsky C, Ganslandt O, Fahlbusch R (2007) Implementation of fiber tract navigation. Neurosurgery 61:306–317, discussion 317–318
12. Nimsky C, Ganslandt O, Hastreiter P, Wang R, Benner T, Sorensen AG, Fahlbusch R (2007) Preoperative and intraoperative diffusion tensor imaging-based fiber tracking in glioma surgery. Neurosurgery 61:178–185, discussion 186
13. Nimsky C, von Keller B, Schlaffer S, Kuhnt D, Weigel D, Ganslandt O, Buchfelder M (2009) Updating navigation with intraoperative image data. Top Magn Reson Imaging 19:197–204
14. Nimsky C, von Keller B, Ganslandt O, Fahlbusch R (2006) Intraoperative high-field magnetic resonance imaging in transsphenoidal surgery of hormonally inactive pituitary macroadenomas. Neurosurgery 59:105–114, discussion 105–114
15. Holly LT, Foley KT (2003) Intraoperative spinal navigation. Spine (Phila Pa 1976) 28:S54–S61
16. Holly LT, Foley KT (2007) Image guidance in spine surgery. Orthop Clin North Am 38:451–461, abstract viii
17. Kim PD, Truwit CL, Hall WA (2009) Three-tesla high-field applications. Neurosurg Clin N Am 20:173–178
18. Lewin JS, Metzger AK (2001) Intraoperative MR systems. Low-field approaches. Neuroimaging Clin N Am 11:611–628
19. Pamir MN, Peker S, Ozek MM, Dincer A (2006) Intraoperative MR imaging: preliminary results with 3 tesla MR system. Acta Neurochir Suppl 98:97–100
20. Pamir MN, Ozduman K, Dincer A, Yildiz E, Peker S, Ozek MM (2010) First intraoperative, shared-resource, ultrahigh-field 3-Tesla magnetic resonance imaging system and its application in low-grade glioma resection. J Neurosurg 112(1):57–69

Multimodal Navigation Integrated with Imaging

Christopher Nimsky, Daniela Kuhnt, Oliver Ganslandt, and Michael Buchfelder

Abstract Intraoperative high-field MRI in combination and close integration with microscope-based navigation serving as a common interface for the presentation of multimodal data in the surgical field seems to be one of the most promising surgical setups allowing avoiding unwanted tumor remnants while preserving neurological function. Multimodal navigation integrates standard anatomical, structural, functional, and metabolic data. Navigation achieves visualizing the initial extent of a lesion with the concomitant identification of neighboring eloquent brain structures, as well as, providing a tool for a direct correlation of histology and multimodal data. With the help of intraoperative imaging navigation data can be updated, so that brain shift can be compensated for and initially missed tumor remnants can be localized reliably.

Keywords Brain shift · Intraoperative MRI · MRI · Neuronavigation

Introduction

The possibility to objectively determine the extent of tumour removal during surgery is highly advantageous. Thus, intraoperative imaging has gained increasing interest in the last decade. If a resection is incomplete, one can attempt to remove the tumour residues that were initially missed during the same operation. In contrast to a subjective estimation by the surgeon, intraoperative imaging allows an objective evaluation of the intraoperative situation, thus acting as quality control during surgery [1–6]. In addition to intraoperative imaging, an integral part of our concept of computer aided surgery is the simultaneous application of navigation [5, 7, 8]. This integrated navigation allows essentially visualizing the results of pre- and intraoperative imaging in the surgical field, so that the image data provide an immediate feedback. The main goal is to prevent increased neurological deficits despite increased resections that might result from the attempt to remove initially overlooked tumor remnants that are detected by intraoperative imaging.

In standard navigation, also known as frameless stereotaxy, the real space of the surgical field is registered to the 3-D image space, which is based on anatomical data only. We prefer the application of microscope-based navigation, where the extent and localization of a tumour is superimposed on the surgical field through contours using the heads-up display technology of the modern operating microscopes. Standard navigation, based on anatomical information only, which has become a routine tool in many neurosurgical departments, was enhanced by the integration of further information from other modalities resulting meanwhile in the so-called multimodal navigation.

Functional navigation, integrating preoperative data from magnetoencephalography (MEG) [9–11] and functional magnetic resonance imaging (fMRI) [5, 12] to define the localization of cortical eloquent brain areas, such as the motor and speech areas, was the first step in the direction of modern multimodal navigation. Functional navigation allowed more thorough resections of tumours in risk zones with low morbidity. Integration of diffusion tensor imaging (DTI) data delineating the course of major white matter tracts extended this concept also to subcortical areas [13–16], while the co-registration of PET data and information from MR spectroscopy (MRS) added metabolic information leading to true multimodal navigation [17–22].

C. Nimsky (✉) and D. Kuhnt
Department of Neurosurgery, University Marburg, Baldingerstrasse 35033 Marburg, Germany
e-mail: nimsky@med.uni-marburg.de

O. Ganslandt and M. Buchfelder
Department of Neurosurgery, University Erlangen-Nuremberg, Erlangen, Germany

Navigation in an Environment with Intraoperative Imaging

There are several concepts implementing the combination of navigation and intraoperative imaging. One possibility is that the MR scanner serves as a navigational device per se, as it was the basic principle in the 0.5 T double-doughnut GE scanner concept, where the patient was operated directly in the scanner [1, 23, 24]. Since surgical space and imaging space are identical, an instrument in the surgical space can be tracked in the image space without much additional effort. Direct navigation in the MR scanner is often based on realtime imaging, like in the so-called prospective stereotaxy, a method for trajectory alignment for placements of catheters or sampling biopsies [25–27].

Alternative attempts to integrate intraoperative MRI and navigation result in a standard navigation setup because image space and surgical space are not identical, necessitating some kind of patient registration. Most setups implement navigation at the 5 G line, so that standard non-MR-compatible instruments can be used. Ceiling mounted solutions of the navigation camera and screens [5] are an optimal solution in the intraoperative scenario, since placing a standard navigation system just close to the MR scanner might increase the risk of potential magnetic accidents. High navigation accuracy is a prerequisite if the navigation information is to be used at critical steps during the resection of a tumor. Among all errors contributing to the overall navigation accuracy, the initial patient registration process is mostly prone to errors. The most common strategy for patient registration relies on placement of skin-adhesive fiducials, which can be detected in the images, so that their position in virtual and real physical space can be correlated to define the registration coordinate system. Automatic registration setups, allowing an user-independent registration of patient space and image space, try to reduce the user dependent errors [28].

Our concept of automatic registration is based on a registration matrix containing markers at predefined positions which are visible during the imaging process. Combining the information where the registration matrix is in relation to the reference array and how the detected markers in the images relate to the actual markers of the registration matrix allows calculating a transformation matrix, so that then the relation between image space and physical/surgical space is defined and navigation can be used. An additional skin fiducial that is not used for the registration process is localized after patient registration to document a target registration error, which is typically in the range between 0.3 and 2.5 mm. Phantom studies resulted in median localization errors between 0.88 and 2.13 mm for the automatic registration approach, which was at least not worse, in most test series even significantly better, than that of the standard registration no matter whether 4 or 7 fiducial markers were used [28].

Integration of Multimodal Data

It is absolutely mandatory to combine the goal of maximum resection with the goal of preservation of function. Intraoperative imaging helps on one side to maximize the extent of resection, but on the other side it also allows in combination with functional multimodal navigation a minimization of postoperative neurological deficits [13, 29]. With the advances in surgical techniques and perioperative technology, it is now possible to maximally resect malignant intrinsic glial neoplasms, even close to functionally critical areas, with minimally increased morbidity. Recent studies have demonstrated a survival advantage of these lesions with a resection extent of 98% or greater, particularly in younger patients with good Karnofsky scores [30].

Functional navigation, i.e. integrating functional data into anatomical navigational datasets, is an important add-on to intraoperative MRI since it prevents too extensive resections, which would otherwise result in new neurological deficits. Meanwhile, data from MEG and fMRI can be routinely integrated in functional navigation allowing identification of eloquent brain areas such as the motor area and speech related areas [10, 12].

In a retrospective study we analyzed how the decision for glioma resection was influenced by MEG [9]. In a time period of 5 consecutive years we had investigated every patient proposed for surgery, harbouring a lesion adjacent to eloquent brain areas. Altogether 191 patients were examined, 119 of them with supratentorial gliomas. About every forth patient (26.8%) yielded a severe possible danger of postoperative neurological morbidity according to MEG and thus was not considered being a good candidate for surgery. This corresponds well to other published data where 12 out of 40 investigated patients (30%) with tumours and vascular malformations underwent non-surgical therapy according to the MEG findings [31]. When functional data were used in combination with frameless stereotactic devices the postoperative morbidity was as low as 2.3%. Overall morbidity however was 6.8%. These data reflect the beneficial effects of functional navigation in comparison to data of other studies with morbidity rates varying from 6 to 31.7% [32–36]. These data can also be interpreted as a result of a more careful patient selection through the help of advanced preoperative brain mapping. Preoperative identification of eloquent brain areas has an impact in the risk evaluation in glioma surgery, as well as functional navigation reduces the risk for postoperative neurological deficits. Besides identification of the motor strip, the localisation of language areas is of great clinical impact [37, 38].

Functional data from MEG and fMRI only localize functional areas at the brain surface. However, neurological deficits can also be caused during tumor resection by damaging of deeper structures, such as major white matter tracts.

Diffusion tensor imaging (DTI) can be used not only to delineate tumor borders, but also to display the course of major white matter tracts, such as the pyramidal tract. The knowledge of the course of these tracts in relationship to a tumor helps to reduce or even prevent new postoperative neurological deficits [39, 40]. The registration of diffusion data with the navigational data [16, 41, 42] facilitates the intraoperative preservation of these eloquent structures. A prerequisite is that intraoperative changes of the brain anatomy, known as brain shift, are taken into account. In contrast to the use of fMRI and MEG, brain shift clinically impacts the DTI data to a much more relevant extent, because the intraoperative shifting of cortical areas during surgery can be well detected by direct observation with the operating microscope, however changes in the depth of a resection cavity, close to major white matter tracts, is nearly undetectable for the neurosurgeon during tumor resection. Intraoperative DTI is a convenient possibility to visualize this shifting during tumor resection [15, 43]. As a consequence of brain shift preoperative functional data are no longer valid during the course of tumor removal, so navigation can no longer relied on, if this shifting is not compensated for. Therefore, it is necessary that not only intraoperative anatomical data are used to compensate for the effects of brain shift but also functional data have to be updated. Intraoperative acquisition of DTI data enables intraoperative fiber tracking to visualize how a tumor remnant is localized in relation to major white matter tracts [15, 43]. Even intraoperative fMRI applying electrical stimulation of median and tibial nerves as a passive stimulation paradigm is possible and enables identification of the somatosensory cortex [44].

Besides functional and structural data further information is available for a multimodal navigation setup. PET, MRS, and diffusion weighted imaging may provide information on the diffuse tumor border. Integration of metabolic maps into the neuronavigation datasets enables a spatial correlation of metabolic data and histopathological findings [19, 45]. Whether these techniques can also be used intraoperatively, so that these data can also be updated, is under investigation. Furthermore, upcoming techniques such as MR-based molecular imaging may find its role in the intraoperative imaging armamentarium.

Navigation Updating by Intraoperative Image Data

Tumor removal, brain swelling, the use of brain retractors, and cerebrospinal-fluid drainage all result in intraoperative brain deformation, which is known as brain shift [24, 46]. Thus, in navigation systems relying on preoperative image data only the accuracy decreases with the course of surgery. Intraoperative imaging offers a possibility to compensate for the effects of brain shift, because it provides a virtual reproduction of the actual intraoperative physical reality, both in regard of brain deformation and on the actual extent of tumor removal [24, 47–49]. Updating of the navigation by intraoperative registration of the intraoperative image data had been a cumbersome process in the initial low-field MRI systems. Bone fiducial markers, which had to be placed around the craniotomy, were hardly detectable in the intraoperative images, as well as the whole update procedure was a quite time-consuming process [48, 49]. This mainly explains why only in 16 out of 330 patients investigated with low-field MRI an actual navigation update was performed, despite intraoperative imaging had detected tumor remnants e.g. in the gliomas that could undergo further resection in about 26% [48, 50].

Integrating high-field MRI and microscope-based navigation allowed facilitating this intraoperative update procedure clearly [5]. One possibility for intraoperative image registration is to apply the automatic registration matrix by attaching it to the upper part of the head coil, like it is done for the initial patient registration process with preoperative image data [28]. Alternatively navigation updating is also possible without repeated patient registration. This approach is based on a rigid registration of the intraoperative image data with the preoperative image data, subsequent segmentation of the tumor remnant, and final restoring of the initial patient registration. Thus, the registration coordinate system of the preoperative image data is applied on the intraoperative images, serving as an immediate intraoperative image update. Updated image data allow a reliable identification of a tumor remnant or correction of a catheter position. Microscope-based image injection with the direct visualization of the segmented tumor remnant in the surgical field plays a crucial role in the precise localization and orientation in the resection cavity. Histological analysis of the extended resections proved pathological tissue in all cases; there were no false positive findings. This is also mainly due to the fact that only areas of reliably identified tumor remnants were segmented and used for updating. The side-by-side analysis of pre- and intraoperative images greatly facilitates image interpretation and excludes misinterpretations due to surgically induced changes at the resection border. Repeated landmark checks have proved that the rigid registration approach is a reliable approach to update the navigation system without a repeated patient registration. The rigid registration algorithm is robust enough to accomplish a registration that is not sensitive to the effects of brain shift and the actual reduction of the tumor mass. This could be shown by analyzing the registration accuracy of structures that are not affected by brain shift. An extensive analysis comparing the automatic registration, which is used to register pre- and intraoperative images, with an independent reference registration showed, that the registration error is below 2 mm even in a worst case scenario [51]. Nevertheless, to prevent a mis-registration a visual control after rigid registration of pre- and intraoperative images is mandatory. Figures 1–3 depict an illustrative example of

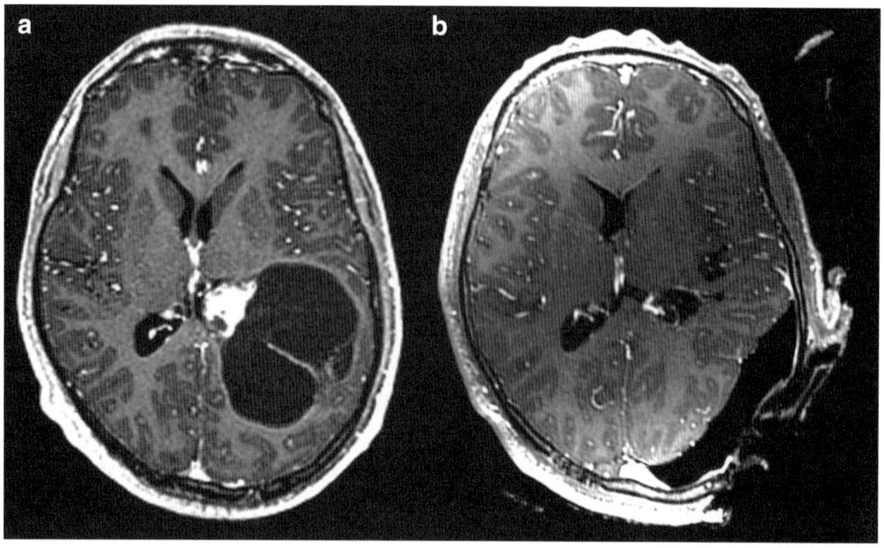

Fig. 1 22-years-old male patient with a left-sided parietal pilocytic astrocytoma, (**a**) preoperative image depicting the large cystic component, (**b**) intraoperative imaging after completion of tumor resection depicting complete tumor removal (both: contrast-enhanced T1-weighted images)

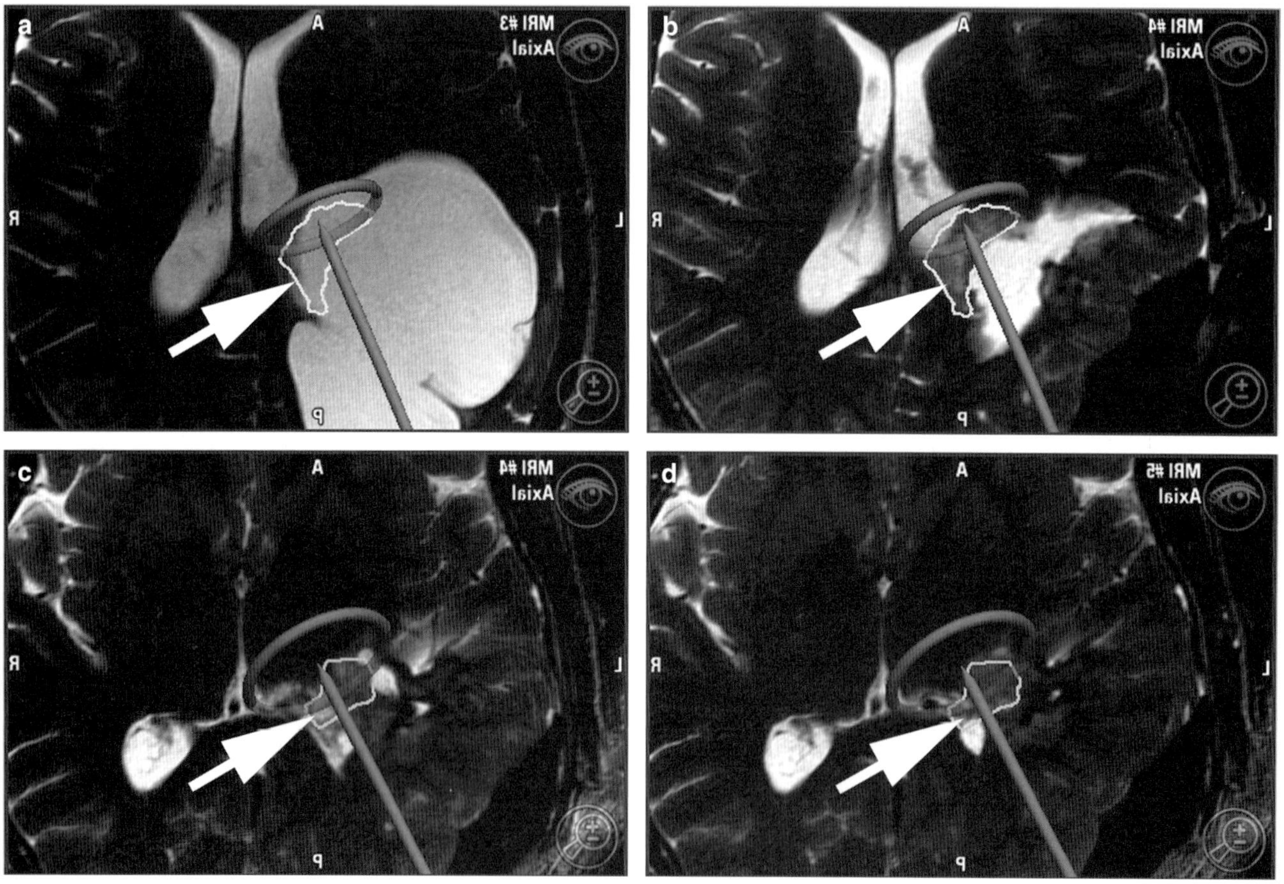

Fig. 2 Same patient as in Fig. 1; an update with intraoperative images was performed twice – **a/b** depict the first intraoperative update with a co-registered display of pre- and first intraoperative (iop1) images, while the tumor remnant was segmented in the iop1 images (**b**) and also displayed in the preoperative images (**a**) visualizing the distinct shift; **c/d** depict the second update after further tumor resection and repeated imaging, co-registered are first and second intraoperative imaging (iop2), the tumor remnant was segmented in the iop2 images (**d**) and also visualized in the iop1 images (**c**) (all images T2-weighted axial scans displayed with the navigation software, *white arrows* depict the segmented tumor remnants)

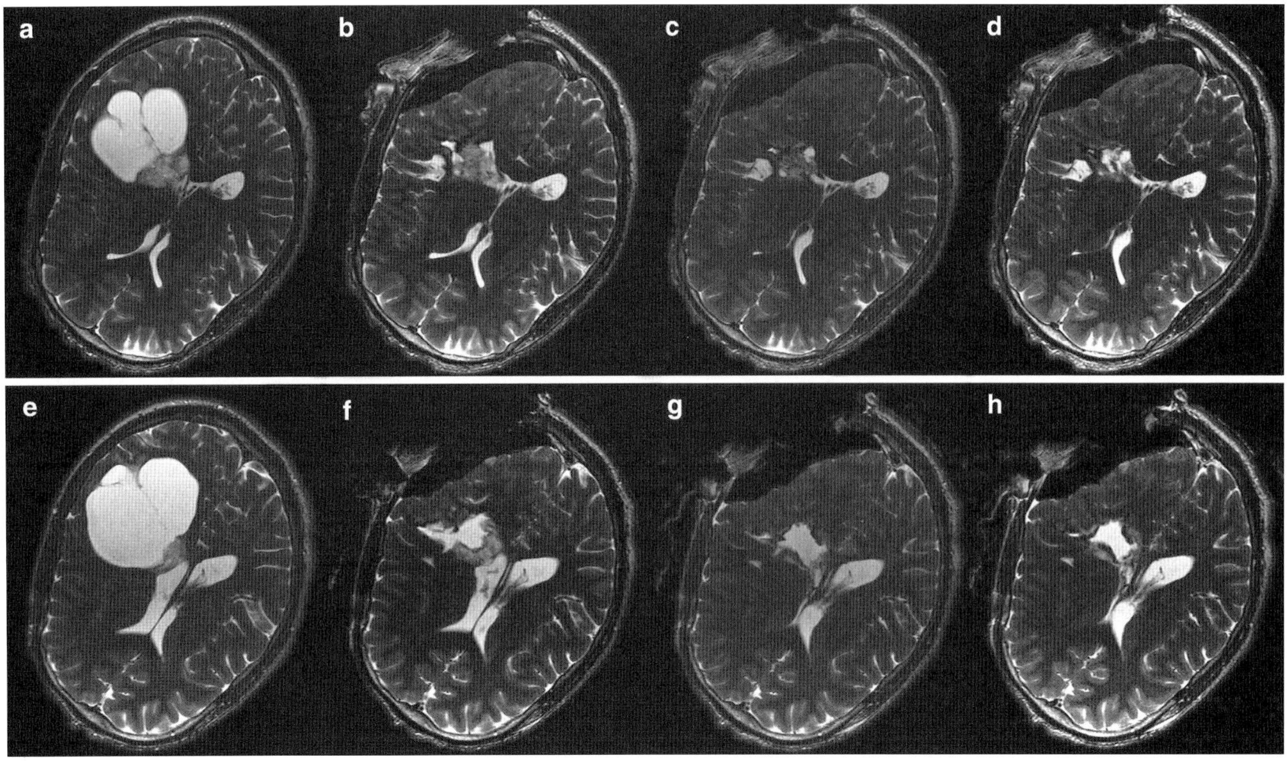

Fig. 3 Same patient as in Figs. 1 and 2 depicting the course of resection in two slice positions that were identical in all 4 imaging sessions (pre: **a/f**, iop1: **b/f**, iop2: **c/g**, iop3 **d/h**, all images axial T2-weighted, slice thickness 3 mm, difference between slice positions row **a–d** to row **e–h**: 9 mm), note the different portions of brain shift first after opening the large tumor cysts (difference **a/e** to **b/f**) and additionally after first updating collapsing of the left frontal ventricular horn (**f** to **g**)

repeated intraoperative updating during resection of a pilocytic astrocytoma.

Updating the navigation system with intraoperative high-field MR image data at the moment seems to be the most reliable method to compensate for the effects of brain shift. In contrast to previous setups this framework is also open to update multimodal information. Functional data, such as fMRI or DTI data can also be acquired intraoperatively and directly used for intraoperative updating, which in the clinical routine might be a time-consuming effort, especially when in case of e.g. visualization of speech connecting fiber tracts some sophisticated time-consuming non-standard tracking algorithms have to be applied.

Alternatively non-linear registration techniques or sophisticated techniques from pattern recognition analysis may allow a matching of preoperative MR data sets containing functional information with intraoperative MR image volumes [52, 53]. This might also be an approach in cases where intraoperative MRI is not available, but other imaging modalities provide intraoperative 3-D information about the brain configuration, so that high-resolution multi-modality data can be registered non-linearly onto the "low-quality" intraoperative data. Such an alternative to intraoperative MRI might be intraoperative ultrasound, especially intraoperative 3-D ultrasound [54–56]. Whether the image quality to evaluate the extent of a glioma resection is really equivalent among the different imaging modalities is still discussed controversially. Mathematical models describing the deformation of the brain during surgery might help in the process of deforming preoperative image data [57–61]. However, it is important that some sparse data describing the actual intraoperative 3-D situation serve as input for the mathematical models, so that they are able to adjust high-quality preoperative data to represent the intraoperative reality [59, 61–63]. If such a workflow is established intraoperative high-field MRI with anatomical and functional imaging possibilities would be the ideal tool to validate and refine these models.

Conclusion

Intraoperative high-field MRI in combination and close integration with microscope-based navigation serving as a common interface for the presentation of multimodal data in the surgical field seems to be one of the most promising surgical setups allowing avoiding unwanted tumor remnants while preserving neurological function. Multimodal navigation integrates standard anatomical, structural, functional, and metabolic data. Navigation achieves visualizing the initial extent of a lesion with the concomitant identification of neighboring eloquent brain structures, as well as, providing a tool for a direct correlation of histology and multimodal data. With the help of intraoperative imaging navigation data can be updated, so that brain shift can be compensated for and initially missed tumor remnants can be localized reliably.

Conflict of interest statement Ch. Nimsky is scientific consultant for Brainlab.

References

1. Black PM, Moriarty T, Alexander E III, Stieg P, Woodard EJ, Gleason PL, Martin CH, Kikinis R, Schwartz RB, Jolesz FA (1997) Development and implementation of intraoperative magnetic resonance imaging and its neurosurgical applications. Neurosurgery 41:831–845
2. Hall WA, Kowalik K, Liu H, Truwit CL, Kucharezyk J (2003) Costs and benefits of intraoperative MR-guided brain tumor resection. Acta Neurochir Suppl 85:137–142
3. Hall WA, Liu H, Martin AJ, Pozza CH, Maxwell RE, Truwit CL (2000) Safety, efficacy, and functionality of high-field strength interventional magnetic resonance imaging for neurosurgery. Neurosurgery 46:632–642
4. Nimsky C, Ganslandt O, Fahlbusch R (2005) Comparing 0.2 tesla with 1.5 tesla intraoperative magnetic resonance imaging analysis of setup, workflow, and efficiency. Acad Radiol 12:1065–1079
5. Nimsky C, Ganslandt O, Von Keller B, Romstock J, Fahlbusch R (2004) Intraoperative high-field-strength MR imaging: implementation and experience in 200 patients. Radiology 233:67–78
6. Sutherland GR, Kaibara T, Louw D, Hoult DI, Tomanek B, Saunders J (1999) A mobile high-field magnetic resonance system for neurosurgery. J Neurosurg 91:804–813
7. Nimsky C, Ganslandt O, Kober H, Buchfelder M, Fahlbusch R (2001) Intraoperative magnetic resonance imaging combined with neuronavigation: a new concept. Neurosurgery 48:1082–1091
8. Steinmeier R, Fahlbusch R, Ganslandt O, Nimsky C, Buchfelder M, Kaus M, Heigl T, Lenz G, Kuth R, Huk W (1998) Intraoperative magnetic resonance imaging with the magnetom open scanner: concepts, neurosurgical indications, and procedures: a preliminary report. Neurosurgery 43:739–748
9. Ganslandt O, Buchfelder M, Hastreiter P, Grummich P, Fahlbusch R, Nimsky C (2004) Magnetic source imaging supports clinical decision making in glioma patients. Clin Neurol Neurosurg 107:20–26
10. Ganslandt O, Fahlbusch R, Nimsky C, Kober H, Möller M, Steinmeier R, Romstöck J, Vieth J (1999) Functional neuronavigation with magnetoencephalography: outcome in 50 patients with lesions around the motor cortex. J Neurosurg 91:73–79
11. Ganslandt O, Steinmeier R, Kober H, Vieth J, Kassubek J, Romstock J, Strauss C, Fahlbusch R (1997) Magnetic source imaging combined with image-guided frameless stereotaxy: a new method in surgery around the motor strip. Neurosurgery 41:621–628
12. Nimsky C, Ganslandt O, Kober H, Moller M, Ulmer S, Tomandl B, Fahlbusch R (1999) Integration of functional magnetic resonance imaging supported by magnetoencephalography in functional neuronavigation. Neurosurgery 44:1249–1256
13. Nimsky C, Ganslandt O, Fahlbusch R (2005) 1.5 T: intraoperative imaging beyond standard anatomic imaging. Neurosurg Clin N Am 16:185–200, vii
14. Nimsky C, Ganslandt O, Fahlbusch R (2006) Implementation of fiber tract navigation. Neurosurgery 58:292–304
15. Nimsky C, Ganslandt O, Hastreiter P, Wang R, Benner T, Sorensen AG, Fahlbusch R (2005) Preoperative and intraoperative diffusion tensor imaging-based fiber tracking in glioma surgery. Neurosurgery 56:130–138
16. Nimsky C, Ganslandt O, Merhof D, Sorensen AG, Fahlbusch R (2006) Intraoperative visualization of the pyramidal tract by diffusion-tensor-imaging-based fiber tracking. Neuroimage 30: 1219–1229
17. Ganslandt O, Stadlbauer A, Fahlbusch R, Kamada K, Buslei R, Blumcke I, Moser E, Nimsky C (2005) Proton magnetic resonance spectroscopic imaging integrated into image-guided surgery: correlation to standard magnetic resonance imaging and tumor cell density. Neurosurgery 56:291–298
18. Stadlbauer A, Ganslandt O, Buslei R, Hammen T, Gruber S, Moser E, Buchfelder M, Salomonowitz E, Nimsky C (2006) Gliomas: histopathologic evaluation of changes in directionality and magnitude of water diffusion at diffusion-tensor MR imaging. Radiology 240:803–810
19. Stadlbauer A, Moser E, Gruber S, Nimsky C, Fahlbusch R, Ganslandt O (2004) Integration of biochemical images of a tumor into frameless stereotaxy achieved using a magnetic resonance imaging/magnetic resonance spectroscopy hybrid data set. J Neurosurg 101:287–294
20. Stadlbauer A, Nimsky C, Buslei R, Pinker K, Gruber S, Hammen T, Buchfelder M, Ganslandt O (2007) Proton magnetic resonance spectroscopic imaging in the border zone of gliomas: correlation of metabolic and histological changes at low tumor infiltration–initial results. Invest Radiol 42:218–223
21. Stadlbauer A, Nimsky C, Buslei R, Salomonowitz E, Hammen T, Buchfelder M, Moser E, Ernst-Stecken A, Ganslandt O (2007) Diffusion tensor imaging and optimized fiber tracking in glioma patients: histopathologic evaluation of tumor-invaded white matter structures. Neuroimage 34:949–956
22. Stadlbauer A, Prante O, Nimsky C, Salomonowitz E, Buchfelder M, Kuwert T, Linke R, Ganslandt O (2008) Metabolic imaging of cerebral gliomas: spatial correlation of changes in O-(2-18F-fluoroethyl)-L-tyrosine PET and proton magnetic resonance spectroscopic imaging. J Nucl Med 49:721–729
23. Black PM, Alexander E III, Martin C, Moriarty T, Nabavi A, Wong TZ, Schwartz RB, Jolesz F (1999) Craniotomy for tumor treatment in an intraoperative magnetic resonance imaging unit. Neurosurgery 45:423–433
24. Nabavi A, Black PM, Gering DT, Westin CF, Mehta V, Pergolizzi RS Jr, Ferrant M, Warfield SK, Hata N, Schwartz RB, Wells WM 3rd, Kikinis R, Jolesz FA (2001) Serial intraoperative magnetic resonance imaging of brain shift. Neurosurgery 48:787–798
25. Hall WA, Liu H, Truwit CL (2000) Navigus trajectory guide. Neurosurgery 46:502–504
26. Truwit CL, Hall WA (2006) Intraoperative magnetic resonance imaging-guided neurosurgery at 3-T. Neurosurgery 58:ONS338–ONS345, discussion ONS345–ONS346
27. Truwit CL, Liu H (2001) Prospective stereotaxy: a novel method of trajectory alignment using real-time image guidance. J Magn Reson Imaging 13:452–457
28. Rachinger J, von Keller B, Ganslandt O, Fahlbusch R, Nimsky C (2006) Application accuracy of automatic registration in frameless stereotaxy. Stereotact Funct Neurosurg 84:109–117
29. Nimsky C, Ganslandt O, Fahlbusch R (2004) Functional neuronavigation and intraoperative MRI. Adv Tech Stand Neurosurg 29:229–263

30. Hentschel SJ, Sawaya R (2003) Optimizing outcomes with maximal surgical resection of malignant gliomas. Cancer Control 10:109–114
31. Hund M, Rezai AR, Kronberg E, Cappell J, Zonenshayn M, Ribary U, Kelly PJ, Llinas R (1997) Magnetoencephalographic mapping: basic of a new functional risk profile in the selection of patients with cortical brain lesions. Neurosurgery 40:936–943
32. Ammirati M, Galicich JH, Arbit E, Liao Y (1987) Reoperation in the treatment of recurrent intracranial malignant gliomas. Neurosurgery 21:607–614
33. Black PM (1999) Surgery for cerebral gliomas: past, present and future. In: Howard MA III, Elliott JP, Haglund MM, McKhann GM II (eds) Clinical neurosurgery, vol 47. Lippincott Williams & Wilkins, Boston, pp 21–45
34. Cabantog AM, Bernstein M (1994) Complications of first craniotomy for intra-axial brain tumour. Can J Neurol Sci 21:213–218
35. Ciric I, Ammirati M, Vick N, Mikhael M (1987) Supratentorial gliomas: surgical considerations and immediate postoperative results. Gross total resection versus partial resection. Neurosurgery 21:21–26
36. Fadul C, Wood J, Thaler H, Galicich J, Patterson RH Jr, Posner JB (1988) Morbidity and mortality of craniotomy for excision of supratentorial gliomas. Neurology 38:1374–1379
37. Grummich P, Nimsky C, Pauli E, Buchfelder M, Ganslandt O (2006) Combining fMRI and MEG increases the reliability of presurgical language localization: a clinical study on the difference between and congruence of both modalities. Neuroimage 32: 1793–1803
38. Kober H, Moller M, Nimsky C, Vieth J, Fahlbusch R, Ganslandt O (2001) New approach to localize speech relevant brain areas and hemispheric dominance using spatially filtered magnetoencephalography. Hum Brain Mapp 14:236–250
39. Clark CA, Barrick TR, Murphy MM, Bell BA (2003) White matter fiber tracking in patients with space-occupying lesions of the brain: a new technique for neurosurgical planning? Neuroimage 20:1601–1608
40. Hendler T, Pianka P, Sigal M, Kafri M, Ben-Bashat D, Constantini S, Graif M, Fried I, Assaf Y (2003) Delineating gray and white matter involvement in brain lesions: three-dimensional alignment of functional magnetic resonance and diffusion-tensor imaging. J Neurosurg 99:1018–1027
41. Coenen VA, Krings T, Mayfrank L, Polin RS, Reinges MH, Thron A, Gilsbach JM (2001) Three-dimensional visualization of the pyramidal tract in a neuronavigation system during brain tumor surgery: first experiences and technical note. Neurosurgery 49:86–93
42. Nimsky C, Grummich P, Sorensen AG, Fahlbusch R, Ganslandt O (2005) Visualization of the pyramidal tract in glioma surgery by integrating diffusion tensor imaging in functional neuronavigation. Zentralbl Neurochir 66:133–141
43. Nimsky C, Ganslandt O, Hastreiter P, Wang R, Benner T, Sorensen A, Fahlbusch R (2005) Intraoperative diffusion-tensor MR imaging: shifting of white matter tracts during neurosurgical procedures – initial experience. Radiology 234:218–225
44. Gasser T, Ganslandt O, Sandalcioglu E, Stolke D, Fahlbusch R, Nimsky C (2005) Intraoperative functional MRI: implementation and preliminary experience. Neuroimage 26:685–693
45. Stadlbauer A, Moser E, Gruber S, Buslei R, Nimsky C, Fahlbusch R, Ganslandt O (2004) Improved delineation of brain tumors: an automated method for segmentation based on pathologic changes of 1H-MRSI metabolites in gliomas. Neuroimage 23:454–461
46. Hastreiter P, Rezk-Salama C, Nimsky C, Lürig C, Greiner G, Ertl T (2000) Registration techniques for the analysis of the brain shift in neurosurgery. Comput Graph 24:385–389
47. Hastreiter P, Rezk-Salama C, Soza G, Bauer M, Greiner G, Fahlbusch R, Ganslandt O, Nimsky C (2004) Strategies for brain shift evaluation. Med Image Anal 8:447–464
48. Nimsky C, Ganslandt O, Hastreiter P, Fahlbusch R (2001) Intraoperative compensation for brain shift. Surg Neurol 56:357–365
49. Wirtz CR, Bonsanto MM, Knauth M, Tronnier VM, Albert FK, Staubert A, Kunze S (1997) Intraoperative magnetic resonance imaging to update interactive navigation in neurosurgery: method and preliminary experience. Comput Aided Surg 2:172–179
50. Nimsky C, Ganslandt O, Tomandl B, Buchfelder M, Fahlbusch R (2002) Low-field magnetic resonance imaging for intraoperative use in neurosurgery: a 5-year experience. Eur Radiol 12: 2690–2703
51. Veyrat A (2005) Automatic fusion of pre-and intraoperative patienta data. A statistical evaluation of accuracy. Diploma thesis, Technical University Munich
52. Archip N, Clatz O, Whalen S, Kacher D, Fedorov A, Kot A, Chrisochoides N, Jolesz F, Golby A, Black PM, Warfield SK (2007) Non-rigid alignment of pre-operative MRI, fMRI, and DT-MRI with intra-operative MRI for enhanced visualization and navigation in image-guided neurosurgery. Neuroimage 35:609–624
53. Wolf M, Vogel T, Weierich P, Niemann H, Nimsky C (2001) Automatic transfer of preoperative fMRI markers into intraoperative MR-images for updating functional neuronavigation. IEICE Trans Inf Syst E84-D:1698–1704
54. Comeau RM, Sadikot AF, Fenster A, Peters TM (2000) Intraoperative ultrasound for guidance and tissue shift correction in image-guided neurosurgery. Med Phys 27:787–800
55. Letteboer MM, Willems PW, Viergever MA, Niessen WJ (2005) Brain shift estimation in image-guided neurosurgery using 3-D ultrasound. IEEE Trans Biomed Eng 52:268–276
56. Tirakotai W, Miller D, Heinze S, Benes L, Bertalanffy H, Sure U (2006) A novel platform for image-guided ultrasound. Neurosurgery 58:710–718
57. Arbel T, Morandi X, Comeau RM, Collins DL (2004) Automatic non-linear MRI-ultrasound registration for the correction of intra-operative brain deformations. Comput Aided Surg 9:123–136
58. Coenen VA, Krings T, Weidemann J, Hans FJ, Reinacher P, Gilsbach JM, Rohde V (2005) Sequential visualization of brain and fiber tract deformation during intracranial surgery with three-dimensional ultrasound: an approach to evaluate the effect of brain shift. Neurosurgery 56:133–141
59. Lunn KE, Paulsen KD, Lynch DR, Roberts DW, Kennedy FE, Hartov A (2005) Assimilating intraoperative data with brain shift modeling using the adjoint equations. Med Image Anal 9:281–293
60. Rasmussen IA Jr, Lindseth F, Rygh OM, Berntsen EM, Selbekk T, Xu J, Nagelhus Hernes TA, Harg E, Haberg A, Unsgaard G (2007) Functional neuronavigation combined with intra-operative 3D ultrasound: initial experiences during surgical resections close to eloquent brain areas and future directions in automatic brain shift compensation of preoperative data. Acta Neurochir (Wien) 149:365–378
61. Roberts DW, Miga MI, Hartov A, Eisner S, Lemery JM, Kennedy FE, Paulsen KD (1999) Intraoperatively updated neuroimaging using brain modeling and sparse data. Neurosurgery 45:1199–1207
62. Cao A, Thompson RC, Dumpuri P, Dawant BM, Galloway RL, Ding S, Miga MI (2008) Laser range scanning for image-guided neurosurgery: investigation of image-to-physical space registrations. Med Phys 35:1593–1605
63. Ding S, Miga MI, Thompson RC, Dumpuri P, Cao A, Dawant BM (2007) Estimation of intra-operative brain shift using a tracked laser range scanner. Conf Proc IEEE Eng Med Biol Soc 2007: 848–851

Multimodality Imaging Suite: Neo-Futuristic Diagnostic Imaging Operating Suite Marks a Significant Milestone for Innovation in Medical Technology

Mitsunori Matsumae, Jun Koizumi, Atsushi Tsugu, Go Inoue, Jun Nishiyama, Michitsura Yoshiyama, Jiro Tominaga, and Hideki Atsumi

Abstract In February 2006, Tokai University Hospital officially opened the imaging operation suite, which is the first hybrid neurosurgical procedure suite to combine magnetic resonance imaging, computed tomography and angiography with a neurosurgical operating room. Here, we describe the concept of the imaging operation suite and the first 4 years' experience using this suite.

Keywords Imaging operation room · Interventional procedure · Intraoperative MRI · MRI

Introduction

The use of magnetic resonance imaging (MRI) in diagnostic radiology has made great strides over the last 20 years. In many hospitals, MRI is no longer used exclusively for diagnostic imaging. It also plays a crucial role during therapy and interventional procedures, and has now been introduced into an operating suite. At the Tokai University Hospital, Kanagawa Japan, seamless integration of MRI and X-ray imaging with a high-end operating table has been accomplished in a futuristic and highly efficient approach to image-guided surgery [1, 2].

Method

The new facility is equipped with ideally-positioned radiological equipment (computed tomography (CT), MRI, and angiography) combined with a fully-functional operating room. Physically, the MRI, CT, and combined operating theater with X-ray angiography components have been installed in three separate bays (Fig. 1), separated by a sliding door lined with lead and copper shielding for X-ray and MR, respectively When the door is closed, each room may be used independently, enabling unsurpassed flexibility and economic efficiency.

For procedures that combine use of MRI and angiography, the angiography table can be rotated in the direction of the MRI room. The connecting bridge is then placed between the MRI table and the angiography table. The tabletop can then be moved in both directions.

For procedures that combine CT and angiography, the angiography table can be rotated in the direction of the CT room. Then, the CT table and angiography table are joined directly, and the tabletop can be moved in both directions. During imaging, the shielding door must be closed to eliminate imaging artifacts.

For procedures that combine surgery and MRI, the operating table can be placed in the direction of the MRI room, and surgery can be performed normally in that position. Intraoperative imaging can be performed at any time, provided that the usual precautions are taken to ensure sterility. When a surgeon calls for mixed modality imaging, the tabletop carrying the patient can be slid in-line through the open door between the two rooms of the suite, allowing reproducible imaging with minimal patient movement and time delay, while the most appropriate modality can be selected at any particular moment during any procedure (Figs. 2 and 3).

The center room is equipped with an operating room-grade, clean air-conditioning system, operating lights, medical gas outlets, and an in-hospital information system; this enables various surgical procedures, including craniotomy, to be undertaken. The adjacent CT and MRI rooms are also equipped with medical gas outlets, an OR-grade, clean air-conditioning system, and operating lights, etc., for the safe transfer of an anesthetized patient to the CT or MRI for diagnosis.

M. Matsumae (✉), J. Koizumi, A. Tsugu, G. Inoue, J. Nishiyama, M. Yoshiyama, J. Tominaga, and H. Atsumi
Department of Neurosurgery, Tokai University School of Medicine, 143 Shimokasuya, Isehara, Kanagawa, 259-1193, Japan
e-mail: mike@is.icc.u-tokai.ac.jp

DOI 10.1007/978-3-211-99651-5_33,

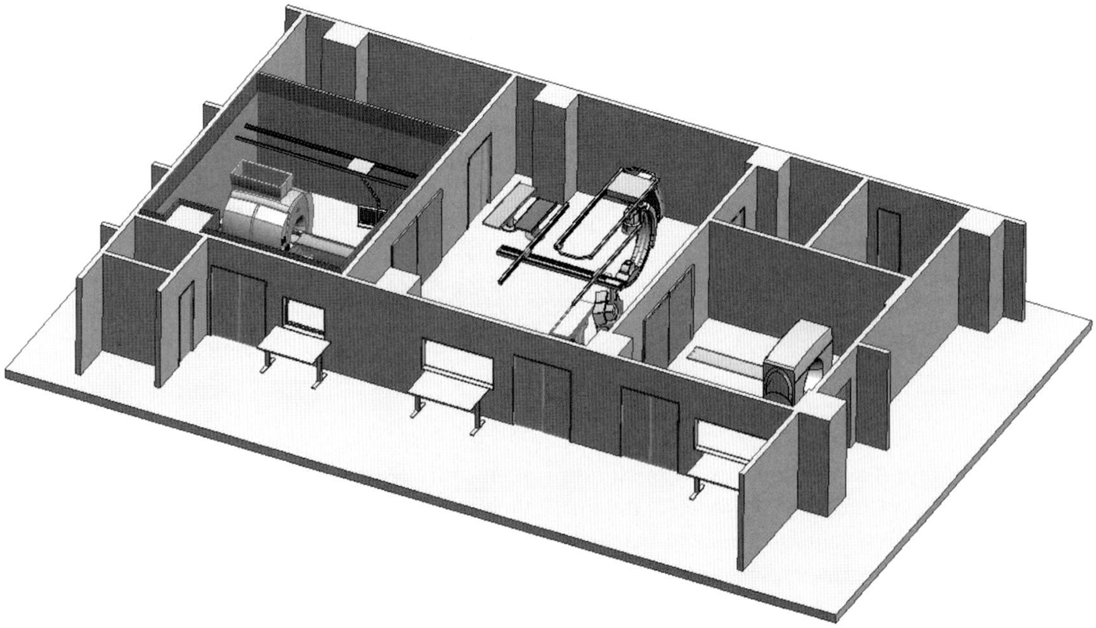

Fig. 1 Schematic diagram of Tokai University's imaging operating suite. *Left*: MR scanner, center: angiography equipment combined with operating room, *right*: CT scanner. Electric sliding doors enable either combined or single use of the separate areas

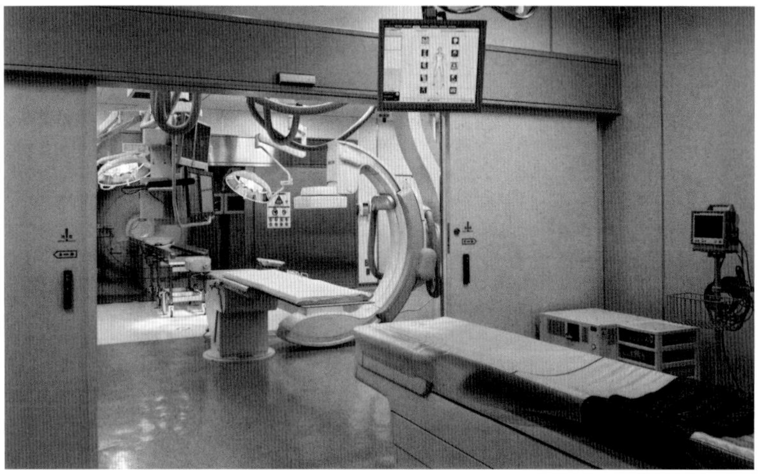

Fig. 2 View from the CT through the angiography with operating room to the MRI scanner of the imaging operating suite at Tokai University Hospital

All ferromagnetic instruments are removed from the surgical field, and the wound is covered with a sterile drape. The patient can, in fact, be moved into and out of the scanner in some 10–20 s, but due account must be taken of the time needed to remove the non-MRI compatible instruments and to adjust the surgical drapes. The results of the imaging can determine the surgical approach by showing the presence of any residual tumor that can be safely removed, often in areas that cannot be directly observed by the surgeon. After the intraoperative imaging, the patient is returned to the primary surgical position, and resection continues.

Results

One or two cases of neurosurgery and two cases of radiological intervention are currently performed per week. In addition, routine diagnosis of a variety of diseases is done when this suite is not being used for interventional procedures. An average of 40 diagnostic CT cases, 16 diagnostic MRI cases, and one angiography case are performed each day using these facilities, both day and night, and also on weekends.

The indications for using this suite for neurosurgical procedures include any type of supratentorial or infraten-

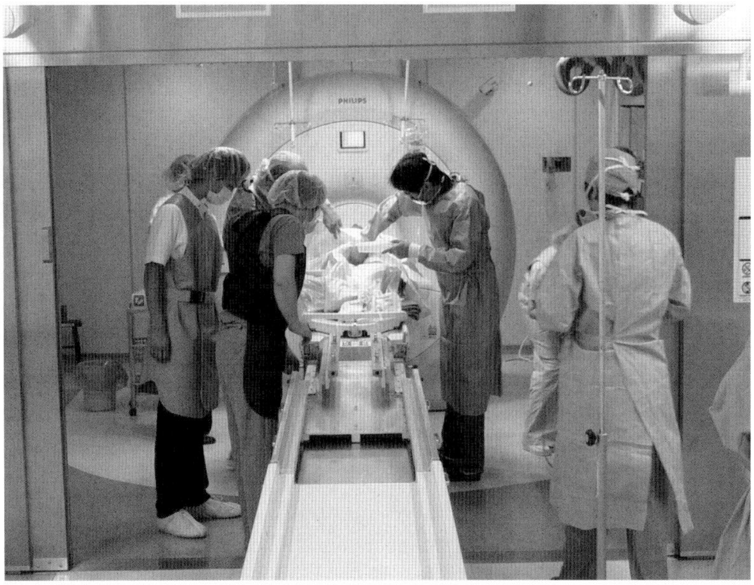

Fig. 3 Interventional radiologist brings his patient into the MR scanner from the angiography bay

torial glioma, and pituitary adenomas that extend superiorly and laterally. MRI scans have been taken an average of 1.2 times per procedure, with a maximum of 5 MR imaging sessions per surgical procedure. Most MRI scans were performed in the final stage of the surgical procedure to identify small residual tumor. The choice of MRI scan sequence depends on the type of tumor.

For interventional radiology procedures, this suite is used for the treatment of stroke, intra-abdominal tumors, and any vascular occlusive diseases. For example, in patients with uterine cervical cancer, chemoinfusion therapy via bilateral internal iliac arteries is performed. To increase drug concentration in the cancer and decrease the infusion of drug into the extrapelvic organs, balloon-occluded arterial infusion therapy is routinely attempted. However, the actual perfusion depends on each patient's anatomy, though angiography does not adequately demonstrate it. The comparison of direct perfusion images during arterial infusion of contrast media with and without balloon-occlusion is helpful to obtain the optimal distribution of anticancer drugs. For patients with portal hypertension or splenomegaly, partial splenic embolization is often performed. Before partial splenic embolization, the gastric or pancreatic branches from the splenic artery should be excluded from the embolization, and CT during splenic arteriography helps discriminate these branches. Because excessive embolization of the splenic artery may induce abscess formation, 60–75% of embolization is thought to be optimal. However, the evaluation of necrotic volume is not easy on angiography or even CT, because congestion of contrast media during embolization disturbs the images. MRI is useful to demonstrate the ischemic foci immediately after the procedure on blood oxygen level-dependent images without any contrast media. Several other indications, such as the evaluation of laser ablation, percutaneous biopsy, abscess drainage, etc., should be included for this state-of-art this system in the future.

Discussion

The present imaging operating suite represents the state of the art in the respective imaging modalities. Together they offer exciting opportunities to explore new fields of interactive and interventional imaging. In the field of intraoperative MRI, in 1993 Brigham and Women's Hospital introduced the world's first intraoperative MRI system, the so-called double doughnut [3]. At Brigham and Women's Hospital, they brought MRI into the operating theater. In the German city of Erlangen, there is a unique intraoperative MRI system, the so-called "twin operating theater", in which an independent MRI scanner and surgical unit are housed in two separate rooms [4]. There are several intraoperative MRI systems currently available in the world, in which the MRI machine is placed in the operating room [5, 6], the MRI machine is placed next to the operating room [2], a small MRI machine is installed under the operating table [7–9], or a mobile MRI scanner is moved into the operating room [10]. With respect to the MRI scanners, there are MRI scanners specially designed for intraoperative MR scanning [3, 7–9], and some are routine diagnostic MRI scanners modified for use as intraoperative MRI scanners [2, 5]; the MR scanner field strength started low and became relatively high, now reaching 3 T [11].

In the present imaging operating suite, special attention has been given to economic issues. Our key phrase is "sharing imaging equipment". The center room is the core of the suite; it contains angiographic equipment within a fully functional operating room. The tabletop enables both imaging and surgical procedures. The most significant feature of this system is the ease of patient transfer between imaging during treatment, e.g., from angiographic examination to MRI or CT without changing beds. The patient can be transferred easily from the operating table to the MRI, and back to imaging once again. Patient transfer during treatment is performed with the utmost care under the direction of a specially trained safety supervisor.

Each of the imaging modalities is capable of performing diagnostic examinations; however, once treatment (for example, surgery) commences in the operating room located in the center of the suite, imaging is easily performed as required to provide intraoperative information using high-performance diagnostic equipment.

Neurosurgical procedures aim to accomplish safe treatment with high precision in a short period of time. Here, the key that governs the progress of the operation is the intraoperative identification of the extent of preoperative planning achieved at a given time. We consider that this suite enables precise patient treatment within a shorter time period than previously possible because the progress of the operation can now be identified using intraoperative imaging as required. In practical terms, the system facilitates intraoperative patient transfer from the treatment room to the MRI examination room for verification of the patient's condition and the degree of procedural progress before returning to the treatment room and return transfer to the examination room for final verification before the operation is completed; surgery proceeds more smoothly and safely than previously possible.

Operating rooms equipped with a CT scanner, MRI, or angiographic equipment have been developed previously; however, this newly-built imaging operating suite at Tokai University Hospital is a more evolved, integrated system of radiological diagnosis/treatment and surgery that represents a "neo-futuristic diagnostic imaging operating suite". Tokai University Hospital will endeavor to enhance the efficacy of treatment by actively using this imaging operating suite. This multimodality imaging intervention suite was developed successfully and is another milestone for innovation in medical technology, which reflects the flexible attitude of our hospital with respect to the needs of all kinds of patients.

This imaging operating suite is not currently used to perform intra-operative angiography. However, it is likely that there will be a need to perform intraoperative angiography (e.g., balloon-assisted aneurysm clipping, identification of perfusion during removal of an arterio-venous malformation nidus) using this suite in the near future. The intraoperative functional techniques that have so far been used for surgical decision-making with this imaging operating suite have been MR spectroscopy, functional MRI, MR angiography and venography, and chemical shift imaging. We are planning to introduce thermoablation therapy for removal of brain tumors under the guidance of MR temperature mapping. Moreover, we are exploring the possibility of applying this imaging operating suite to other fields, such as otorhinology and orthopedics. There are many possibilities for this unique interventional suite in various medical fields.

Conflict of interest statement We declare that we have no conflict of interest.

Reference

1. Matsumae M, Fukuyama H, Osada T, Baba T, Mizokami Y, Atsumi H, Ishizaka H, Tsugu A, Tominaga J, Shiramizu H, Shimoda M (2008) Fully functional MR-compatible flexible operating table resolves the neurosurgeon's dilemma over use of intraoperative MRI. Tokai J Exp Clin Med 33:57–60
2. Matsumae M, Koizumi J, Fukuyama H, Ishizaka H, Mizokami Y, Baba T, Atsumi H, Tsugu A, Oda S, Tanaka Y, Osada T, Imai M, Ishigura T, Yamamoto M, Tominaga J, Shimoda M, Imai Y (2007) World's first hybrid interventional procedure suite; MRI/X-ray/Operation suite (MRXO) marks a significant milestone in improvement of neurosurgical diagnosis and treatment. J Neurosurg 107:266–273
3. Black PM, Moriarty T, Alexander E III, Stieg P, Woodard EJ, Gleason PL, Martin CH, Kikinis R, Schwartz RB, Jolesz FA (1997) Development and implementation of intraoperative magnetic resonance imaging and its neurosurgical applications. Neurosurgery 41:831–845
4. Steinmeier R, Fahlbusch R, Ganslandt O, Nimsky C, Buchfelder M, Kaus M, Heigl T, Lenz G, Kuth R, Huk W (1998) Intraoperative magnetic resonance imaging with the magnetom open scanner: concepts, neurosurgical indications, and procedures: a preliminary report. Neurosurgery 43:739–747
5. Hall WA, Liu H, Martin AJ, Pozza CH, Maxwell RE, Truwit CL (2000) Safety, efficacy, and functionality of high-field strength interventional magnetic resonance imaging for neurosurgery. Neurosurgery 46:632–642
6. Nimsky C, Ganslandt O, Von Keller B, Romstöck J, Fahlbusch R (2004) Intraoperative high-field-strength MR imaging: implementation and experience in 200 patients. Radiology 233:67–78
7. Ahn JY, Jung JY, Kim J, Lee KS, Kim SH (2008) How to overcome the limitations to determine the resection margin of pituitary tumours with low-field intra-operative MRI during trans-sphenoidal surgery: usefulness of Gadolinium-soaked cotton pledgets. Acta Neurochir 150:763–771
8. Hadani M, Spiegelman R, Feldman Z, Berkenstadt H, Ram Z (2001) Novel, compact, intraoperative magnetic resonance imaging-guided system for conventional neurosurgical operating rooms. Neurosurgery 48:799–809
9. Schulder M, Catrambone J, Carmel PW (2005) Intraoperative magnetic resonance imaging at 0.12 T: is it enough? Neurosurg Clin N Am 16:143–154
10. Sutherland GR, Kaibara T, Louw D, Hoult DI, Tomanek B, Saunders J (1999) (1999) A mobile high-field magnetic resonance system for neurosurgery. J Neurosurg 91:804–813
11. Pamir MN, Peker S, Ozek MM, Dinçer A (2006) Intraoperative MR imaging: preliminary results with 3 Tesla MR system. Acta Neurochir Suppl 98:97–100

Improving Patient Safety in the Intra-operative MRI Suite Using an On-Duty Safety Nurse, Safety Manual and Checklist

Mitsunori Matsumae, Yasuhiro Nakajima, Eiji Morikawa, Jun Nishiyama, Hideki Atsumi, Jiro Tominaga, Atsushi Tsugu, and Isao Kenmochi

Abstract This paper describes the use of an on-duty safety nurse, a surgical safety manual and a checklist as an essential precursor to evaluating how these approaches affect surgical quality, communication in surgery crews and contribute to the safety of surgical care in the intra-operative magnetic resonance imaging (MRI) suite.

Keywords Checklist · Intra-operative magnetic resonance imaging · Manual · On-duty safety nurse · Surgical safety

Introduction

The use of intra-operative imaging is gradually increasing in the field of neurosurgery. In February 2006, our hospital officially opened the Magnetic Resonance/X-ray/Operation Suite (MRXO) which is a novel surgical suite that includes an interventional radiology system for intra-operative MRI. This imaging operation suite represents a major advance in the field of neurosurgery, and will facilitate the development of many new clinical techniques. The details of this imaging operation suite were reported previously [1, 2].

We introduced an on-duty safety nurse, a surgical safety manual and a checklist in this imaging operation suite. There are several reasons for introducing this safety system into this imaging operation suite. During interventional procedure specially designed for the intra-operative MRI, the surgical crew must pay special attention to both surgical and MRI safety. Intra-operative MRI is not a routine surgical procedure, and the surgical crew is not as accustomed to this kind of special procedure. There are many steps required to take an MR image during surgery. Additionally, teamwork in the intra-operative MRI suite is an important component of operation room efficiency, quality of surgical care, and patient safety. For this reason, the surgical safety manual and checklist and the on-duty safety nurse are needed to manage concerns or ambiguities related to procedures, promote team building, and keep the surgical workflow smooth.

M. Matsumae (✉), J. Nishiyama, H. Atsumi, J. Tominaga, and A. Tsugu
Department of Neurosurgery, Tokai University School of Medicine, 143 Shimokasuya, Isehara, Kanagawa 259-1193, Japan
e-mail: mike@is.icc.u-tokai.ac.jp

Y. Nakajima, E. Morikawa, and I. Kenmochi
Division of Emergency and Critical Care Unit, Tokai University Hospital, 143 Shimokasuya, Isehara, Kanagawa 259-1193, Japan

Materials and Methods

On-Duty Safety Nurse

The aim of the on-duty safety nurse is to focus only on safety issues. The on-duty safety nurse functions independently from nurses involved in the surgical procedure, and behaves as a third person in the imaging operation room. During preparation for the intra-operative MRI, the on-duty safety nurse reads aloud a surgical safety manual and checklist (Fig. 1). The on-duty safety nurse is requested to speak up and provide clear instructions during the surgery. The surgical safety checklist is read aloud by the on-duty safety nurse and requires oral confirmation by all other crew in the intra-operative suite. All crew in the operation room, including the surgeon, anesthesiologist, scrub and circulation nurses, and radiology technician, are required to follow the on-duty safety nurse's instructions.

Surgical Safety Manual

The surgical safety manual defines six phases of the surgery: preoperative inspection (42 items), before skin incision (16 items), preparation for the intra-operative MRI (75 items), after taking the intra-operative MRI (53 items),

DOI 10.1007/978-3-211-99651-5_34, © Springer-Verlag/Wien 2011

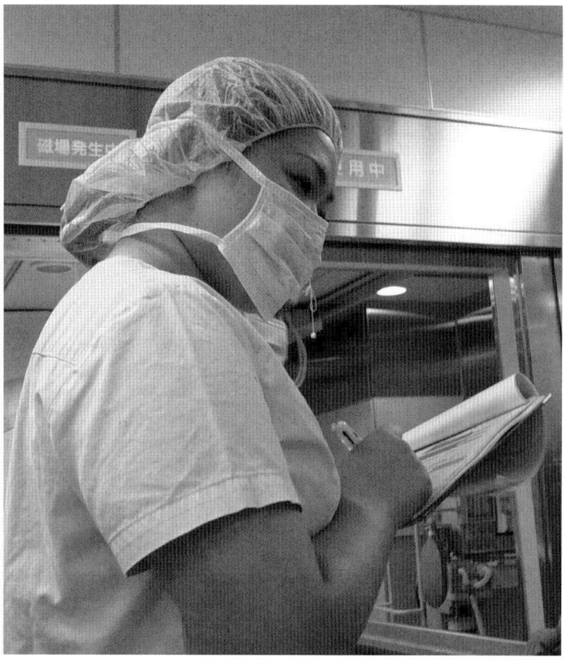

Fig. 1 The safety checklist is orally implemented by the on-duty safety nurse with oral confirmation by other crew members. The on-duty safety nurse improves team communication and enables smooth workflow during surgery

after the operation (20 items), and non-normal (emergency) condition (32 items). The surgical safety manual and checklist identifies each phase corresponding to a specific period in the workflow of the intra-operative MRI. In each phase, the surgical safety manual and checklist help surgical crews confirm that the critical safety steps are completed before proceeding with the operation and other activities.

The phase of *preoperative inspection* includes: confirmation of the conditions of all surgical and imaging facilities, identification of the surgical procedure, verification of the patient's name, and introduction of the crew to each other.

The phase of *before skin incision* includes: a clearance check for the MRI bore (Fig. 2), and verification of whether the right procedure is being performed on the right patient at the right head site.

The *preparation for the intra-operative MRI* phase has many points. For intra-operative MRI, surgery can be performed in the usual fashion with usual surgical instruments (not MRI compatible). Intra-operative imaging can be performed at any time. Once the surgeon wants to take the intra-operative MRI, the on-duty safety nurse takes control of the procedure. The on-duty safety nurse instructs the surgeons and scrub nurse to remove all ferromagnetic instruments from the surgical field, and the surgical wound is covered with a sterile drape while the tabletop is placed in a flat position. The circulation nurse places the patient transfer system between the operating table and the MRI table on the order of the on-duty safety nurse. Once the on-duty safety nurse checks the patient's transfer system, the locking system that unlocks the tabletop from the operation table base can be released. After the safety checklist is completed, the on-duty safety nurse allows the patient to be moved into the MRI scanner.

The phase of *after taking intra-operative MRI* includes: replacing the patient transfer system between the MRI table and operation table; the on-duty safety nurse repeats the patient moving step in reverse order of the phase of *preparation for the intra-operative MRI* process.

The phase of *after surgery* includes: confirming the patient's vital signs and verifying the type of procedure,

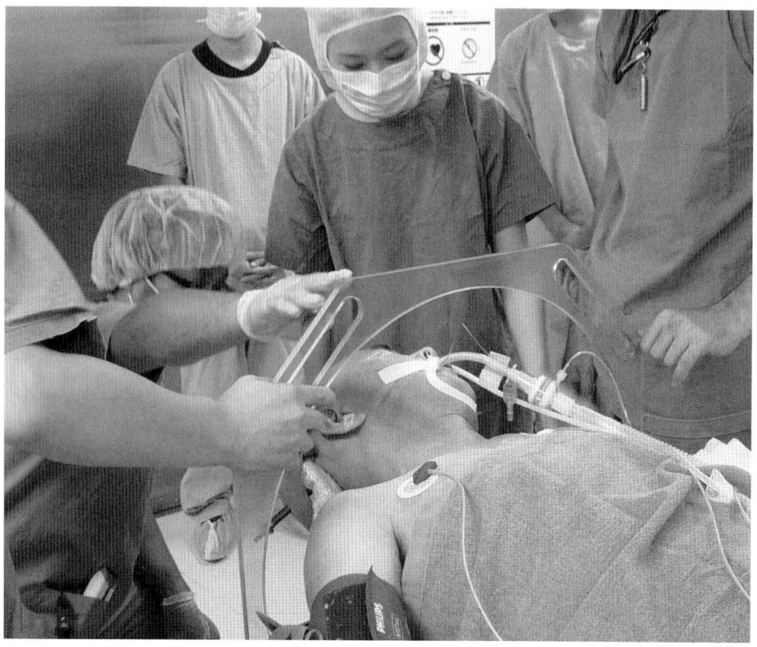

Fig. 2 After the patient position is set, and the head is secured and fixed, both the neurosurgeon and on-duty safety nurse check the clearance between the patient's body and the MRI bore to avoid a collision. The on-duty safety nurse is applying the dummy MRI bore above the patient. The surgeon makes sure the patient position allows an approach into the MRI bore before starting the operation

specimen labels, instrument counts, and liaison points from operation room to intensive care unit.

Non-normal events may include: emergency stop of the MRI, emergency opening of the shielded door, alerts from the oxygen monitor and vital sign checks, handling problems with the patient transfer system, shielded door, or the operation table, and handling the emergency communication system.

Surgical Safety Check List

At each workflow key point, the surgical safety checklist provides specific checkpoints to be verified by the surgical on-duty safety nurse. The specific checkpoints in the workflow are: phase of preoperative inspection (4 points), before skin incision (4 points), preparation for the intra-operative MRI (10 points) (Table 1), after taking intra-operative MRI (6 points), after surgery concluded (4 points), and non-normal (4 points).

Results

In the present series of patients, there was no incident or accident during patient transport or intra-operative imaging in the 3 years since the intra-operative imaging operation suite opened. The time required for the phase of *preparation for the intra-operative MRI* process was an average of 22 min, and the phase of *after taking intra-operative image* was 12 min on average. The intra-operative MRI required an average of 13 min. The total extra time required for completing the safety manual and intra-operative MRI averaged 47 min. There has been some minor modification of the surgical safety manual in the last 3 years. It was noted that the learning curve over the past 3 years showed that the time required for the safety protocol has gradually shortened by about 8 min. There were no significant differences in time required for the safety protocol and in the workflow pattern for each on-duty safety nurse.

Table 1 Elements of the surgical safety checklist

Checklist for preparation to the intraoperative MRI		
Check points	Response	Responder
All ferromagnetic materials removed from the operation table	Removed	CN
Surgical instruments count	Completed	SN
Bed position	Flat	CN
MRI bore clearance	Clear	NS
Surgical field covered by sterilized cap	Covered	NS
Shielded door open	Opened	RT
Patient transfer system	Clear	RT
Anyone dose not have any ferromagnetic materials	Clear	All crew
Vital signs check	Normal	AN
Safety lock	Unlocked	CN
Check list completed	Cleared for transfer	SON

CN circulaqtion nurse, *SN* scrub nurse, *NS* neurosurgeon, *RT* radiation technician, *AN* anesthesiologist, *SON* safety on-duty nurse

The on-duty safety nurse behaved as a sophisticated crew leader, and maintained workflow during the surgery. The surgical safety manual eradicated ambiguous working processes for intra-operative MRI. We successfully developed good communication and a well organized intra-operative MRI crew using this safety tool.

Discussion

Neurosurgical care has seen rapidly increasing technology advances worldwide for more than a century, including the introduction of a navigation system and an imaging operation system. Today, we can easily introduce new technology into our operation room. However, introducing a new technology may drive a patient into an unsteady condition. To prevent this situation, we needed a new tool which works well in the field of patient safety, especially surgical safety.

Not only surgeons, but all humans are fallible; therefore, relying solely on memory to carry out all tasks may cause people to commit errors that could result in adverse events [3]. There are many causes for human errors, including several psychological factors such as anxiety, ambiguousness, impatience, fear, interruptions, and time stress [4, 5]. These psychological factors should be eliminated in all crew members in the operation room. Teamwork in the operation room is an important component of operation room efficiency, and the quality of surgical care and patient safety is generally emphasized [6, 7]. Careless and inadvertent mistakes usually occur in routine workflow. It is important to verbalize instructions using simple and standardized words, especially when the speaker and listener are physically separated [8, 9]. Surgical crews require explicit communication with each other, and should understand the role of standardization in effective team functioning as it relates to policies and procedures [9]. The scientific literature indicates that adverse events can be avoided if proper tools are available in working environments [9]. Process manuals and checklists are some of the tools that have been successful in other high-risk industries, such as airline cockpits and nuclear power plants, as well as in the medical field [10, 11].

In 2008, the World Health Organization launched a new safety checklist for surgical teams to use in operating theatres as part of a major drive to make surgery safer around the world [12]. This safety checklist worked 19 points into a simple one-page checklist developed in consultation with international experts in surgery, anesthesiology, nursing and patient safety, and divides surgical procedures into three phases. This surgical safety checklist was used in eight hospitals in eight cities around the world for 1 year. The results of this study showed that a checklist-based program was associated with a significant decline in the rate of complications and death from surgery in a diverse group of institutions around the world [13]. In each region and country, institutions can modify this list to fit each type of surgical procedure. Our intra-operative MRI team introduced a surgical safety checklist in our imaging operation suite. Our safety surgical checklist has many checkpoints when compared with that of the World Health Organization, but the concept and aim are similar. In the 3 years since the opening of our imaging operation suite, we have not had an incident or accident related to items in the surgical safety manual and checklist.

While intra-operative MRI is a relatively new technique, its use has gradually increased in the neurosurgical field over the past 15 years [14], even though it requires extra operation time to perform MRI. When introducing this kind of new imaging technique into surgery, there are many processes needed to keep the workflow smooth. This is the reason we introduced the on-duty safety nurse and the surgical safety manual into our imaging operation room. Our on-duty safety nurse plays a very powerful role as a third person. The surgical safety manual is implemented by the on-duty safety nurse step by step, and the surgical safety checklist is called by the on-duty safety nurse at key points in the process. The surgical safety manual provides a defined set of steps to remove ambiguities in work processes. These new approaches lead to sustainable team building, provide education for new surgical crew staff, and keep the imaging surgical procedure workflow smooth.

Conflict of interest statement We declare that we have no conflict of interest.

References

1. Matsumae M, Koizumi J, Fukuyama H, Ishizaka H, Mizokami Y, Baba T, Atsumi H, Tsugu A, Oda S, Tanaka Y, Osada T, Imai M, Ishiguro T, Yamamoto M, Tominaga J, Shimoda M, Imai Y (2007) World's first magnetic resonance imaging/x-ray/operating room suite: a significant milestone in the improvement of neurosurgical diagnosis and treatment. J Neurosurg 107:266–273
2. Matsumae M, Fukuyama H, Osada T, Baba T, Mizokami Y, Atsumi H, Ishizaka H, Tsugu A, Tominaga J, Shiramizu H, Shimoda M (2008) Fully functional MR-compatible flexible operating table resolves the neurosurgeon's dilemma over use of intraoperative MRI. Tokai J Exp Clin Med 33:57–60
3. Leape LL (1994) Error in medicine. JAMA 272:1851–1857
4. Gibbs VC (2005) Patient safety practices in the operating room: correct-site surgery and nothing left behind. Surg Clin North Am 85:1307–1319
5. Perazzelli M (2007) Operating room working procedures: a good tool for patient safety? Perioper Nurs Clin 2:255–257
6. Makary MA, Sexton JB, Freischlag JA, Holzmueller CG, Millman EA, Rowen J, Operating Room Teamwork among Physicians and Nurses (2006) Teamwork in the eye of the beholder. J Am Coll Surg 202:746–752
7. Sexton JB, Makary MA, Tersigni AR, Pryor D, Hendrich A, Thomas EJ (2006) Teamwork in the operating room: frontline perspectives among hospitals and operating room personnel. Anesthesiology 105:877–884
8. Pronovost P, Berenholtz S, Dorman T, Lipsett PA, Simmonds T (2003) Improving communication in the ICU using daily goals. J Crit Care 18:71–75
9. Sexton BJ, Grote G, Naef W, Straeter O, Helmreich RL (eds) (2004) The better the team the safer the world: golden rules of group interaction in high risk environments: evidence based suggestions for improving performance. Gottlieb Daimler and Karl Benz Foundation, Ladenburg, pp 1–58
10. Lingard L, Espin S, Rubin B, Whyte S, Colmenares M (2005) Getting teams to talk: development and pilot implementation of a checklist to promote interprofessional communication in the OR. Qual Saf Health Care 14:340–346
11. Lingard L, Regehr G, Orser B, Reznick R, Baker GR, Doran D, Espin S, Bohnen J, Whyte S (2008) Evaluation of a preoperative checklist and team briefing among surgeons, nurses, and anesthesiologists to reduce failures in communication. Arch Surg 143: 12–17
12. World Health Organization World Alliance for Patient Safety (2009) Implementation manual surgical safety checklist, 1st edn. http://www.who.int/patientsafety/safesurgery/tools_resources/SSSL_Manual_finalJun08.pdf. Accessed 21 Sept 2009
13. Haynes AB, Weiser TG, Berry WR, Breizat LSR, AS DEP, Herbosa T, Joseph S, Kibatala PL, Lapitan MCM, Merry AF, Moorthy K, Reznick RK, Taylor B, Gawande AA (2009) Surgical safety checklist to reduce morbidity and mortality in a global population. N Engl J Med 360:491–499
14. Black PM, Moriarty T, Alexander E III, Stieg P, Woodard EJ, Gleason PL, Martin CH, Kikinis R, Schwartz RB, Jolesz FA (1997) Development and implementation of intraoperative magnetic resonance imaging and its neurosurgical applications. Neurosurgery 41:831–845

Operating Room Integration and Telehealth

Richard D. Bucholz, Keith A. Laycock, and Leslie McDurmont

Abstract The increasing use of advanced automated and computer-controlled systems and devices in surgical procedures has resulted in problems arising from the crowding of the operating room with equipment and the incompatible control and communication standards associated with each system. This lack of compatibility between systems and centralized control means that the surgeon is frequently required to interact with multiple computer interfaces in order to obtain updates and exert control over the various devices at his disposal. To reduce this complexity and provide the surgeon with more complete and precise control of the operating room systems, a unified interface and communication network has been developed. In addition to improving efficiency, this network also allows the surgeon to grant remote access to consultants and observers at other institutions, enabling experts to participate in the procedure without having to travel to the site.

Keywords Integration · Interface · Remote access · Surgical communication network · SurgON

Introduction

In recent decades, the introduction of computer-based imaging and navigation systems has revolutionized many aspects of neurosurgery, resulting in improved precision and control and enhanced ability to make adjustments to the surgical plan during the course of a procedure.

A representative neurosurgical procedure that benefits from these advances is the placement of a deep brain electrode to help control a movement disorder such as Parkinson's disease. In such cases, the location of the electrode is dictated by the patient anatomy and data from intraoperative recording of brain activity using microelectrodes. Once the device has been placed, its position must then be confirmed by recordings from the electrode and intraoperative imaging.

The first step in planning such a procedure is to obtain image data of the target in order to determine its exact location. Using scan data acquired in multiple planes, a virtual 3D model of the patient's neuroanatomy can be constructed using a computer navigation system such as the Medtronic StealthStation, allowing the optimum path to the target to be determined.

Before surgery begins, the 3D space of the navigation system is registered with the patient anatomy to ensure precise localization of the target and surgical instruments. The surgical procedure then commences with the insertion of the electrode into the skull, followed by its advancement to the target under guidance from the navigation system. Though the preoperative planning ensures accurate positioning of the electrode with respect to the target, it is necessary to fine-tune the position of the electrode by reference to electrophysiological recordings acquired during the procedure itself. Once the optimum position is determined, the recording microelectrode is withdrawn and replaced with the stimulation electrode, whose position is then verified with further imaging.

A neurosurgical procedure of this type thus involves (at least) six distinct steps:

- Imaging
- Planning
- Navigation
- Recording
- Therapy (the stimulation electrode)
- Confirmation by imaging

Each of these steps involved a computer, networking and clinician interaction. However, current operating rooms are poorly designed to support such complex procedures, while

R.D. Bucholz (✉), K.A. Laycock, and L. McDurmont
Division of Neurosurgery, Department of Surgery, Saint Louis University Health Sciences Center, 3635 Vista Avenue, Saint Louis, MO 63110, USA
e-mail: Richard@bucholz.org

DOI 10.1007/978-3-211-99651-5_35,

personnel and economic constraints further interfere with optimal performance.

An obvious problem is that the various systems and devices in the operating room (OR) are developed and manufactured by unrelated companies and are not designed to interact efficiently. On the personnel front, the perennial shortage of trained staff has been exacerbated in recent years by economic considerations. OR staff must be able to support a variety of cases – staff specialization in one particular field of surgery is not practical at many hospitals – and this requires appropriate levels of training and experience. Unfortunately, having acquired the requisite experience, they tend to seek more attractive appointments, resulting in constant turnover. Likewise, experienced neurophysiologists are also hard to find and may have to be brought in from other institutions to assist with certain cases, often at significant cost.

Just as the OR staff must be able to support various types of procedures, so the ORs themselves are expected to be able to accommodate any kind of case. Few hospitals can dedicate ORs to a single purpose; an open-heart procedure may follow a craniotomy case in the very same OR. Needless to say, with such a bewildering variety of procedures being performed in rapid succession in a given location, often involving many of the same support staff, a significant proportion of medical errors occur in the OR.

Despite the variety of procedures which may be scheduled for a given OR, there are certain requirements common to all surgical interventions:

- Shielding (against microbial contamination and to protect information)
- Documentation (in the form of audio, video and still image records)
- Life support
- Visualization
- Therapeutics
- Plasticity

Devices and systems that are required for most surgical procedures can be left in place in the OR, but when additional equipment is introduced for particular procedures, this can result in crowding and obstruction of the OR staff. Furthermore, the various incompatible systems require the surgeon and his team to monitor and interact with multiple control interfaces and displays, impairing their efficiency and increasing the risk of unforeseen complications. Consequently, there is intense pressure to integrate devices, both to reduce the number of visualization and control displays and to permit more effective control [1].

As it is, the plasticity required of a modern OR places tremendous stress on the system. Complex devices must be easy to move, capable of instant integration with the systems already in use in the OR, robust and fault-tolerant, and easily dissociated for use elsewhere. Integration of a device within a given procedure requires interactions between devices in terms of control, data (video, audio) and automation (with respect to positional information). Furthermore, the aforementioned turnover in OR personnel dictates that control interfaces must be relatively simple. To facilitate this, a standard for communication is clearly required [2].

The rise of a similar problem in the field of radiology resulted in the development of the DICOM standard. This allowed hospitals to connect multiple different diagnostic and treatment devices and have them interact and share information. Unfortunately, the standard is constantly evolving, with various add-on specialties (such as dosimetry and image guidance) having being introduced after the initial standards had been established. Furthermore, it has been discovered that many devices theoretically capable of being integrated through DICOM actually communicate in different "dialects", thus impairing the reliability and practicality of communication.

Nevertheless, despite these limitations, it is time to introduce a similar standard for communication between and control of surgical devices. Such a system would greatly relieve the technological chaos that currently prevails in the OR, and if properly designed would be able to satisfy the needs of all users, regardless of their particular surgical specialty. The result would be less expensive, more efficient, and higher quality medical care.

An Integrated Surgical Communication Network: SurgON

Our group has developed a prototype of an integrated surgical communication network as outlined above in the form of SurgON (SURGical Operative Network) [3]. In this system, each device acts as a web server, storing the web pages that serve as control panels for that particular device. These web pages are used locally to control the devices, each of which has an Ethernet port. An IP address is assigned upon attaching a device to the SurgON local area network (LAN), and the appropriate web page is transmitted as requested. The surgeon's controller allows secure routing of data and control streams via a firewall to the hospital and beyond.

For such an approach to be effective, several design objectives must be met. First, each device must be assured of a specific bandwidth, and every type of surgical device must be controllable locally, even in the event of complete network failure. It is also desirable that devices can be connected and removed with instant recognition, while data streams can be shared over the Internet using a graphic user interface.

With respect to the control of devices, three classes of control have been identified:

- Simple control (request-based control and telemetry)
- Compound control (synchronized control and telemetry; shareable bidirectional datastreams)
- Complex control (synchronized control and feedback to multiple users; automated interaction with other devices)

When a device to be controlled is plugged in, it becomes available on the OR network through its web page. Alternatively, radio frequency shielding in the OR will allow a wireless device to be recognized as it is brought into the shielded room. The web control page is transmitted to control devices when selected, and the device becomes controllable locally or remotely (as permitted).

This approach offers several benefits, the most obvious of which is the ability to use one cable connection for multiple data streams. The surgeon can monitor any data source during a procedure, and the video stream is also viewable by nursing and anesthesia staff. Control of complex diagnostic equipment would be simplified, and the surgeon's own control preferences could be distributed in an automated fashion over many devices. For optimum efficiency, each device could be automatically aligned to a chosen surgical path, and a high dedicated bandwidth would ensure precise control. If desired, one or more other control systems could be implemented as a separate surgical controller (voice, gesture, etc.), and a remote assistant or expert can be given access to the systems as needed [4].

Figure 1 shows a schematic layout for a network controlling multiple devices from the surgeon's console. This console would display a dynamic list of available devices, each represented by an icon. Clicking on the icon for a particular device would bring up its controls. Similarly,

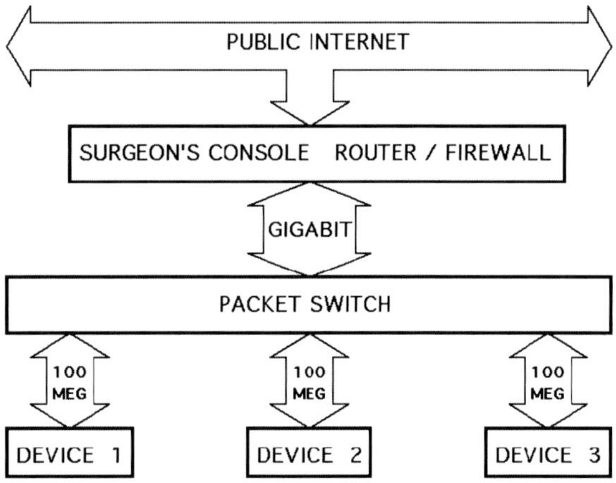

Fig. 1 Schematic layout for a network controlling multiple devices from the surgeon's console

remote consultants could also be represented as icons, with their observation or participation being enabled by a drag-and-drop interface. Figure 2 shows a screenshot of the surgeon's console as configured to control a Möller VM900 microscope, a bipolar coagulator and a Tetrad ultrasound imaging system. A surgeon's particular preferences can be stored on appropriate media and uploaded prior to surgery.

The single unified multi-source display system would avoid the need for multiple computer monitors in the OR. The display device could take one of several forms as long as it is compatible with a sterile cover for use in the OR. Our current test model uses an LCD panel on wheels, but wall-mounted plasma screens or head-mounted displays would be equally practical, and even a personal data assistant (PDA) could be used.

Devices producing information would have a streaming web server; pertinent information would be digitalized and

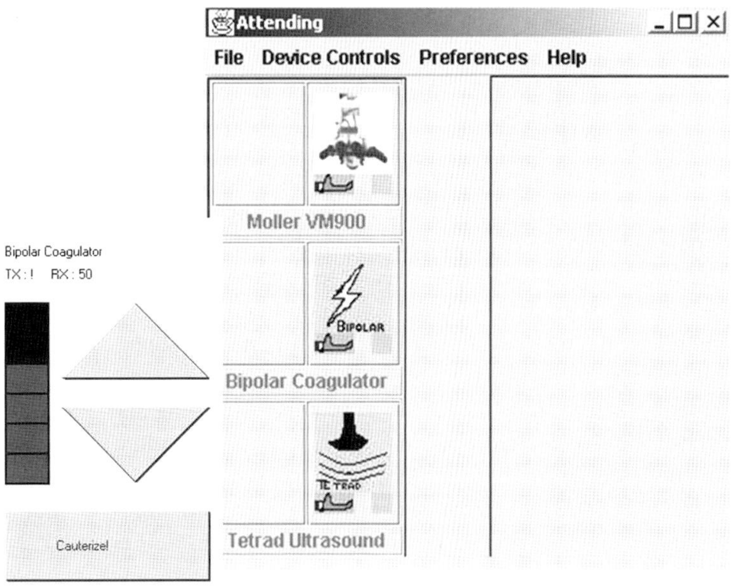

Fig. 2 Screenshot of the surgeon's console as configured to control a Möller VM900 microscope, a bipolar coagulator and a Tetrad ultrasound imaging system

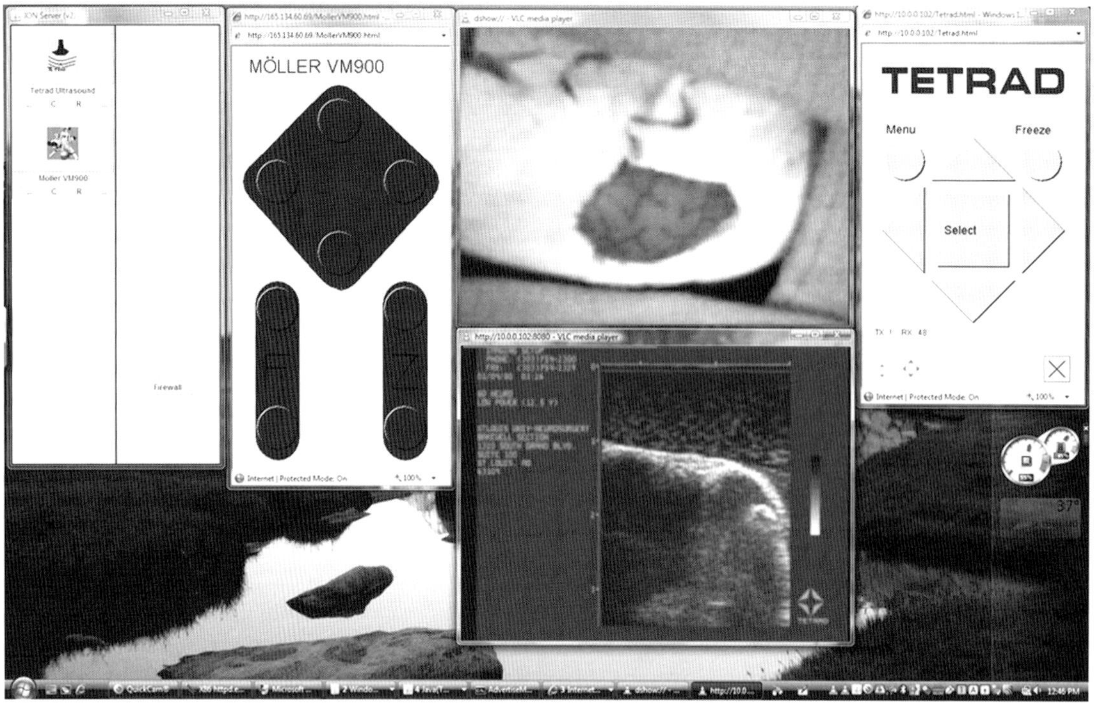

Fig. 3 Representative screen shot of a remote station displaying control interfaces for a Möller VM900 microscope and Tetrad ultrasound system

sent out as a data stream. Thus, a microscope would produce a video stream, the life-support equipment would generate EKG readouts, and the neurophysiological monitor would produce an audio stream.

Every control panel and information stream can be shared outside the operating room as required. To facilitate such remote access, the dynamic firewall software provides a graphic interface that allows sharing of information with a remote consultant equipped with nothing but a PC. It isolates local network traffic from the wide area network (WAN) and guarantees bandwidth to the surgeon. The local surgeon retains complete control over external connections into the OR: upon logging in, a remote consultant only sees the locations of surgeons currently using the system. Controls could also be shared to maximize device optimization (image quality, etc.).

The local surgeon can grant outside viewing or control as needed. By dragging the selected device icon over the remote consultant's icon, a logical connection is established. The local surgeon can also stipulate the type of access to each device, e.g., data sharing, joint control or autonomous control by the remote surgeon. The control and/or connection can also be revoked as needed. Figure 3 shows a representative screen shot of a remote station, displaying the control interfaces for the microscope and the Tetrad ultrasound system.

For the SurgON system to work with a remote workstation, a suitable network connection is required. For control signals and audio, a modem is fast enough, and standard Internet software (Internet Explorer, Java plug-in, NetMeeting, etc.) should be adequate. Thus, almost any current computer is capable of being used as a remote controller.

Conclusion

It is our belief that SurgON addresses the needs of surgery of the future. It provides the requisite shielded space, empowering the surgeon to control all informational streams. It fulfills life support requirements through its ability to be networked and displayed on request to all clinicians involved with a case, while the associated display devices allow seamless communication between the clinicians. There is a protocol for instant recognition of all devices entering the protected space, and the system provides the option to share control of intraoperative devices with remote consultants and assistants.

Conflict of interest statement We declare that we have no conflict of interest.

References

1. Healthcare Financial Management Association (2003) Achieving operating room efficiency through process integration. Healthc Financ Manage 57(3):Suppl 1–7, following 112

2. Gallagher AG, Smith CD (2003) From the operating room of the present to the operating room of the future. Human-factors lessons learned from the minimally invasive surgery revolution. Semin Laparosc Surg 10(3):127–139
3. Bucholz RD (2000) SurgON: a standard for networked communication between surgical devices (keynote presentation). Third international conference on medical image computing and computer-assisted intervention (MICCAI 2000), Pittsburgh, Pennsylvania, October 2000
4. Feussner H (2003) The operating room of the future: a view from Europe. Semin Laparosc Surg 10(3):149–156

Other Intraoperative Imaging Technologies and Operative Robotics

Intra-operative Robotics: NeuroArm

Michael J. Lang, Alexander D. Greer, and Garnette R. Sutherland

Abstract This manuscript describes the development and ongoing integration of neuroArm, an image-guided MR-compatible robot.

Methods: A neurosurgical robotics platform was developed, including MR-compatible manipulators, or arms, with seven degrees of freedom, a main system controller, and a human-machine interface. This system was evaluated during pre-clinical trials and subsequent clinical application, combined with intra-operative MRI, at both 1.5 and 3.0 T.

Results: An MR-compatible surgical robot was successfully developed and merged with ioMRI at both 1.5 or 3.0 T. Image-guidance accuracy and microsurgical capability were established in pre-clinical trials. Early clinical experience demonstrated feasibility and showed the importance of a master-slave configuration. Surgeon-directed manipulator control improved performance and safety.

Conclusion: NeuroArm successfully united the precision and accuracy of robotics with the executive decision-making capability of the surgeon.

Keywords Human-machine interface · Image-guided surgery · Microsurgery · Robotic surgery · Stereotaxy

Introduction

Robotic technology has been applied to surgery for many years [1–3]. As with industrial manufacturing applications, robotics has demonstrated precision and accuracy that exceeds human ability, particularly for repetitive tasks [4]. Meanwhile, human capacity for non-linear processing incorporates incomplete data sets and prior experience, and is necessary for anticipatory action [5]. At the human-machine interface (HMI), the unique attributes of robots and humans may well result in improved surgical intervention and outcome. These advantages are exploited in the master-slave configuration of most medical robotic devices [6], and are why automation, in order to be safe, would require a fundamental change to processing architecture and software design.

Following the modification of an industrial robot (Programmable Universal Machine for Assembly (PUMA), Advance Research and Robotics, Oxford, Connecticut) for neurosurgical use, various robotic systems have been adapted to or created for neurosurgery [2]. These systems have seen only isolated acceptance, largely due to a combination of safety concerns, complexity of use, intra-operative imaging incompatibility, cost, and restricted range of application. In 2002, development of an MR-compatible robot was initiated at the University of Calgary in an effort to integrate the precision and accuracy of robotics with the imaging capabilities of an innovative intra-operative MRI (ioMRI) system based on a moveable magnet [7, 8]. The master-slave dynamic governing neuroArm is discussed, together with the neurobiological mechanisms which separate human and computer decision-making capability.

Materials and Methods

The design and manufacture of neuroArm has been previously reported [3, 9]. In summary, the system consists of two MR-compatible manipulators mounted on a mobile base, a main system controller, and a human-machine interface (HMI), or workstation. The manipulators, or arms, have seven degrees of freedom (DOF), and are able to grasp and manipulate a variety of neurosurgical instruments. The main system controller processes the computational needs of

M.J. Lang, A.D. Greer, and G.R. Sutherland (✉)
Department of Clinical Neurosciences, University of Calgary, Calgary, AB, Canada
e-mail: garnette@ucalgary.ca

M.N. Pamir et al. (eds.), *Intraoperative Imaging*, Acta Neurochirurgica Supplementum, Vol. 109,
DOI 10.1007/978-3-211-99651-5_36, © Springer-Verlag/Wien 2011

robotic manipulation, and mediates the reciprocal exchange of information between surgeon and machine. Finally, the HMI provides the sensory milieu in which the surgeon is able to perform surgery within an image-guided environment.

To develop an image-guided robotic system, manipulator arms were constructed from MR-compatible materials, such as titanium and polyetheretherketone. Piezoelectric motors were chosen for their MR-compatibility, 20,000-h lifetime, and intrinsic braking characteristics in the event of sudden power loss. The system includes dual-redundant rotary electric encoders, which record joint position to an accuracy of 0.01 degrees. The end-effector incorporates a unique mechanism for tool grasping, roll, and actuation, such as opening or closing bipolar forceps or scissors. In addition, the configuration maintains sterility via end-effector attachments which pierce the manipulator drapes while capping the break in the sterile field (Fig. 1). Two titanium six-axis force/torque sensors in contact with the tool generate force data in three translational DOF, which is fed back to the surgeon via two handcontrollers. For microsurgery, both manipulators are transferred to a mobile base, along with a 6-DOF digitizing arm. The digitizing arm is used to register the manipulators to fiducials located within the radiofrequency (RF) coil, and hence to pre- or intra-operatively acquired MR images. For stereotaxy, one manipulator is transferred to a polyetheretherketone platform attached to the gradient insert within the bore of the magnet. The platform includes two MR-compatible cameras, which allow visualization of the operative site and manipulator from the workstation monitors. In this configuration, the manipulator is registered to the magnet isocenter.

The main system controller governs the transmission of input signals to the robot, as well as position and force data returning to the HMI. The software currently being utilized in the main system controller took over four years to develop, given the requirements of image guidance, quantified force feedback, and safety. This software not only acts as a throughput for data, but actively monitors all aspects of the system. In the event of divergence from intended manipulator motion, the embedded safety mechanisms halt further movement. However, while system software can recognize positional error, the surgeon may be able to recognize the context of unintended movement more rapidly, and thus avoid injury to adjacent neural tissue. This is particularly relevant given the speed of surgery, in which small variations in reaction time can result in substantially different outcomes. To avoid such a critical event, a foot-pedal, used as a dead-man switch and wired directly into the process logic controller, was added to allow the surgeon to rapidly halt the manipulators in the event of unintended movement.

Union of the precision and accuracy of machine technology and human executive capacity is made possible by the HMI apparatus [10]. The surgeon is immersed in sensory data, including 3D intra-operative MR images with tool overlay, virtual position of the manipulators relative to the RF coil, stereoscopic display of the surgical field from the operating microscope, an image of the operative area, and recreated sense of touch, which is displayed in Newtons and

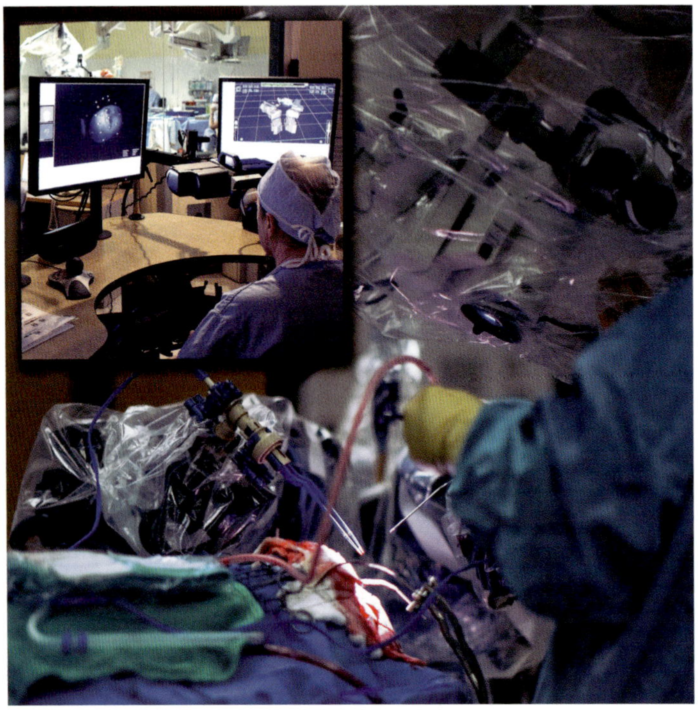

Fig. 1 Integration of human and machine: the figure shows neuroArm positioned for removal of an olfactory groove meningioma. The right arm holds a bipolar forcep and the left a bayonet-shaped sucker. Stereoscopic images from two high-definition cameras attached to the operating microscope are projected to the surgeon at the workstation (*insert*). Also shown in the *insert*, are the 3D MRI display (*left*) and virtual manipulators registered to the RF-coil (*right*)

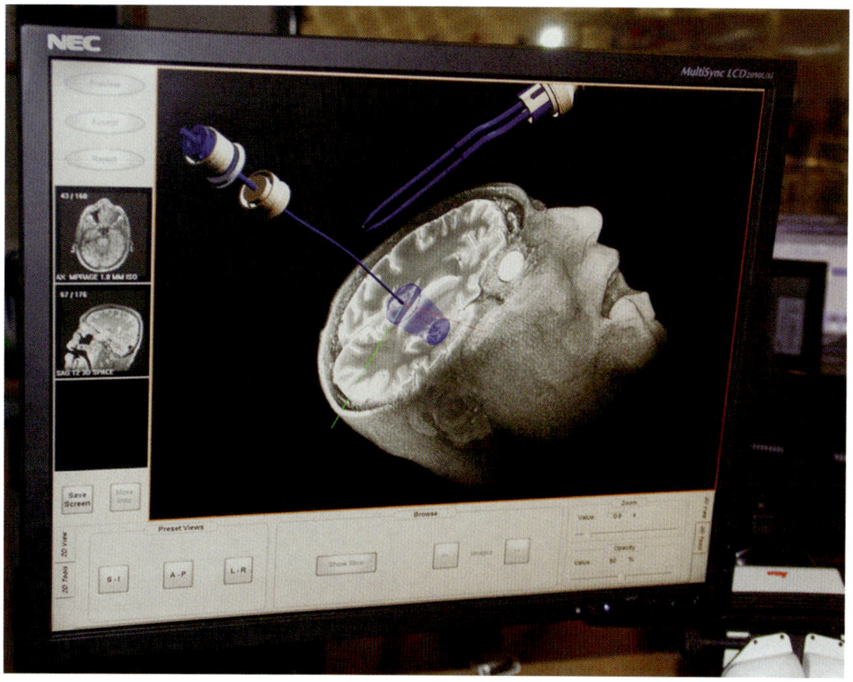

Fig. 2 Three-dimensional MRI display: the image demonstrates a selected surgical corridor with tool overlay. Once delineated, the tools may only pass within the limits of the pre-defined corridor

also pictorially represented. Force feedback, essential for microsurgery, permits quantification of the forces of dissection and the potential to set explicit limits to applied force. In addition, the surgeon can construct virtual surgical corridors on the MRI display (Fig. 2). Once established, tool manipulation may occur only within the limits of these pre-determined pathways. Within this sensory immersive environment, the surgeon is able to safely control the manipulators.

Results

As previously published, the surgical robotic system was designed, manufactured, and integrated into a neurosurgical operating room over a 6-year interval [3]. During the subsequent 18 months, deficiencies in both hardware and software were identified and resolved. The foot-pedal, added during this interval, was found to increase manipulator control, further enhancing safety. With usage, errors related to positioning data and image registration were likewise identified and resolved.

Pre-clinical trials were performed using rats and cadavers [9]. To establish microsurgical application, two qualified microsurgeons achieved comparable results using either established microsurgical techniques or neuroArm. The tested procedures consisted of splenectomy, nephrectomy, and submandibular gland resection in a rodent model. Navigational accuracy was established by means of nanoparticle implantation into predetermined targets using a cadaveric model. Accuracy was found to be equal or better to existing surgical navigation technology. Unlike traditional navigation technology, location of the implanting device was confirmed with real-time imaging prior to nanoparticle release.

Clinical application was initially demonstrated in five patients with various intracranial neoplasms [9]. NeuroArm was progressively introduced in a staged manner, so as to isolate specific issues relating to its use in the operating room. Early cases focused on the positioning and draping of the manipulators for use within the sterile field. Assessment of image-guidance accuracy was then performed, followed by initial use during neoplasm resection. During the fifth case, an encoder failure occurred, resulting in uncontrolled motion causing the suction tool to come into contact with a retractor. This event triggered a safety review, out of which the aforementioned foot-pedal was developed and incorporated. Despite the occurrence of minor technical complications, patient safety remained uncompromised.

Sample size during initial clinical use was limited by the decision to upgrade the 1.5 T ioMRI system to 3.0 T. This was complicated by the decision to shift from local to whole-room RF-shielding. NeuroArm was integrated into this new ioMRI environment. To avoid RF-interference from electronic cables controlling neuroArm, a penetration panel was constructed. At the site of shield penetration, RF-noise is eliminated with line filtration and copper to fiber-optic converters. Conversion to whole-room shielding simplified the method for registration during stereotaxy. Manipulator placement on a polyetheretherketone platform, attached to

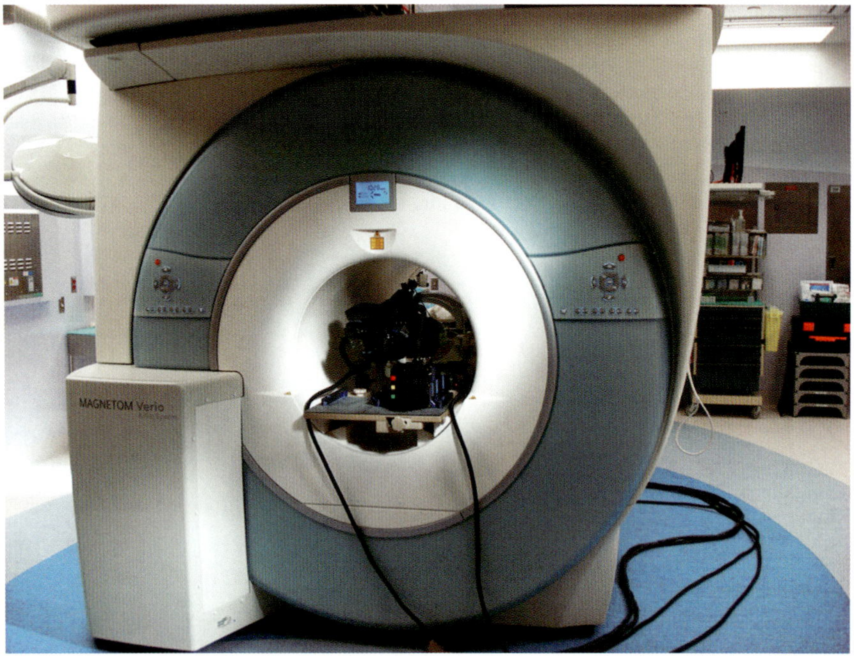

Fig. 3 Image-guided robotic-assisted stereotaxy at 3.0 T: this photograph shows the right manipulator, located on a platform attached to the gradient insert within the bore of the moveable 3.0 T magnet. Cables are connected to two MR-compatible cameras, allowing visualization of the manipulator and surgical field

the gradient insert within the magnet bore, allows image registration to be based on the magnet isocenter (Fig. 3).

Discussion

Pre-clinical trials and initial clinical experience with neuroArm have demonstrated that the system safely unites robotic precision and accuracy with human decision-making. This connection is based on a master-slave configuration, similar to most surgical robotic systems. Such a design was chosen largely due to limitations in contemporary computer technology, but was fortuitous nonetheless. Indeed, the master-slave dynamic is indispensable to the practice of robotic surgery, owing to the nature of human decision-making. While the superior precision and accuracy of robotic movement is accepted [2], the mechanisms separating human and computer decision-making capability in the surgical setting have not been well-studied.

Human decision-making has been studied extensively in the fields of neuroscience, psychology, and economics [11–13]. In vivo experiments have been able to demonstrate the neurobiological underpinnings of decision-making processes during simple sensory-motor tasks [14]. Researchers have delineated complex neural circuits involved in the processes of choice valuation and decision execution; within associated regions, distinct populations of neurons respond independently to each available option [15]. The result is a non-linear computational system capable not only of evaluating multiple choice alternatives simultaneously, but also continued processing and modification of such choices after the action has been initiated. Consequences of a decision are then incorporated as experience into future heuristics. Presently, computers, which do not rely on the relatively slow synaptic connections of neuronal transmission, utilize computational circuitry and software designed with inherent linearity, although this may change [16]. The surgeon controlling neuroArm can evaluate the context of unintended motion, resulting in a much faster reaction than the main system controller.

In addition to differences at the level of basic computation, higher-level data processing is critical to human executive functioning. Step-by-step deduction in computer processing requires the evaluation of all possible choices to conclusion or a pre-determined fail condition, prior to selecting a single option with the highest likelihood of success. When applied to surgery, these distinctions have substantial impact as decision complexity increases. At a given point in time, there exist almost infinite possible actions within the surgical field, organized in ascending levels of importance and complexity. Were true automation attempted, so-called *combinatorial explosion* would result. The surgeon, presented with immersive sensory data at the workstation, can rapidly combine multiple incomplete data sets in order to execute manipulator motion. This is the basis for efficacy during pre-clinical studies and success in the early clinical use of neuroArm.

Small-scale anatomical variability further complicates the process of automation by adding layers of ambiguity and disorganization to the surgical data set, thereby increasing computational density. Though intra-operative imaging and intuitive HMI design attempt to minimize this uncertainty, the surgeon's decision-making is not paralyzed by incomplete data, as some degree of sensory uncertainty is tolerated. Surgeons routinely apply knowledge of anticipated structural relationships to actively guide dissection, prior to full visualization of the relevant anatomy. Such action is predicated on computation that allows the brain to both infer probability from uncertain data and determine the threshold of sensory certainty required to initiate action [17]. The use of a foot-pedal to halt unintended manipulator motion takes advantage of the human capacity to evaluate the error in the setting of contextual dissonance, though the system software may not recognize technical failure. While neuroArm is capable of extremely basic automation in the form of a partially-automated tool exchange, it is capable of producing only a single solution to generate a given movement. Surgeons, on the other hand, can intuitively alter speed, force, and hand position efficiently and effectively in order to complete a task in a variety of approaches.

Technological developments have presented neurosurgeons with increasingly informative imaging modalities and tools that have substantially altered the scope and nature of neurosurgical intervention. NeuroArm combines advanced image guidance, robotic accuracy and precision, and the neural processing mechanisms employed during human control. The master-slave organization of this system links human executive function and robotic accuracy in a way that may generate surgical outcomes beyond those currently possible.

Conflict of interest statement Dr. G.R. Sutherland and A.D. Greer hold shares in IMRIS (Winnipeg, Canada). M.J. Lang declares no conflict of inerest.

Acknowledgements This work was supported by grants from the Canada Foundation for Innovation, Western Economic Diversification, and Alberta Advanced Education and Technology.

References

1. Ballantyne GH, Moll F (2003) The da Vinci telerobotic surgical system: the virtual operative field and telepresence surgery. Surg Clin North Am 83:1293–1304, vii
2. Lwu S, Sutherland GR (2009) The development of robotics for interventional MRI. Neurosurg Clin N Am 20:193–206
3. Sutherland GR, Latour I, Greer AD, Fielding T, Feil G, Newhook P (2008) An image-guided magnetic resonance-compatible surgical robot. Neurosurgery 62:286–292
4. Stefanidis D, Wang F, Korndorffer JR Jr, Dunne JB, Scott DJ (2009) Robotic assistance improves intracorporeal suturing performance and safety in the operating room while decreasing operator workload. Surg Endosc 18:18
5. Yang T, Shadlen MN (2007) Probabilistic reasoning by neurons. Nature 447:1075–1080
6. Ewing DR, Pigazzi A, Wang Y, Ballantyne GH (2004) Robots in the operating room–the history. Semin Laparosc Surg 11:63–71
7. Sutherland GR, Kaibara T, Louw D, Hoult DI, Tomanek B, Saunders J (1999) A mobile high-field magnetic resonance system for neurosurgery. J Neurosurg 91:804–813
8. Sutherland GR, Latour I, Greer AD (2008) Integrating an image-guided robot with intraoperative MRI: a review of the design and construction of neuroArm. IEEE Eng Med Biol Mag 27:59–65
9. Pandya S, Motkoski JW, Serrano-Almeida C, Greer AD, Latour I, Sutherland GR (2009) Advancing neurosurgery with image-guided robotics. J Neurosurg 17:17
10. Greer AD, Newhook PM, Sutherland GR (2008) Human-machine interface for Robotic surgery and stereotaxy. IEEE ASME Trans Mechatron 13:355–361
11. Dehaene S, Spelke E, Pinel P, Stanescu R, Tsivkin S (1999) Sources of mathematical thinking: behavioral and brain-imaging evidence. Science 284:970–974
12. Padoa-Schioppa C, Assad JA (2006) Neurons in the orbitofrontal cortex encode economic value. Nature 441:223–226
13. Platt ML, Huettel SA (2008) Risky business: the neuroeconomics of decision making under uncertainty. Nat Neurosci 11:398–403
14. Resulaj A, Kiani R, Wolpert DM, Shadlen MN (2009) Changes of mind in decision-making. Nature 461:263–266
15. Furman M, Wang XJ (2008) Similarity effect and optimal control of multiple-choice decision making. Neuron 60:1153–1168
16. Denning PJ, Tichy WF (1990) Highly parallel computation. Science 250:1217–1222
17. Knill DC, Pouget A (2004) The Bayesian brain: the role of uncertainty in neural coding and computation. Trends Neurosci 27:712–719

Clinical Requirements and Possible Applications of Robot Assisted Endoscopy in Skull Base and Sinus Surgery

K.W.G. Eichhorn and F. Bootz

Abstract Functional Endoscopic Surgery of Paranasal sinuses (FESS) and Skull Base surgery is one of the most frequent surgeries performed at the ENT department of the Bonn University, Germany. Beside of surgical Navigation Robotic is one of the upcoming fields of Computer assisted Surgery developments. This work presents novel research and concepts for Robot Assisted Endoscopic Sinus Surgery (RASS) of the Paranasal sinuses and the anterior Skull Base containing the analysis of surgical workflows, the segmentation and modelling of the Paranasal sinuses and the anterior Skull Base and the development of the robotic path planning. An interdisciplinary group of software engineers and surgeons in Braunschweig and Bonn, Germany are approximate to solutions by a clinical and technical research program financed through the DFG (Deutsche Forschungsgemeinschaft, German research Community).

Keywords Computer assisted surgery · Endoscopic surgery · Endoscopy · FESS · Paranasal sinuses · Robot assisted surgery · Robotic · Skull base

Introduction

Over the past years Functional Endoscopic Sinus Surgery (FESS) has been established as one of the important standard techniques in the field of Otorhinolaryngology and Skull base Surgery. The major disadvantage of this technique is that the surgeon has to hold the Endoscope by himself in one hand. He has only his second hand free for surgical instruments, suction or navigation devices. This can result in unsteady endoscope images caused by tiredness or in frequent instrument changes. Since this is also true for other endoscopic operations like laparoscopy, robot systems are developed taking control of the endoscope during surgical procedures (some of them are listed in [1–3]).

Our aim in Robot Assisted Endoscopic Sinus Surgery (RASS) is that the robot guides the endoscope during an operation as autonomous as possible. One of the main challenges is the close proximity of critical regions like the anterior skull base, orbits, carotid arteries and optical nerves to the work space of the robot.

Clinical Requirements

Parts of these requirements are that

1. the tip of the instrument is always in the centre of the endoscopic view
2. the surgeon has enough free space for his instruments
3. the motion of the robot harmonize with the motion of the surgeon
4. the robot can automatically clean the camera lens and
5. the surgeon can direct the robot to (e.g. in CT data) specified locations.

Especially the last two points require a path planning algorithm. In contrast to most industrial applications we have to deal with partly soft structures. And due to the limited space in the nasal and paranasal cavities, the robot has to deform some of these elastic structures like the middle turbinates to reach the ethmoid complex. The amount of these deformations should be restricted in such a way that the risk of an injury is minimal for the patient. Moreover, some anatomical structures (soft or hard) are removed for most of the surgical approaches, which requires dynamic data structures.

K.W.G. Eichhorn (✉) and F. Bootz
Klinik und Poliklinik fuer HNO-Heilkunde/Chirurgie, Universitätsklinikum Bonn, Sigmund-Freud-Strasse 25, 53105 Bonn, Germany
e-mail: klaus.eichhorn@ukb.uni-bonn.de

Modelling the Endoscopic Sinus Surgery

The primer experiments were analysing regular FESS operations done by clinical specialist in a conventional two handed operation (One hand for the endoscope and the second hand for an instrument or navigation pointer or the suction device).

Methods/Material

During 23 FESS procedures (five cadaver dissection and 18 in vivo FESS) we mounted force/torque sensor (Nano 43 SI-36-0.5, Schunk GmbH &Co. KG, Lauffen, Neckar; Germany) between the camera/handle and the endoscope while operating to monitor the forces and torques occurring at the endoscope in six degrees of freedom. In addition we added in four FESS marker spheres at the patient, the endoscope and the instruments to determine the position of these three by a self developed passive navigation system and collected the endoscope images and took a camcorder video from the hole procedure from a half bird view (Fig. 1).

Results

As result we determine an amount of points where the endoscope tip is located during FESS which builds nearly the whole nasal cavity. We defined a geometrical centre as a standard position for the robot to have the shortest distance to reach all positions in the shortest time. Furthermore we reduced our data to 50% of the points lying close to the balance center and designed so a cube defining the ground work space of the endoscope tip. The dimension of the cube in our FESS was 16.59 mm × 11.38 mm × 6.30 mm and 1.19 cm^3.

As a main result we get the pose (position and orientation) of the endoscope in relation to the patients head and the points of passage into the nose. So we defined a plane we call pivot plane where all poses of the endoscope entering the nose are located. We also reduce these points to the closed 50% of points to a balance center. So we get a pivot plane of 3.93 mm × 2.31 mm or rather 9.07 mm^2 surface. The surface of 9.07 mm^2 is the surface of the lateral cut of all standard endoscope used in sinus surgery. So in technical terms we define a pivot point at the nasal entrance (Fig. 2).

Our force/torque senor delivers a force/operation time diagram for every FESS and we calculated the average force and the maximum force and thus we found the 94.9%

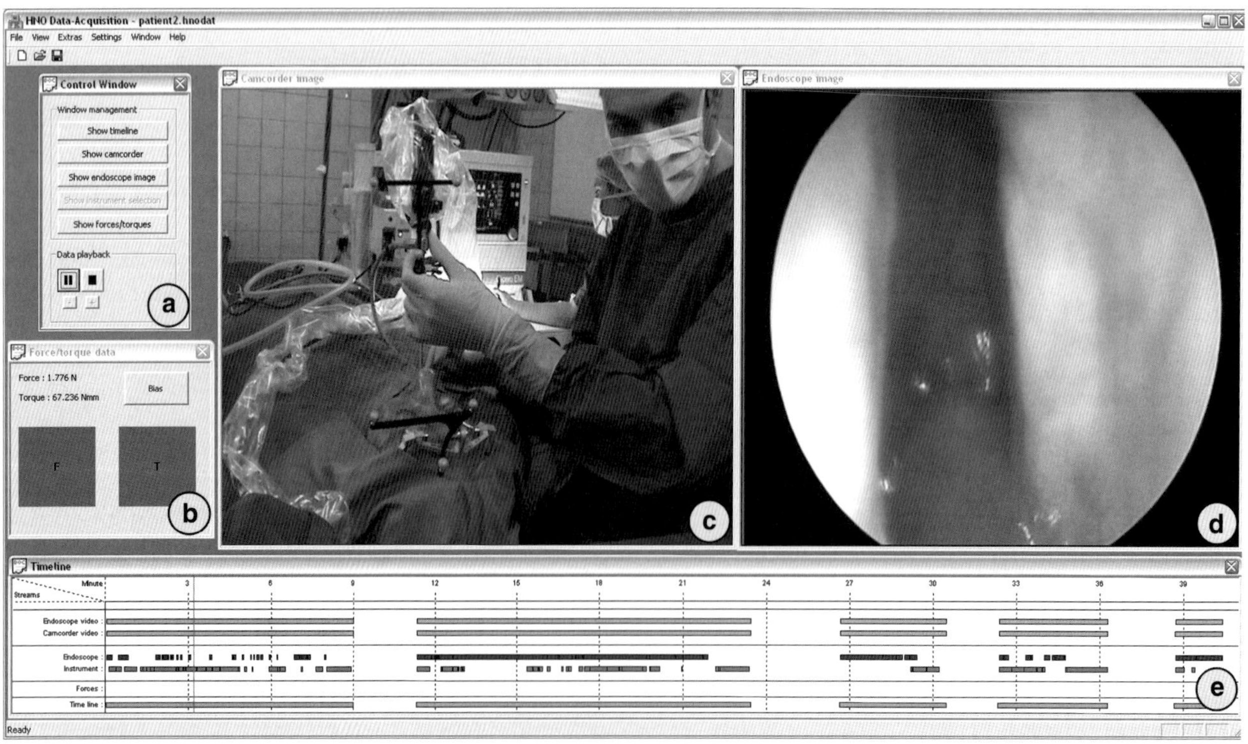

Fig. 1 Screenshot of the data acquire software during conventional endoscopic sinus surgery with explanatory notes: (**a**) control window, (**b**) force/torque data, (**c**) camcorder view, (**d**) endoscope image, (**e**) time line

percentile lying by 7.1 N. So most of the times the forces occurring at the endoscope tip are below 7 N and in average 3.3 N.

Technical Developments

To describe the soft tissue and bone properties we designed different experiments on human soft tissue and cadaver specimen. Elasticity and tissue properties were measured.

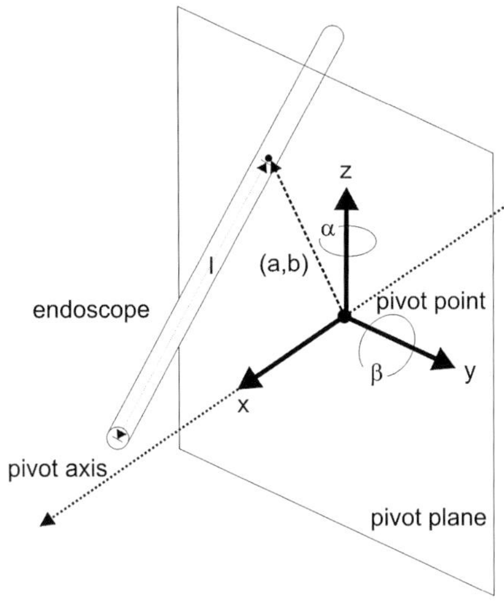

Fig. 2 Diagram of pivot plane, pivot point and the endoscope rotations and translations around the pivot point at the nasal entrance: l is the distance between the tip and the intersection point of the endoscope axis and the pivot plane, (a, b) is a displacement vector within the pivot plane, α is the rotation angle around the z-axis (*yaw*), β is the rotation angle around the y-axis

Also we used the software ANSYS for creating a FEM-(Finite Element Model)-Simulation.

In our experiments we have seen that the amounts of data's need for the FEM-Model are to complex for an online calculation. So we go ahead and designed a total new model for the path planning which will be introduced in following.

In our work we distinguish between the interior and the exterior environment. The interior environment describes the inner structures of the patients head. So far we concentrated on modelling the interior environment [4]. This interior environment we divided into voxels according to the CT-scans and defined for each voxel three different properties: HARD, SOFT and FREE.

HARD structures and other critical regions (e.g. brain, eyes) can be treated as prohibitive zones for the robot. Contacts with SOFT structures can not be avoided. But the amount of deformation should be limited so that the risk of injuries is minimal for the patient. In FREE Region the maximum speed for FESS endoscope movements is allowed.

Discussion

After throwbacks in medical robotics a few years ago [5], there are new interdisciplinary groups [6] working at the development of new systems to relieve surgeons during complex operations. In our work the assistance of the robot in FESS is the main topic. The surgeon would have two hands free to perform saver and more precise manipulations at the patient [7]. On the market there are so far only systems for telemanipulation available for example the DaVinci-System [8], but partly autonomous working machines are

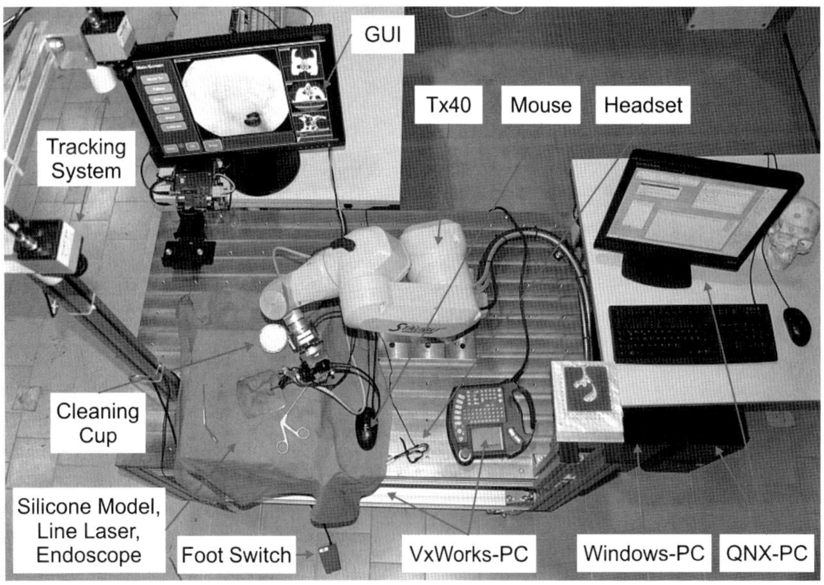

Fig. 3 Prototype for robot assisted endoscope guidance for surgery of the paranasal sinuses and the anterior skull base (*GUI* Graphical User Interface, *Tx 40* Robotor Type Tx40)

still missed. In technical ways we defined a ground work space and a fixed pivot point at the nasal entrance. We are able to reduce the movements of the robot to guide the endoscope in the nose to one translation and two rotation directions. By the use of limits of the work space to a cube of 1.19 cm^3 and the limiting of the forces to 7 N at the endoscope tip we can protect critical regions like the anterior skull base, orbits, carotid arteries and optical nerves by injuries belonging to the endoscope tip and the robot movements [4, 9]. Limits for translations and rotations of the endoscope and simplification of the voxel based interior environment make the run time for a path planning request at about 1 s for the worst case (single threaded, E6600 CPU, unoptimized code). The paths were smooth with a good balance between limited deformations and straight driving to the goal positions of the endoscope tip (Fig. 3).

Perspectives

In our work we developed different approaches for the realization of the partly autonomous robot assisted endoscope guidance in functional endoscopic sinus surgery and the surgery of the anterior skull base. In the future we start new experiments with our prototype (seen in Fig. 3) and RASS on cadaver heads.

Conflict of interest statement We declare that we have no conflict of interest.

References

1. Dario P, Hannaford B, Menciassi A (2003) Smart surgical tools and augmenting devices. IEEE Trans Rob Autom 19(5):782–792
2. Pott P (2008) Meroda, the medical robotics database. http://www.ma.uni-heidelberg.de/apps/ortho/meroda/
3. Taylor RH, Stoianovici D (2003) Medical robotics in computer-integrated surgery. IEEE Trans Rob Autom 19(5):765–781
4. Tingelhoff K, Eichhorn KWG, Wagner I, Kunkel ME, Moral AI, Rilk M, Wahl FM, Bootz F (2008) Analysis of manual segmentation in paranasal CT images. Eur Arch Otorhinolaryngol 265:1061–1070
5. Schulz AP, Seide K, Queitsch C, von Haugwitz A, Meiners J, Kienast B, Tarabolsi M, Kammal M, Jürgens C (2007) Results of total hip replacement using the Robodoc surgical assistant system: clinical outcome and evaluation of complications for 97 procedures. Int J Med Robot 3(4):301–306
6. Federspil PA, Plinkert PK (2004) Robotic surgery in otorhinolaryngology. Otolaryngol Pol 58:237–242
7. Briner HR, Simmen D, Jones N (2005) Endoscopic sinus surgery: advantages of the bimanual technique. Am J Rhinol 19:269–273
8. Palep JH (2009) Robotic assisted minimally invasive surgery. J Minim Access Surg 5(1):1–7
9. Wagner I, Tingelhoff K, Westphal R, Kunkel ME, Wahl FM, Bootz F, Eichhorn KWG (2008) Ex vivo evaluation of force data and tissue elasticity for robot-assisted FESS. Eur Arch Otorhinolaryngol 265:1335–1339

Robotic Technology in Spine Surgery: Current Applications and Future Developments

Carsten Stüer, Florian Ringel, Michael Stoffel, Andreas Reinke, Michael Behr, and Bernhard Meyer

Abstract Medical robotics incrementally appears compelling in nowadays surgical work. The research regarding an ideal interaction between physician and computer assistance has reached a first summit with the implementation of commercially available robots (Intuitive Surgical's® *da Vinci*®). Moreover, neurosurgery – and herein spine surgery - seems an ideal candidate for computer assisted surgery. After the adoption of pure navigational support from brain surgery to spine surgery a meanwhile commercially available miniature robot (Mazor Surgical Technologies' The Spine Assist®) assists in drilling thoracic and lumbar pedicle screws. Pilot studies on efficacy, implementation into neurosurgical operating room work flow proved the accuracy of the system and we shortly outline them. Current applications are promising, and future possible developments seem far beyond imagination. But still, medical robotics is in its infancy. Many of its advantages and disadvantages must be delicately sorted out as the patients safety is of highest priority. Medical robots may achieve a physician's supplement but not substitute.

Keywords Spinal robotics · Computer assisted surgery · Medical robotics · Robotic neurosurgery · Spine surgery · Robotic assisted screw placement

Introduction

Medical robotics has tremendous potential for improving the precision and capabilities of neurosurgical, and therein spinal surgical procedures. The intrinsic characteristics of robots, such as high precision, repeatability and endurance make them ideal surgeon's assistants [1]. During the last two decades, important efforts have been made between academic and industry partnerships to develop robots suitable fur use in the operating room environment. Although some applications have been successful in areas of laparoscopic surgery at cardiac and urologic procedures, such as Intuitive Surgical's *da Vinci*®, cerebral and spinal Neurosurgery still presents a major challenge due to the eloquence of the surrounding anatomy. The development of minimally invasive surgery and introduction of medical imaging techniques (virtual reality) is a paradigm shift for the surgical application of medical robots for reproducibility and improved precision in surgical procedures. In many ways, spinal surgery is ideally suited for the integration of robotic-assisted surgical procedures [2]. Spinal procedures commonly require fine manipulation of trajectories to deeply seated, critical bony structures that are accessed through a small corridor. Since spinal procedures – in terms of implanting screws and rods constructs accompanying intervertebral fusion – can be quite lengthy and tedious, spinal surgeons may experience fatigue, hand tremor, and a scaled down hand motion regarding further decompressive, more eloquent work at the spinal cord and nerve roots. Ideally, robots are indefatigable, able to perform repetitious tasks with precision and reproducible outcomes.

C. Stüer (✉), F. Ringel, M. Stoffel, A. Reinke, M. Behr, and B. Meyer
Department of Neurosurgery, Klinikum rechts der Isar, Technische Universität München, Ismaningerstr. 22, 81675 München, Germany
e-mail: carsten.stueer@lrz.tu-muenchen.de

Current Applications

To date, medical robotics is still in its infancy and only a few commercial companies and their products are available. Especially for spinal surgery, only one commercial CE- and FDA-approved product exists (The SpineAssist®, Mazor Surgical Technologies, Caesarea, Israel), and the number of scientific publications is scarce.

The SpineAssist® is a bone mounted hexapod miniature robot (Fig. 1). It is firmly connected to the patient's body through one of three platforms: a clamped bridge attached to the spinous process, a Hover-T bridge attached through three

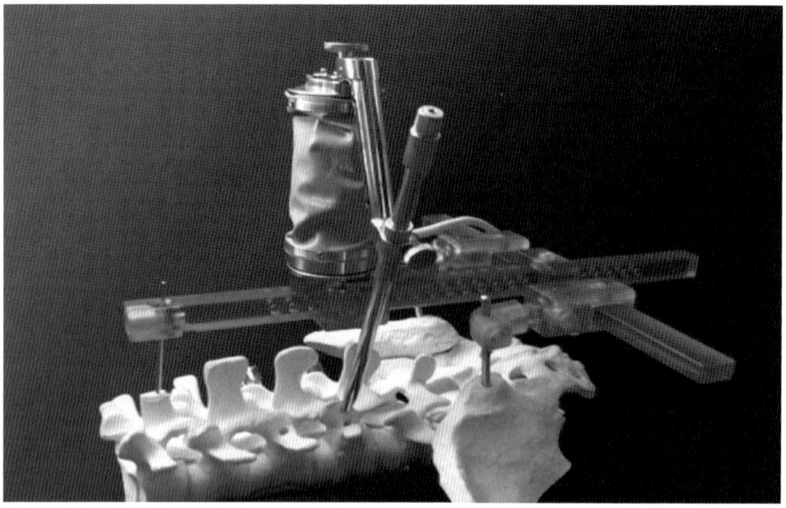

Fig. 1 Picture of The SpineAssist® (Mazor Surgical Technologies, Caesarea, Israel), the only commercial robotic system available for spine surgery. It is a hexapod miniature robotic device that places preoperatively planned trajectories for drilling screw canal into in vivo. As shown, it hovers above the spine via the Hover-T, which might be attached for minimally invasive procedures to a spinous process and the iliac crest

pins to the patient's bony anatomy or a bed mount device with only one pin connecting the Hover-T to the patient's spine. According to the medical robot classification of Nathoo et al. [3] this system, as the majority of robot-assistants, serves as a shared-control system, which allows both the surgeon and the robot to directly control the instruments at the same time. Prior to surgery, there are a few basic steps in the operation:

1. Preoperative planning on a reformatted CT scan of the operated area imported to the software.
2. Calibration of the fluoroscopy c-arm.
3. Intra-operative fluoroscopy images of the operated field with targets mounted to the robotic platform.
4. Merging of the intra-operative fluoroscopy images with the pre-operative CT scan (registration).
5. Execution of the pre-operative plan.

Further information on the system can be found elsewhere [4–7]. Thus, the system provides with navigation and guidance, and assists via the trajectories with drilling prior to screw implantation, translaminar facet screws, vertebral biopsies or kypho- and vertebroplasties. Safety and accuracy have been shown in clinical pilot studies [8, 9].

Results of a pilot study with this system regarding clinical feasability, safety and integration into operative workflow at our institution confirm an excellent accuracy with a deviation <2 mm to the surgeons plan in 97%. 100 lumbar pedicle screws were inserted in 19 patients (average age 66.81; range 47–86) with degenerative disease in 25 motion segments (Figs. 1 and 2). Only one patient underwent revision according to malposition of two screws (Fig. 3). After a steep learning curve, easy use of the system and unconventional integration into the work flow was possible, as shown in a previous study at another institution [9]. Furthermore, superiority over fluoroscopy guidance in terms of radiation exposure was proven. Since its introduction into the field of spinal surgery some studies have been published and besides good feasability and accuracy those authors warranted prospective randomized controlled trials. Preliminary results of such a study currently done at our institution point to:

1. Considerably less radiation exposure of the surgeon
2. An improvement of the accuracy and less pedicle breach with spinal instrumentation
3. An increase of the total duration of the spinal procedure due to preoperative planning, intraoperative hardware and software breakdown and therefore
4. An increase of annoying factors around spinal surgery

Future Projects

In future, as this system currently is not only in lumbar but in thoracic pedicle screw insertion service The SpineAssist will guide with placing cervical pedicle screws. First attempts with this approach have been done at several institutions in Europe, so far. Complex cranio-cervical, atlanto-axial and subaxial pathologies (i.e. rheumatoid cases, complex cervical trauma, ankylosing spondylitis) still are challenging to the spine surgeon, as the risk of neurological damage to the spinal cord or nerve roots is quoted as 0.2–1.0%, and vascular injury may occur in up to 5% with possibly devastating consequences [10, 11]. Image guidance in such procedures is supposed to offer an increased margin of safety for lateral mass, isthmic or transarticular screw placement [12]. To our mind, robotic assistance in guidance-optimized placement of cervical and lumbar total disc replacements with disc arthroplasty seems to be a further ideal area of a robotic supplement.

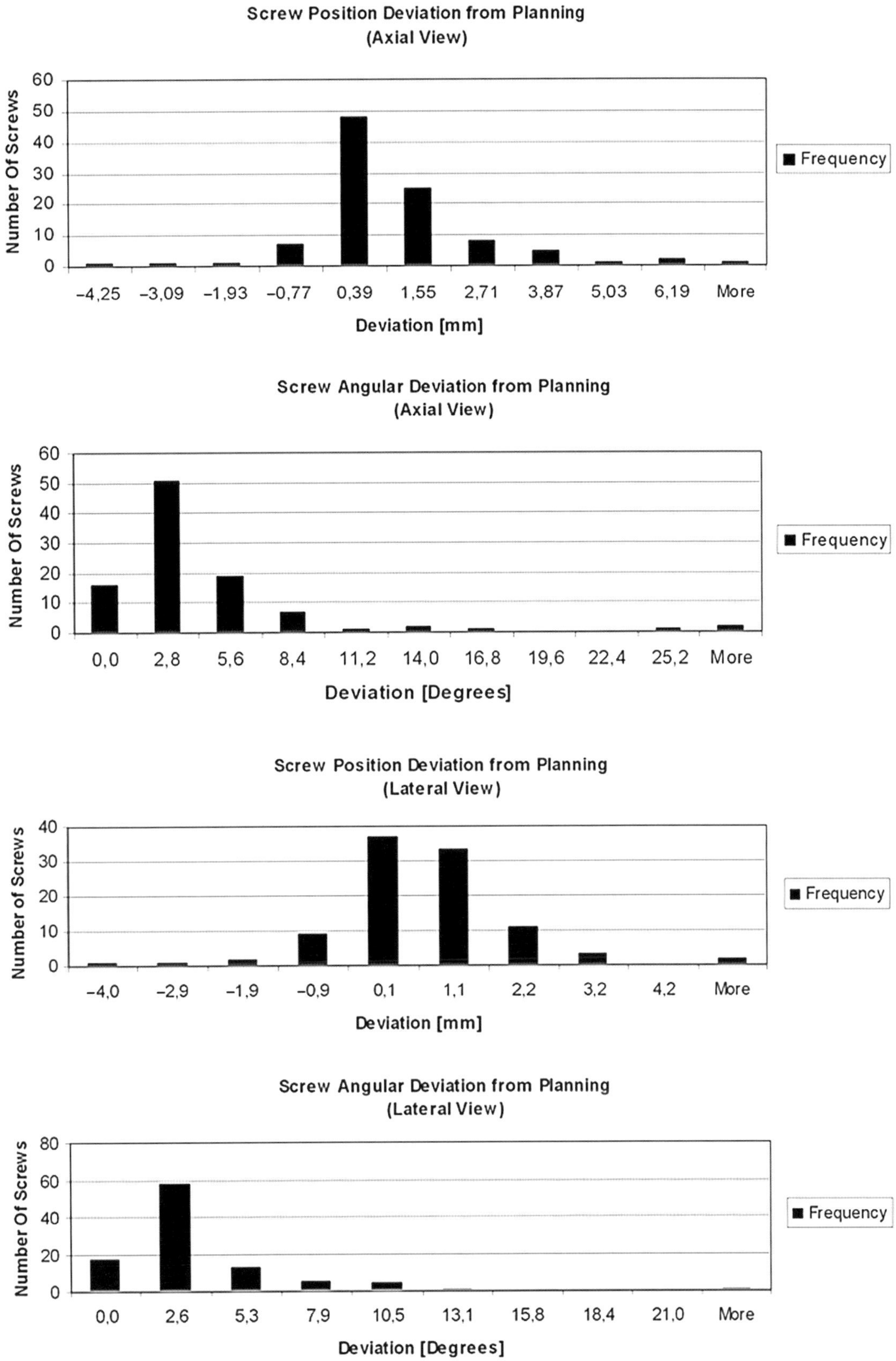

Fig. 2 The total average position deviation was 0.34 mm from the preoperative plan, Standard deviation = 1.49; total average angular deviation was 2.7° from the preoperative plan, Standard deviation = 4.22. Average position deviation was calculated also for 2 sub-groups: First 9 out of 19 procedures (*solid screws*) – 0.5 mm; Last 10 out of 19 procedures (*cannulated screws*) – 0.24 mm. Average angular deviation was calculated also for 2 sub-groups: First 9 out of 19 procedures (*solid screws*) – 3.4°; Last 10 out of 19 procedures (*cannulated screws*) – 2.23°

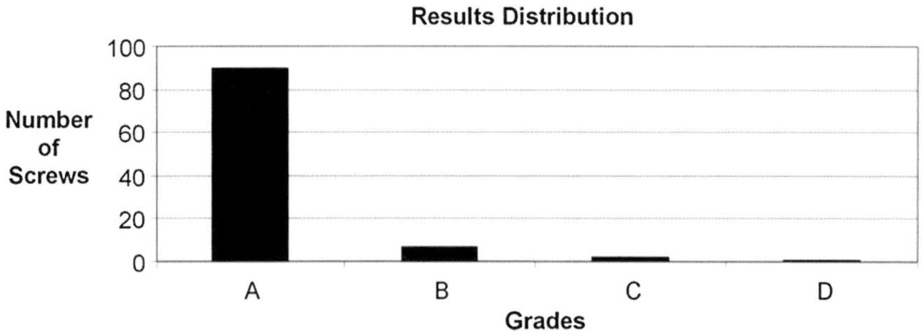

Fig. 3 The relative position of the screw to the pedicle was assessed and graded according to the ABC-method analysis: A=completely within the pedicle; B=pedicle wall breach less than 2 mm; C=pedicle wall breach equal to 2–4 mm; D=pedicle wall breach more than 4 mm. 90 of 100 screws were graded as A; 7 of 100 screws were graded as B; 2 of 100 screws were graded as C and one screw was graded as D

Future Prospects and Developments

Generally, still some disadvantages of medical robotics have to be counteracted. To some extent, medical robots (and herewith especially its hardware) are bulky and space occupying – characteristics that are of major concern within the setup and work flow in an operation room. So there is need for improvement of usability and practicability around bringing it into clinical application which yet is fulfilled with the SpineAssist. Another main disadvantage that accompanies almost every medical robotic system is that it still requires a fixed position of the patient in relation to the robot base. This seems of major concern in spinal surgery, as for navigation and guidance on bony structures direct contact to such anatomy and avoidance of soft tissue (muscles, subcutaneous fat tissue) is warranted in at least one fixing point. Thus, approaches to refine such procedures and to overcome the intra-operative movement-dependent inaccuracy have been made by developing a spine frame [13] or by interfacing infrared systems allowing dynamic referencing and complementarities [1]. Thus, in future, medical robotics will be increasingly linked to imaging modalities, while these systems are, for the most part, still under the direct control of the physician. This is based on the popularity and necessity of the image-guided interventions and the requirement of the robotic systems to work within the constraints of such various modalities as CT, MRI and PET. Repeatability and accuracy are of major concern regarding safety issues facing spinal surgery. Since the robotics' excellent accuracy in in vivo spinal procedures could be proven, medical robotics in general will never be a supplant but always be a supplement to the surgeon. Medical robots must operate in cooperation with physicians to be fully effective [14, 15]. Safety measures that can be taken include the use of redundant sensors, the design of special-purpose robots whose capabilities are tailored to the task at hand and the use of fail-safe techniques so that if the robot does fail it can be removed and the procedure can be completed by the surgeon. For the surgeon naturally is very concerned about the safety of the application of medical robotics in the operating room and therefore has to cope his responsibility following the fundamental principle in any surgeons training, which is "DO NO HARM". The "growth" of the medical robots from nowadays' childhood to tomorrow's adolescence will possibly follow a hierarchical scheme or the host of tools available to surgeons, ranging from hand-held tools to fully powered autonomous robots. As this hierarchy moves towards autonomous robots, the surgeon is less and less in control, and more dependent on the mechanical and software systems of the robot [14]. These technological challenges need further research areas focussing system architecture, software design, mechanical design, user interface and imaging-compatible designs. Thus, the development of application test beds is critical to move the field forward, and the completion of such medical robotics projects require a close partnership between engineers and clinicians that usually is not easy to establish.

Future development of medical robotics will base on integrated systems with a single interface to switch between planning, navigation, and robotic mode enabling the surgeon to have direct access to the surgical field and control of the integrated system [1]. But it is at this stage we must take into account, that the surgeon does become more of an observer than a controller, and from a purely neurosurgical soulful point of view one might put this development into question. Nevertheless, as with the society of our countries, the neurosurgical field is technology-driven and technology-dependent. Future generations of neurosurgeons will satisfy the immensely fast growing market for medical robotics and computer-assisted surgical equipment (average annual growing rate in the U.S. in 2004 of 32.6%) with a demand we can only imagine at this point. Who would have suspected 30 years ago that we can navigate endoscopically within our third ventricle or a bulging disc at the segment L4/5?

Conflict of interest statement We declare that we have no conflict of interest.

References

1. Zamorano L, Li Q, Jain S, Kaur G (2004) Robotics in neurosurgery: state of the art and future technological challenges. Int J Med Robot 1:7–22
2. Barzilay Y, Kaplan L, Libergall M (2008) Robotic assisted spine surgery – a breakthrough or a surgical toy? Int J Med Robot 4:195–196
3. Nathoo N, Cavusoglu MC, Vogelbaum MA, Barnett GH (2005) In touch with robotics: neurosurgery for the future. Neurosurgery 56:421–433
4. Barzilay Y, Liebergall M, Fridlander A, Knoller N (2006) Miniature robotic guidance for spine surgery – introduction of a novel system and analysis of challenges encountered during the clinical development phase at two spine centres. Int J Med Robot 2:146–153
5. Shoham M, Lieberman IH, Benzel EC, Togawa D, Zehavi E, Zilberstein B, Roffman M, Bruskin A, Fridlander A, Joskowicz L, Brink-Danan S, Knoller N (2007) Robotic assisted spinal surgery – from concept to clinical practice. Comput Aided Surg 12:105–115
6. Sukovich W, Brink-Danan S, Hardenbrook M (2006) Miniature robotic guidance for pedicle screw placement in posterior spinal fusion: early clinical experience with the SpineAssist. Int J Med Robot 2:114–122
7. Togawa D, Kayanja MM, Reinhardt MK, Shoham M, Balter A, Friedlander A, Knoller N, Benzel EC, Lieberman IH (2007) Bone-mounted miniature robotic guidance for pedicle screw and translaminar facet screw placement: part 2 – evaluation of system accuracy. Neurosurgery 60:ONS129–139
8. Lieberman IH, Togawa D, Kayanja MM, Reinhardt MK, Friedlander A, Knoller N, Benzel EC (2006) Bone-mounted miniature robotic guidance for pedicle screw and translaminar facet screw placement: part I – technical development and a test case result. Neurosurgery 59:641–650
9. Pechlivanis I, Kiriyanthan G, Engelhardt M, Scholz M, Lucke S, Harders A, Schmieder K (2009) Percutaneous placement of pedicle screws in the lumbar spine using a bone mounted miniature robotic system: first experiences and accuracy of screw placement. Spine (Phila Pa 1976) 34:392–398
10. Graham JJ (1989) Complications of cervical spine surgery. A five-year report on a survey of the membership of the Cervical Spine Research Society by the Morbidity and Mortality Committee. Spine (Phila Pa 1976) 14:1046–1050
11. Zeidman SM, Ducker TB, Raycroft J (1997) Trends and complications in cervical spine surgery: 1989–1993. J Spinal Disord 10:523–526
12. Kelleher MO, McEvoy L, Nagaria J, Kamel M, Bolger C (2006) Image-guided transarticular atlanto-axial screw fixation. Int J Med Robot 2:154–160
13. Thomale UW, Kneissler M, Hein A, Maetzig M, Kroppenstedt SN, Lueth T, Woiciechowsky C (2005) A spine frame for intra-operative fixation to increase accuracy in spinal navigation and robotics. Comput Aided Surg 10:151–155
14. Davies B (1996) A discussion of safety issues for medical robots. In: Taylor RH, Lavallée S, Burdeaa GC, Mösges R (eds) Computer-integrated surgery: technology and clinical applications. MIT Press, Cambridge, MA, pp 287–296
15. Elder MC, Knight JC (1995) Specifying user interfaces for safety-critical medical systems. Medical robotics and computer assisted surgery. Wiley-Liss, New York, pp 148–155

Microscope Integrated Indocyanine Green Video-Angiography in Cerebrovascular Surgery

Reza Dashti, Aki Laakso, Mika Niemelä, Matti Porras, and Juha Hernesniemi

Abstract Microscope integrated indocyanine green video-angiography (ICG-VA) is a new technique for intraoperative assessment of blood flow that has been recently applied to the field of Neurosurgery. ICG-VA is known as a simple and practical method of blood flow assessment with acceptable reliability. Real time information obtained under magnification of operating microscope has many potential applications in the microneurosurgical management of vascular lesions. This review is based on institutional experience with use of ICG-VA during surgery of intracranial aneurysms, AVMs and other vascular lesions at the Department of Neurosurgery at Helsinki University Central Hospital.

Keywords Arteriovenous malformations · Indocyanine green · Intracranial aneurysm · Intraoperative angiography · Surgery

Introduction

Intra-operative monitoring of blood flow may play an important role during microneurosurgical management of vascular lesions. Various available methods of intraoperative blood flow measurement can provide real time information and improve the efficacy of treatment. Intraoperative angiography is known as the gold standard and its role during microneurosurgical management of intracranial aneurysms and arteriovenous malformations is well known [1–12]. Microvascular Doppler and ultrasonic perivascular flowmetry are among other methods widely used [13–16]. Indocyanine green video-angiography (ICG-VA) is a safe, and reliable method for assessment of blood flow which is recently introduced to the field of cerebrovascular surgery [17].

This review is based on institutional experience with use of ICG-VA during microneurosurgical management of cerebrovascular lesions. Microscope integrated ICG-VA (Opmi Pentero Carl Zeiss Ltd. Oberkochen, Germany) has been in routine use for the last four years in the Department of Neurosurgery at Helsinki University Central Hospital. During this period ICG-VA was used during microneurosurgical management of more than 1,200 intracranial aneurysms, 120 AVMs and some other vascular lesions.

Indocyanine Green Video-Angiography

The use of indocyanine green video-angiography in cerbrovascular surgery was introduced by Raabe et al. in 2003 [17]. The technique is based on obtaining high-resolution and high-contrast images detected by near infrared (NIR) camera integrated to operating microscope. After intravenous injection of the ICG dye its florescence is induced and detected by the NIR video camera. The result is a real time assessment of cerebral vasculature under magnification of operating microscope. ICG-VA has arterial, capillary and venous phases [17–19]. A dose of 0.2–0.5 mg/kg is recommended for ICG-VA, with a maximum daily dose limit of 5 mg/kg.

ICG-VA is now available and in routine use in many centers. The technique is believed to be a safe, practical and cost-effective method of real time assessment of blood flow. ICG-VA can be used during microneurosurgical management of intracranial aneurysms, AVMs, and other vascular lesions of brain and spinal cord. Similarly, together

R. Dashti
Department of Neurosurgery, Helsinki University Central Hospital, 00260 Helsinki, Finland
Department of Neurosurgery, Istanbul University, Cerrahpaşa Medical Faculty Hospital, Istanbul, Turkey

A. Laakso, M. Niemelä, and J. Hernesniemi (✉)
Department of Neurosurgery, Helsinki University Central Hospital, 00260 Helsinki, Finland
e-mail: juha.hernesniemi@hus.fi

M. Porras
Department of Radiology, Helsinki University Central Hospital, 00260 Helsinki, Finland

M.N. Pamir et al. (eds.), *Intraoperative Imaging*, Acta Neurochirurgica Supplementum, Vol. 109,
DOI 10.1007/978-3-211-99651-5_39, © Springer-Verlag/Wien 2011

with microvascular Doppler and intraoperative angiography, ICG-VA can be a useful tool during surgery of vascular tumors and skull base lesions with close relation to major arteries. One of the unique advantages of the ICG-VA is its ability to assess the blood flow in perforating arteries [18–21]. The venous phase of the ICG-VA is another important feature which is particularly helpful in preserving the veins during various steps of dissection and/or retraction [17, 18]. This may play the key role during surgical resection of vascular malformations [22].

ICG-VA During Surgery of Intracranial Aneurysms

Microneurosurgical clipping is known as a durable method of treating for intracranial aneurysms (IAs). A perfect clip should occlude the aneurysm completely while the blood flow in the major and perforating branches is preserved. Detection of neck remnant or inadvertent vessel occlusion necessitates re-exploration if not already late. Intraoperative detection of improperly placed clip brings the advantage of immediate replacement to achieve complete occlusion of or to enhance the blood flow in a compromised vessel. Intraoperative angiography is suggested as the gold standard and the most reliable method to control the quality of clipping. However, limited routine availability, relatively high cost and [2, 4–6, 8, 9, 12, 23, 24] a complication rate of up to 3.5% are the major limitations [12, 25, 26]. Microvascular Doppler and ultrasonic perivascular flow probe are other methods of blood flow assessment [13–16]. Patency of perforating arteries, however, cannot be detected by above techniques.

The first application of microscope integrated ICG-VA during aneurysm surgery was described by Raabe et al. [17]. ICG-VA was used during microneurosurgical clipping of 12 intracranial aneurysms and two patients with dural fistulas. They reported postoperative imaging studies to be comparable with ICG-VA findings in all patients (100%). The technique was reported as a simple and safe alternative to other intraoperative methods of blood flow assessment. In their next study Raabe and colleagues [19] compared the findings of ICG-VA with intra- or postoperative DSA during surgical treatment of 114 patients with 124 aneurysms in two neurosurgical centers. Their results revealed 90% correlation between ICG-VA and intraoperative DSA in 60 aneurysms. Intraoperative findings of the technique were reported to be comparable with 90% of postoperative DSA for another 45 aneurysms [19]. de Oliveira and colleagues [20] demonstrated the advantage of ICG-VA in intraoperative assessment of the patency of perforating arteries around the aneurysm.

Recently we published our experience with ICG-VA during microneurosurgical treatment of 239 intracranial aneurysms in 190 patients [18]. Intraoperative ICG-VA assessment of total occlusion of the aneurysms and patency of major or perforating arteries were retrospectively compared with postoperative CTA and/or digital subtraction angiography (DSA). A total of 457 ICG-VA applications were performed (1–5 for each aneurysm). Technical quality of ICG-VA was optimal for 218 aneurysms (91%) (Fig. 1). Deep location, giant size, and arachnoid scarring due to previous operations were responsible for inadequate quality in the rest of them.

In 14 aneurysms (6%), unexpected neck residuals were detected. This rate was significantly higher in deep seated aneurysms (anterior communicating or basilar artery locations). The effect of deep location of the aneurysm in the surgical field was statistically significant. However, this was not the case with the size or ruptured status of the aneurysm. Unexpected occlusion of major branching or perforating

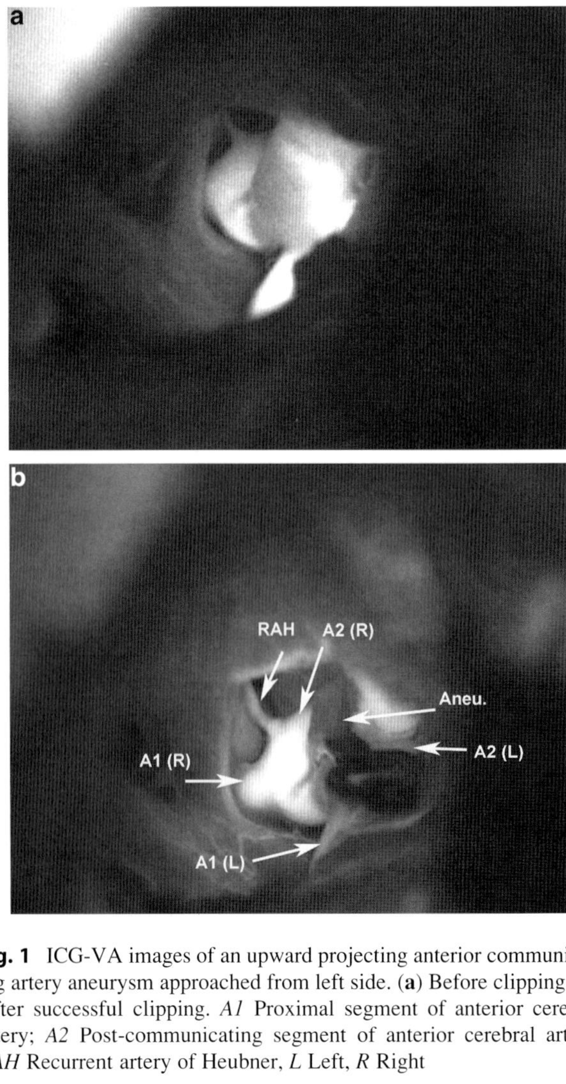

Fig. 1 ICG-VA images of an upward projecting anterior communicating artery aneurysm approached from left side. (**a**) Before clipping, (**b**) After successful clipping. *A1* Proximal segment of anterior cerebral artery; *A2* Post-communicating segment of anterior cerebral artery; *RAH* Recurrent artery of Heubner, *L* Left, *R* Right

arteries was found in 15 aneurysms (6%). Aneurysms located on middle cerebral artery surprisingly constituted the majority of them (n:10=67%). Other locations were anterior communicating, internal carotid-posterior communicating, and ICA posterior wall. Location, size and ruptured status of the aneurysm did not significantly affect the rate of unexpected branch occlusions [18]. Usefulness of ICG-VA was concluded in two other recent reports by Ma et al. [27] and Li et al. [28].

ICG-VA has limited ability to visualize the part of the base behind the aneurysm dome in deeply located aneurysms. Presence of blood clots in the field or arachnoid scarring are further restrictions. Based on our experience intraoperative DSA and or microvascular Doppler should be considered for verification of ICG-VA findings for deep sited, giant, thick walled and complex aneurysms.

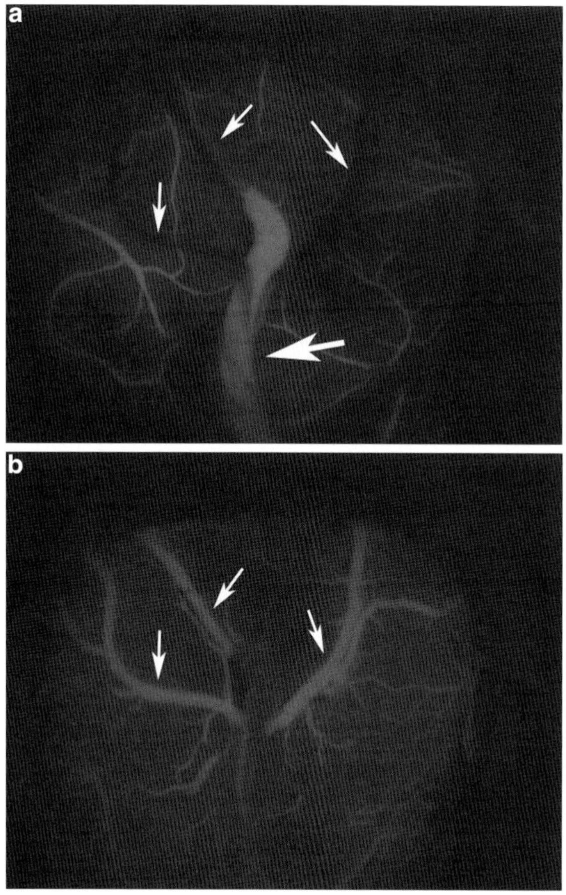

Fig. 2 ICG-VA images of an AVM located at right posterior temporal lobe. At the beginning of intradural part superficial veins are identified. (**a**) Early draining vein (*large arrow*), (**b**) Late filling of cortical veins (*small arrows*)

ICG-VA During Surgery of Brain Arteriovenous Malformations

During microneurosurgical treatment of brain AVMs, intradural strategy includes various steps of intraoperative orientation, localization of the lesion, identification of the arterial feeders, and preservation of the draining veins [29]. In our opinion ICG-VA can serve well during early stages of intraoperative orientation and localization of the vessels. The technique is able to demonstrate the superficial arterial feeders, early draining veins as well as normal ones (Fig. 2). Obtained images can be compared carefully with preoperative angiographic studies. This helps the orientation of surgeon under magnification of operating microscope. However, use of this technique during AVM surgery is limited to that part of lesion which is already exposed and illuminated in the field of microscope. We find ICG-VA very helpful in case of AVMs with cisternal component such as paracallosal or parasylvian ones where the major feeding arteries are in close relation to draining veins as well as the normal vessels. Here the early identification of large arterial feeder(s) and their temporary occlusion can facilitate the later steps of dissection. Comparison of the transit time of the ICG dye between the arterial and venous phases can also give an idea about the state of blood flow in the AVM during surgery. ICG-VA can be repeated safely within the limits of daily dose. We have not encountered any ICG related complications during surgery of AVMs.

Importantly, in AVM surgery, the technique can be only useful in early stages of superficial and sulcal dissection. We do not recommend using ICG-VA in detection of residual AVMs. Intraoperative or postoperative DSA remains the gold standard method in detecting residual AVMs.

Recently, Killory et al., reported their experience with the use of ICG-VA during surgical resection of 10 brain AVMs [22]. The technique was found to be useful in early detection of feeding arteries and veins in nine out of ten cases (90%). The authors reported the ICG-VA to be not useful in detecting the nidus residuals or early draining veins.

We use ICG-VA during micro-neurosurgical management of various other vascular lesions and as well vascular tumors. During surgery of spinal AVMs the technique is helpful in identification of arterialized veins and fistula sites. Similar findings are indicated in the reports by Colby et al. [30] and Hettige et al. [31]. The usefulness of ICG-VA in assessment of the patency of EC-IC bypass procedures was studied by Woitzik et al. [32] and Penã-Tapia et al. [33].

In conclusion, ICG-VA can be used as a simple and practical method intraoperative blood flow assessment. A careful interpretation of the real time information obtained by ICG-VA can serve as a useful tool to improve the quality of microneurosurgical management of various cerebrovascular lesions.

Conflict of interest statement We declare that we have no conflict of interest.

References

1. Anegawa S, Hayashi T, Torigoe R, Harada K, Kihara S (1994) Intraoperative angiography in the resection of arteriovenous malformations. J Neurosurg 80:73–78
2. Barrow D, Boyer K, Joseph G (1992) Intraoperative angiography in the management of neurovascular disorders. Neurosurgery 30:153–159
3. Batjer H, Frankfurt A, Purdy P, Smith S, Samson D (1988) Use of etomidate, temporary arterial occlusion, and intraoperative angiography in surgical treatment of large and giant cerebral aneurysms. J Neurosurg 68:234–240
4. Bauer BL (1984) Intraoperative angiography in cerebral aneurysm and AV-malformation. Neurosurg Rev 7:209–217
5. Chiang V, Gailloud P, Murphy K, Rigamonti D, Tamargo R (2002) Routine intraoperative angiography during aneurysm surgery. J Neurosurg 96:988–992
6. Derdeyn C, Moran C, Cross D, Grubb RJ, Dacey RJ (1995) Intraoperative digital subtraction angiography: a review of 112 consecutive examinations. AJNR Am J Neuroradiol 16:307–318
7. Katz JM, Gologorsky Y, Tsiouris A, Wells-Roth D, Mascitelli J, Gobin YP, Stieg PE, Riina HA (2006) Is routine intraoperative angiography in the surgical treatment of cerebral aneurysms justified? A consecutive series of 147 aneurysms. Neurosurgery 58:719–727
8. Klopfenstein J, Spetzler R, Kim L, Feiz-Erfan I, Han P, Zabramski J, Porter RW, Albuquerque FC, McDougall CG, Fiorella DJ (2004) Comparison of routine and selective use of intraoperative angiography during aneurysm surgery: a prospective assessment. J Neurosurg 100:230–235
9. Martin N, Bentson J, Vinuela F, Hieshima G, Reicher M, Black K, Dion J, Becker D (1990) Intraoperative digital subtraction angiography and the surgical treatment of intracranial aneurysms and vascular malformations [see comment]. J Neurosurg 73:526–533
10. Munshi I, Macdonald RL, Weir BK (1999) Intraoperative angiography of brain arteriovenous malformations. Neurosurgery 45:491–497
11. Peeters FL, Walder HA (1973) Intraoperative vertebral angiography in arteriovenous malformations. Neuroradiology 6:169–173
12. Tang G, Cawley C, Dion J, Barrow D (2002) Intraoperative angiography during aneurysm surgery: a prospective evaluation of efficacy. J Neurosurg 96:993–999
13. Amin-Hanjani S, Meglio G, Gatto R, Bauer A, Charbel F (2006) The utility of intraoperative blood flow measurment during aneurysm surgery using an ultrasonic perivascular flow probe. Neurosurgery 58:ONS 305–ONS 312
14. Bailes J, Tantuwaya L, Fukushima T, Schurman G, Davis D (1997) Intraoperative microvascular Doppler sonography in aneurysm surgery. Neurosurgery 40:965–970
15. Charbel FT, Hoffman WE, Misra M, Ostergren LA (1998) Ultrasonic perivascular flow peobe: technique and application in neurosurgery. Neurol Res 20:439–442
16. Firsching R, Synowitz HJ, Hanebeck J (2000) Practicability of intraoperative microvascular Doppler sonography in aneurysm surgery. Minim Invasive Neurosurg 43:144–148
17. Raabe A, Beck J, Gerlach R, Zimmermann M, Seifert V (2003) Near-infrared indocyanine green video angiography: a new method for intraoperative assessment of vascular flow. Neurosurgery 52:132–139
18. Dashti R, Laakso A, Porras M, Niemelä M, Hernesniemi J (2009) Microscope integrated Near-infrared indocyanine green video angiography during surgery of intracranial Aneurysms: Helsinki experience. Surg Neurol 71:543–550
19. Raabe A, Nakaji P, Beck J, Kim L, Hsu F, Kamerman JD, Seifert V, Spetzler RF (2005) Prospective evaluation of surgical microscope-integrated intraoperative near-infrared indocyanine green videoangiography during aneurysm surgery. J Neurosurg 103:982–989
20. de Oliveira M, Beck J, Seifert V, Teixeria M, Raabe A (2007) Assessment of blood in perforating arteries during intraoperative near-infrared indocyanine green videoangiography. Neurosurgery 61:ONS 63–ONS 73
21. Raabe A, Beck J, Seifert V (2005) Technique and image quality of intraoperative indocyanine green angiography during aneurysm surgery using surgical microscope integrated near-infrared video technology. Zentralbl Neurochir 66:1–6
22. Killory B, Nakaji P, Gonzales L, Ponce F, Wait S, Spetzler R (2009) Prospective evaluation of surgical microscope-integrated intraoperative near-infrared indocyanine green angiography during cerebral arteriovenous malformation surgery. Neurosurgery 65: 456–462
23. Bailes J, Deeb Z, Wilson J, Jungreis C, Horton J (1992) Intraoperative angiography and temporary balloon occlusion of the basilar artery as an adjunct to surgical clipping: technical note. Neurosurgery 31:603
24. Kallmes DF, Kallmes MH (1997) Cost-effectiveness of angiography performed during surgery for ruptured intracranial aneurysms. AJNR Am J Neuroradiol 18:1453–1462
25. Origitano TC, Schwartz K, Anderson D, Azar-Kia B, Reichman OH (1999) Optimal clip application and intraoperative angiography for intracranial aneurysms. Surg Neurol 51:117–124
26. Payner TD, Horner TG, Leipzig TJ, Scott JA, Gilmor RL, DeNardo AJ (1998) Role of intraoperative angiography in the surgical treatment of cerebral aneurysms. J Neurosurg 88:441–448
27. Ma C, Shi J, Wang H, Hang C, Cheng H, Wu W (2009) Intraoperative indocyanine green angiography in intracranial aneurysm surgery: microsurgical clipping and revascularization. Clin Neurol Neurosurg 111:840–846
28. Li J, Lan Z, He M, You C (2009) Assessment of microscope-integrated indocyanine green angiography during intracranial aneurysm surgery: a retrospective study of 120 patients. Neurol India 57:453–459
29. Yaşargil MG (1988) Microneurosurgery, vol 3-B. Georg Thieme Verlag, Stuttgart, New York, pp 25–53
30. Colby GP, Coon AL, Sciubba DM, Bydon A, Gailloud P, Tamargo RJ (2009) Intraoperative indocyanine green angiography for obliteration of a spinal dural arteriovenous fistula. J Neurosurg Spine 11:705–709
31. Hettige S, Walsh D (2010) Indocyanine green video-angiography as an aid to surgical treatment of spinal dural arteriovenous fistulae. Acta Neurochir (Wien) 152(3):533–536
32. Woitzik J, Horn P, Vajkoczy P, Schmiedek P (2005) Intraoperative control of extracranial-intracranial bypass patency by near-infrared indocyanine green videoangiography. J Neurosurg 102:692–698
33. Pena-Tapia PG, Kemmling A, Czabanka M, Vajkoczy P, Schmiedek P (2008) Identification of the optimal cortical target point for extracranial-intracranial bypass surgery in patients with hemodynamic cerebrovascular insufficiency. J Neurosurg 108:655–661

Application of Intraoperative Indocyanine Green Angiography for CNS Tumors: Results on the First 100 Cases

P. Ferroli, F. Acerbi, E. Albanese, G. Tringali, M. Broggi, A. Franzini, and G. Broggi

Abstract *Purpose*: To investigate the application of indocyanine green (ICG) videoangiography during microsurgery for central nervous system (CNS) tumors.

Methods: One hundred patients with CNS tumors who underwent microsurgical resection from December 2006 to December 2008 were retrospectively analyzed. The diagnosis was high grade glioma in 54 cases, low grade in 17 cases, meningioma in 14 cases, metastasis in 12 cases and hemangioblastoma in 3 cases. Overall, ICG was injected intraoperatively 194 times. The standard dose of 25 mg of dye was injected intravenously and intravascular fluorescence from within the blood vessels was imaged through an ad hoc microscope with dedicated software (Pentero, Carl Zeiss Co., Oberkochen, Germany). Pre-resection and post-resection arterial, capillary and venous ICG videoangiographic phases were intraoperatively observed and recorded.

Results: ICG videangiography allowed for a good evaluation of blood flow in the tumoral and peritumoral exposed vessels in all cases. No side effects due to ICG were observed.

Conclusions: ICG video-angiography is a significant method for monitoring blood flow in the exposed vessels during microsurgical removal of CNS tumors. Pre-resection videoangiography provides useful information on the tumoral circulation and the pathology-induced alteration in surrounding brain circulation. Post-resection examination allows for an immediate check of patency of those vessels that are closely related to the tumor mass and that the surgeon does not want to damage.

Keywords Indocyanine green (ICG) videoangiography · Intracranial tumors · Surgical resection · Venous drainage

Ferroli, Acerbi and Albanese equally contributed to the paper.

P. Ferroli (✉), F. Acerbi, E. Albanese, G. Tringali, M. Broggi, A. Franzini, and G. Broggi
Department of Neurosurgery, Fondazione Istituto Neurologico Carlo Besta, Via Celoria 11, 20133 Milano, Italy
e-mail: ferrolipaolo@hotmail.com

Introduction

Angiography with ICG has been first developed in the seventies in Ophthalmology to evaluate choroidal microcirculation [1–6]. Recently, microscope-integrated near-infrared ICG videoangiography has been introduced in Neurosurgery in order to visualize cerebral vessels in case of aneurysm clipping, bypasses and vascular malformations. It has been proven that intraoperative videoangiography with ICG may help to evaluate cerebral vessels that are visible in the surgical field in order to get a real time diagnose of the degree of aneurysm occlusion, vessel patency including the perforating arteries and, in vascular malformations, to distinguish pathologic vessels from normal vessels and arteries from veins based on the timing of fluorescence with the dye [7–20].

To our knowledge, there are no studies in the literature evaluating the potential role of ICG videoangiography during resection of CNS tumors. Therefore, our investigation focused on whether this technique could be used as an intraoperative diagnostic tool to study vascular physiopathology in CNS tumors and whether the information retrieved could be integrated in the decision making-process during surgical removal.

Patients and Methods

In the period between December 2006 and December 2008, almost 1,200 patients affected by CNS tumors were admitted at the III Neurosurgical Unit of the Department of Neurosurgery at the Fondazione IRCCS Istituto Neurologico Carlo Besta in Milan. One hundred of these patients, 67males and 33 females (mean age of 56 years), underwent intraoperative ICG videoangiography and were retrospectively reviewed (Table 1). All patients gave their written informed consent.

DOI 10.1007/978-3-211-99651-5_40, © Springer-Verlag/Wien 2011

Table 1 Types of tumors evaluated by Intraoperative ICG videoangiography in our series

Tumor	# Cases
Meningioma	14
Low-grade glioma	17
High-grade glioma	54
Metastasis	12
Hemangioblastoma	3

Surgery was performed using a near-infrared videointegrated microscope (Pentero, Carl Zeiss Co., Oberkochen, Germany). The video records images from the operating microscope, illuminated with a light source including the ICG excitation wavelength, through an optical filter that allows only fluorescence in the ICG emission wavelength. Only vessels directly visible in the surgical field can be visualized. The ICG video angiography was performed before and after tumor removal, following the standard protocol described elsewhere [14–17, 21–29]. Briefly, ICG was administered intravenously by the anesthesiologist (25 mg in 5 ml of saline). Vessel fluorescence appeared after a few seconds and was cleared within 10 min, allowing for additional injections. The resultant video was shown on the microscope screen in the operative room during surgery and recorded for further visualizations.

Histological diagnoses were obtained in all cases and were analyzed together with the intraoperative findings in order to investigate the tumor-related videangiographic features.

Results

ICG Videoangiography was performed before tumor removal in all cases. In 6 cases the operating surgeon avoided to repeat post-resection ICG injection because it was considered useless. No adverse reaction was observed.

ICG videoangiography allowed intra-operative realtime assessment of the exposed vessel with excellent image quality and resolution. Arterial, capillary, and venous phase could be always recognized.

The post-resection arterial phase was able to show, as already demonstrated for vascular cases [7, 8, 12, 14–17, 19, 20], patency of big cerebral arteries that underwent manipulation for the removal of tumors in contact with or fully encasing them (1 planum sphenoidalis meningioma, 2 lesser wing meningiomas, and 2 sylvian metastases). In addition, the arterial phase was considered particularly useful to confirm patency of small arteries dissected free and preserved during tumor removal because they were traversing the surgical field and nourishing at least in part the normal brain parenchyma (Fig. 1). This occurred in 3 out of 54 cases of high grade gliomas and in 4 out of 17 cases of low-grade gliomas. Furthermore, both arterial and capillary phases were useful to diagnose fronto-temporal ischemia after removal of a huge right frontal high grade glioma encasing the middle cerebral artery, due to its intra-operative thrombosis (Fig. 2).

The ICG videoangiographic pre-operative late arterial-capillary phase provided good quality images and videos of the vascular pattern of the CNS area exposed by surgery, well depicting both specific tumor-related alterations and aspecific mass-effect changes. In particular, when the tumor abutted the CNS surface, ICG videoangiography evidenced the pathologic characteristic of the tumor vasculature, both in cases of neo-angiogenic vascular pattern and in cases in which the tumor showed hypoperfused or avascular areas such as in cystic or necrotic masses. In addition, in this context, it was possible to identify artero-venous fistulas, which were common in high grade gliomas, and were identified in 45 out of 54 cases (Fig. 3), typical of hemangioblastomas (3 out of 3 cases) and sometimes observed in metastases (2 out of 12 cases) and rarely in meningiomas (1 out of 14 cases). Aspecific mass-effect changes i.e. brain gyri compressed by the tumor and edema, and congested, were evident in a greater number of cases (all the 71 cases of low and high grade tumors and 5 out of 12 cases of metastases, 5 out of 14 cases of meningiomas).

Regarding the venous phase of ICG videoangiography, this was found useful to identify impaired venous outflow and consequent congestion. This was evident in case of arterovenous fistulae, as detailed above, and in case of direct venous compression by the tumor itself (5 out of 54 cases of high-grade gliomas, 1 out of 12 cases of metastases, 3 out of 14 cases of meningiomas). In addition, ICG videoangiography allowed to identity, when present, the retrograde outflow trough anastomotic veins. These data were useful to decide whether or not to cut a draining vein in order to provide a wider and safer surgical corridor to the tumor itself (10 cases) or to obtain a radical tumor resection (8 cases). Specifically, in case of arterovenous fistulae, when normal veins afferent to the arterialized vein did not show a retrograde flow, these veins were considered the only outflow for the peri-tumoral CNS area. Therefore they were preserved in all cases in order to re-establish a physiologic pre-tumoral condition. On the contrary, when a collateral flow through an anastomotic circle was evident, the arterialized vein was considered un-needed and therefore was cut, without any related post-operative complication. The same considerations were made in cases of a direct venous compression by the tumor.

ICG videoangiography was also used to perform occlusion test with temporary clipping of veins that showed an

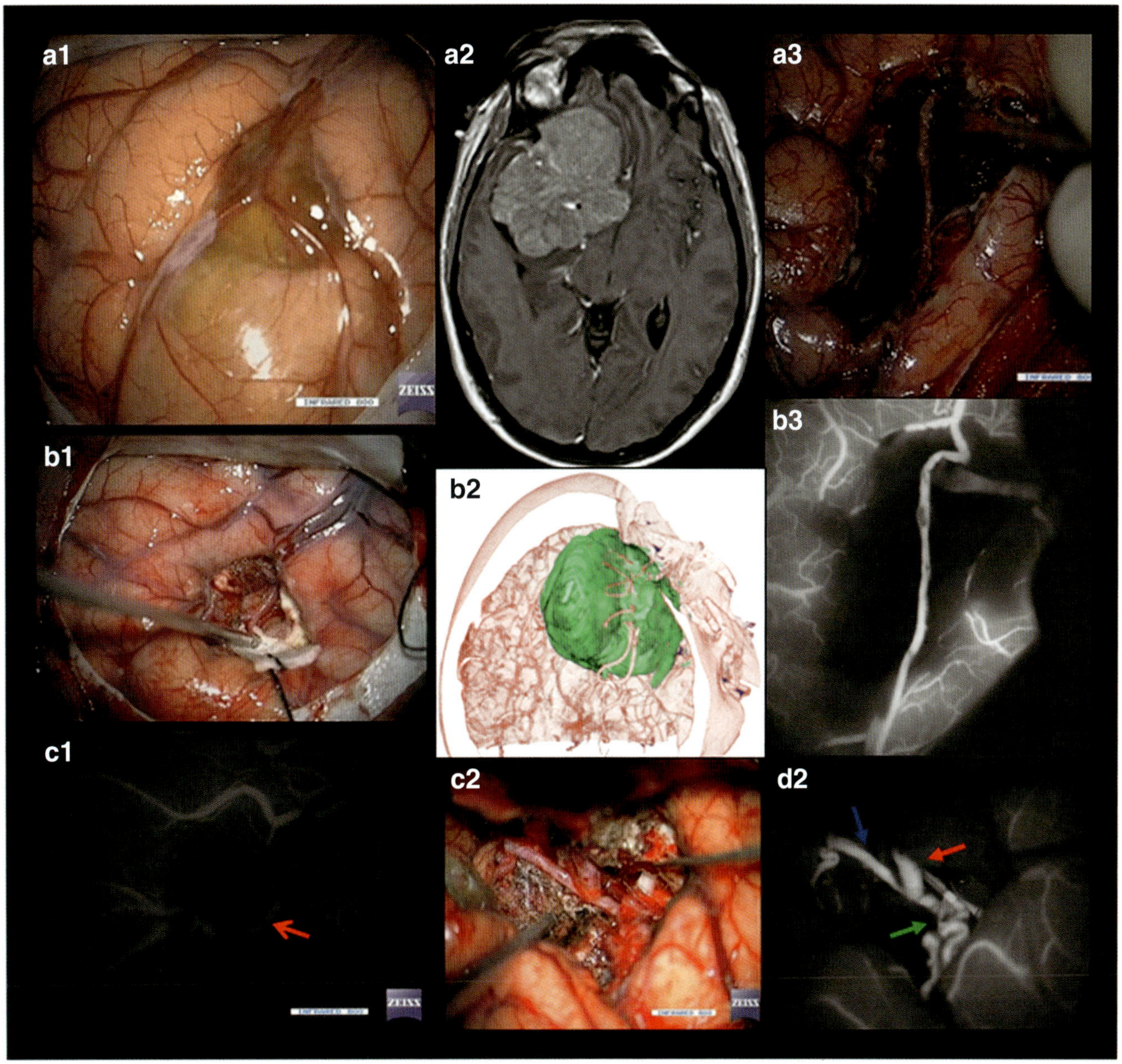

Fig. 1 **a1.** Cystic metastasis: intraoperative view. **b1.** *Post resection view*: the middle cerebral artery and its branches (*arrow*) are visible under the microscope. **c1.** Post-resection ICG videoangiography, arterial phase: the middle cerebral artery (MCA) is well injected (*arrow*). **a2.** Pre-operative MRI (cT1): right etmoido-sphenoidal meningioma with MCA encasement. **b2.** Dextroscope 3D reconstruction to emphasize the encasement of the MCA. **c2.** *Intraoperative view*: post-resection image showing the right internal carotid artery, the anterior and middle cerebral arteries. **d2.** ICG videoangiography, arterial phase: the right internal cerebral artery (*red arrow*), the anterior (*blue arrow*) and middle (*green arrow*) cerebral arteries are patent. **a3.** Post-resection microscopic view in a case of righ rolandic high-grade glioma: the artery over the resected tumor is picked up. **b3.** Post-resection ICG videoangiography: the artery is well injected and patent

intimate relationships with the tumors. This test was used to evaluate the presence of anastomotic circle allowing for venous sacrifice in order to increase the degree of tumor resection.

A summary of videoangiographic results in different tumors is shown in Table 2.

Discussion

The intraoperative ICG videoangiography is a relatively new technique of intraoperative investigation that has been recently applied in the field of Vascular Neurosurgery. Routine or selective use of this technique during surgery of

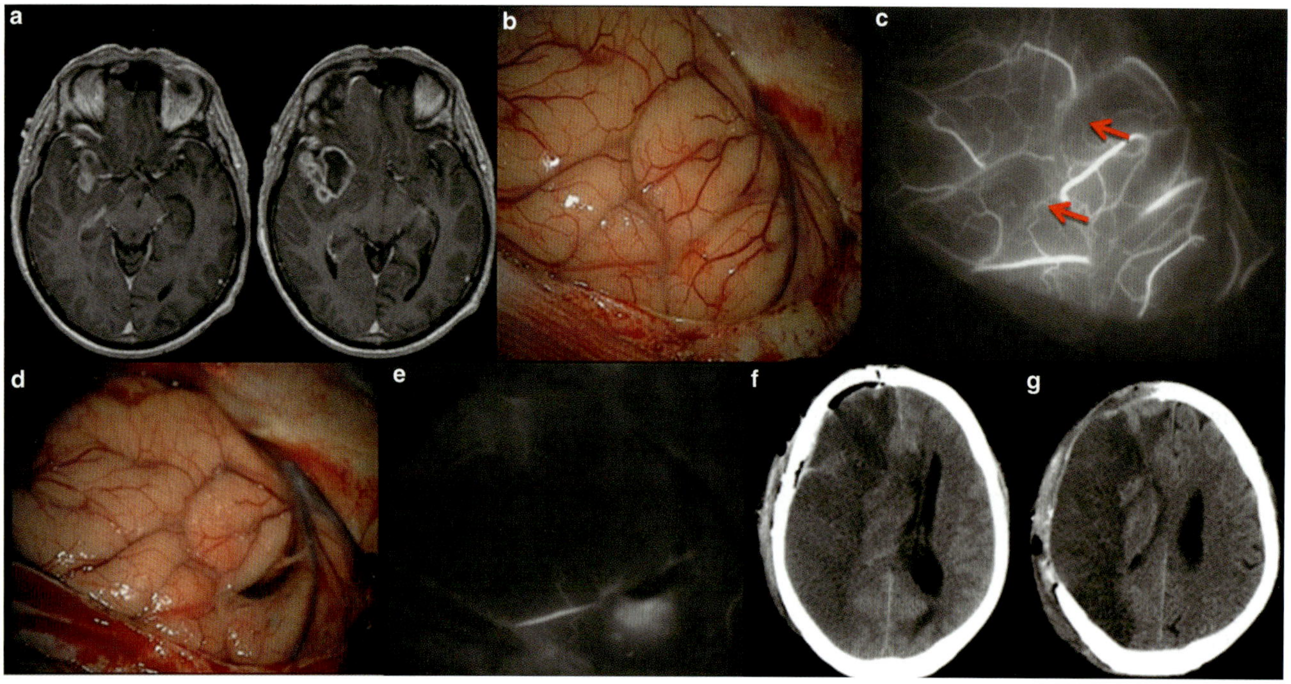

Fig. 2 (**a**) Pre-operative MRI (cT1) showing a fronto-temporal GBM on the right side in close relation with the homolateral middle cerebral artery (MCA). (**b**) Intraoperative view after right fronto-temporal approach and dural opening. Although mannitol was given to the patient, under the microscope the exposed cortex appears congested due to the edema. (**c**) Pre-resection ICG videoangiography: a stagnant flow within the cortical vessels is detected (*arrows*). (**d**) Post-resection view. After tumor removal the surrounding brain appears decompressed. (**e**) Post-resection ICG videoangiography showing no injection of the exposed area of the frontal lobe. An ICP monitoring was therefore positioned (**f**) Due to the increasing of the ICP the patient underwent an early post-operative CT scan. A huge ipodensity of the right hemisphere associated with shift of the structure of the midline was detected. An hemicraniectomy was therefore performed. (**g**) Post-operative CT after decompressive craniectomy

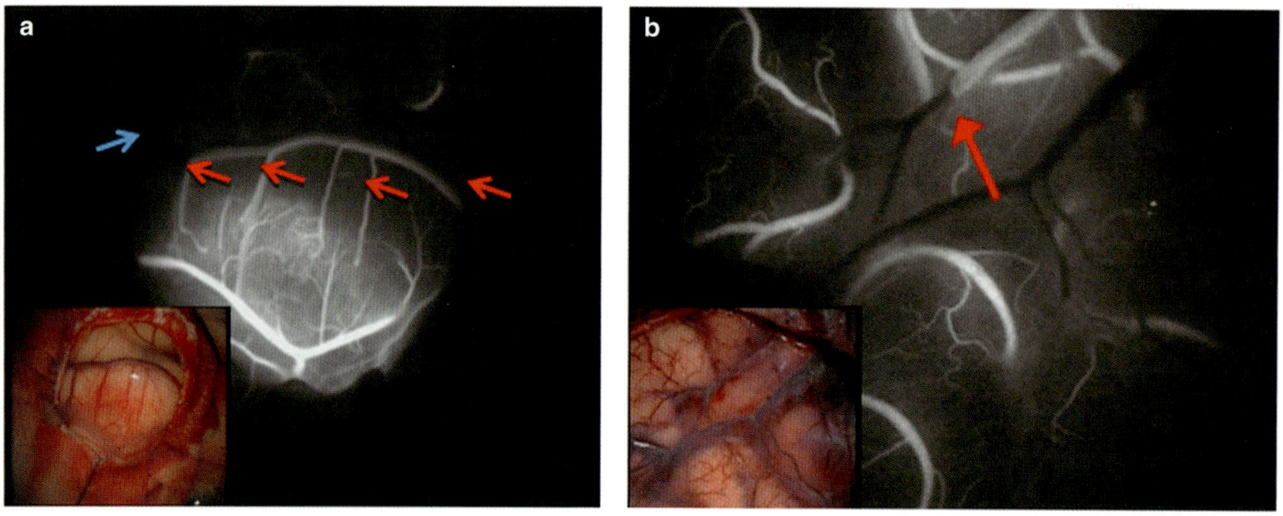

Fig. 3 (**a**) Pre-resection ICG videoangiography in one case of right frontal metastasis (intraoperative microscopic picture in the left corner): in late arterial/capillary phase early injection of arterialized venous vessels (*red arrows*), artero-venous (A-V) fistula, together with physiologic injection of the capillars are visible. The dye is not yet filling the non-arterialized vein (*blue arrow*). (**b**) Pre-resection ICG videoangiography in one case of left frontal high-grade glioma (intraoperative microscopic picture in the left corner): in late arterial/capillary phase an A-V fistula is present (*red arrow*)

vascular malformations and revascularization procedures has been suggested by many authors. It has been proven that intraoperative videoangiography with ICG may help to evaluate cerebral vessels that are visible in the surgical field in order to get a real time diagnose of the degree of aneurysm occlusion and vessel patency including the perforating arteries. In cases of vascular malformations, it can be used to distinguish pathologic vessels from normal vessels and

Table 2 ICG videoangiographic characteristics identified in the three phases, specified for each tumor

Tumor	Arterial phase	Capillary phase	Venous phase
Meningioma	Post-resection vessel patency (3/14)	Pre-resection A-V shunt (1/14)	Pre-resection A-V shunt (1/14)
Low-grade glioma	Post-resection vessel patency (4/17)		
High-grade glioma	Post-resection vessel patency (3/54) Post-resection ischemia (1/54)	Pre-resection A-V shunt (45/54)	Pre-resection A-V shunt (45/54)
Metastasis	Post-resection vessel patency (2/12)	Pre-resection A-V shunt (2/12)	Pre-resection A-V shunt (2/12)
Hemangioblastoma		Pre-resection A-V shunt (3/3)	Pre-resection A-V shunt (3/3)

arteries from veins based on the timing of fluorescence with the dye [7–20].

To our knowledge, there are no studies in the literature investigating the potential role of ICG videoangiography during resection of CNS tumors. The angiographic evaluation of CNS tumor vasculature before surgical removal was the only pre-operative radiological information before the advent of Computerized Tomography and, more recently, Magnetic Resonance. In the early 1920s, Egas Moniz introduced and developed the idea of utilizing X-rays as a method of making visible the blood vessels of the brain and to locate brain tumors. After mapping the normal distribution of the intracranial blood vessels, he clinically used his method in 1927, outlining with X rays the location and size of a patient's brain tumor by the tumor's displacement of injected arteries[25–27]. At that time he defined the angiographic phases that are still used today: arterial, capillary, early and late venous phase. Direct and indirect signs were used to diagnose a brain tumor. The direct signs, i.e. morphological features of the pathological vessels, were utilized to define the nature of the lesion and the indirect signs, i.e. the displacement of the cerebral arteries due to the lesion, were used to locate the tumor [22, 28–31]. Nowadays, the diagnosis of CNS tumors is based mainly on computed tomography and magnetic resonance imaging, however, selective cerebral angiography is still utilized when the neurosurgeon is considering a combined endovascular-surgicalstrategy of treatment in selected cases and it's still the gold standard to evaluate the patency of the dural sinus in oncological cases [32–36].

In this study we had the opportunity to evaluate whether ICG videoangiography could provide some information regarding vascular physiopathology of CNS tumors. We studied a heterogeneous population consisting mainly on high grade gliomas, but including also low grade gliomas, meningiomas, metastases and hemangioblastomas. As already known from previous studies on vascular cases, ICG videoangiography allowed intra-operative real time assessment of the exposed vessel with excellent image quality and resolution. Therefore, we could evaluate only the area exposed by the craniotomy, which, especially for minimally invasive approaches that we routinely use for most of our cases, not always represented the entire area with direct and indirect signs of the tumor's presence. However, arterial, capillary, and venous phase could be recognized in all cases. Therefore, the neovascular architecture, alteration of the calibre, morphology and course of vessels, and the haemodynamic patterns could be studied. The ICG transit time in tumoral vessels was found to be normal or shortened such as in case of malignant tumor (i.e. high grade gliomas and metastases). A short flow-time, due to pathological low-resistance vessels that results in arteriovenous shunting, was found to be common in high grade gliomas, as is the presence of neovascular architecture, dysplastic vessels and thrombosed veins, as previously demonstrated with traditional cerebral angiography [21, 37, 38]. Although the arteriovenous shunts were not always found (45 out of 54 high grade gliomas), an early visualization of the venous compartment was always present. Because arteriovenous shunting causes an arterial steal that leads to hypoperfusion of the surrounding parenchyma, it has been speculated that this mechanism could contribute to local ischemia, eventually causing tissue necrosis. The presence of multiple areas of necrosis suggests that the neovasculature fails to supply the rapidly growing tumor tissue [24]. Sometimes, superficial avascular areas in case of high grade glioma and metastasis, have been seen during pre-resection ICG videoangiography. Although the presence of these vascular characteristics of GBMs have been known for decades, in the last WHO classification there are still controversies on arteriovenous shunts and particularly on the presence/absence of necrosis in GBMs [23, 39]. Although the number of cases studied is low, all the hemangioblastomas, which are peculiar types of tumor, showed the presence of superficial pathologic vessel architecture, with arterovenous fistulae, and arterialized and dilated vein draining the tumor nodule.

Despite the permeability of the blood–brain barrier, the dye does not penetrate the membrane and we were unable to define the margins of the tumor in gliomas and metastases.

Another opportunity offered by this study was to investigate whether the information retrieved by the use of intraoperative ICG videoangiography could be integrated in the decision making process during surgical removal.

First of all, apart from direct visual observation and microvascular Doppler, intraoperative ICG videoangiography was found to be a useful tool for intraoperative assessment of post-resection vessel patency. Microscope-integrated near-infrared ICG videoangiography can confirm the presence of good flow through the arteries that have been exposed during tumor resection. In addition, in the case of intra-operative diagnosis of stroke, as happened for one of the patient in this series (Fig. 2), the early evidence of this complication leaded to ICU admission with ICP monitoring that allowed for further diagnosis and immediate decompressive craniectomy to reduce intracranial hypertension.

Particularly interesting were the pieces of information provided by ICG videoangiography during the venous phase. The possibility of post-operative complications in case of venous sacrifice during neurosurgical procedures has always been debated [40, 41]. However, there are not definite data on post-operative complications rate, related to the sacrifice of single veins in every patient. Although this risk can be related to the variability of individual pattern of venous drainage, which could be evaluated by pre-operative angiography, it is not possible to investigate the real entity of anastomotic circles because an occlusive test on single veins can not be performed. Our data on ICG videoangiography provide some insights into this discussion. In fact, we could evaluate the pattern of venous drainage of the tumor and the surrounding brain parenchyma in every patient. When vein outflow was impaired, as in case of arterovenous fistulae or direct vein compression by the tumor, ICG videoangiography could offer a unique possibility to intraoperatively evaluate the presence of anastomotic circulation. This result could be achieved through a temporary clipping test of veins closely related to the tumor that evaluated the ICG clearance time of the tested vein. We used this information to evaluate whether vein sacrifice could safely be performed. Interestingly, even if these data have been retrieved on few patients, the favourable outcome in these cases is encouraging and the ICG videoangiography seems to add useful information regarding individual venous variability.

Conflict of interest statement We declare that we have no conflict of interest.

References

1. Benson RC, Kues HA (1978) Fluorescence properties of indocyanine green as related to angiography. Phys Med Biol 23:159–163
2. Cochran ST, Bomyea K, Sayre JW (2001) Trends in adverse events after IV administration of contrast media. AJR Am J Roentgenol 176:1385–1388
3. Flower RW, Hochheimer BF (1976) Indocyanine green dye fluorescence and infrared absorption choroidal angiography performed simultaneously with fluorescein angiography. Johns Hopkins Med J 138:3–42
4. Fox IS, Wood EH (1960) Indocyanine green: physical and pathological properties. Proc Mayo Clinic 35:732
5. Hochheimer BF (1971) Angiography of the retina with indocyanine green. Arch Ophthalmol 86:564–565
6. Hope-Ross M, Yannuzzi LA, Gragoudas ES, Guyer DR, Slakter JS, Sorenson JA, Krupsky S, Orlock DA, Puliafito CA (1994) Adverse reactions due to indocyanine green. Ophthalmology 101:529–533
7. Dashti R, Laakso A, Niemelä M, Porras M, Hernesniemi J (2009) Microscope-integrated near-infrared indocyanine green videoangiography during surgery of intracranial aneurysms: the Helsinki experience. Surg Neurol 71:543–550
8. de Oliveira M, Beck J, Seifert V et al (2007) Assessment of flow in perforating arteries during intracranial aneurysm surgery using intraoperative near-infrared indocyanine green videoangiography. Neurosurgery 61:ONS 63–ONS 73
9. Ferroli P, Acerbi F, Broggi M, Broggi G (2010) Arterovenous micro-malformation of the trigeminal root: intraoperative diagnosis with ICG videoangiography. Neurosurgery (in press)
10. Ferroli P, Tringali G, Albanese E, Broggi G (2008) Developmental venous anomaly of petrous veins: intraoperative findings and indocyanine green video angiographic study. Neurosurgery 62(5 suppl 2):ONS418–ONS421
11. Hettige S, Walsh D (2010) Indocyanine green video-angiography as an aid to surgical treatment of spinal dural arteriovenous fistulae. Acta Neurochir (Wien) 152(3):533–536
12. Imizu S, Kato Y, Sangli A, Oguri D, Sano H (2008) Assessment of incomplete clipping of aneurysms intraoperatively by a near-infrared indocyanine green-video angiography (Niicg-Va) integrated microscope. Minim Invasive Neurosurg 51:199–203
13. Killory BD, Nakaji P, Gonzales LF, Ponce FA, Wait SD, Spetzler RF (2009) Prospective evaluation of surgical microscope-integrated intraoperative near-infrared indocyanine green angiography during cerebral arteriovenous malformation surgery. Neurosurgery 65(3):456–462
14. Li J, Lan Z, He M, You C (2009) Assessment of microscope-integrated indocyanine green angiography during intracranial aneurysm surgery: a retrospective study of 120 patients. Neurol India 57(4):453–459
15. Raabe A, Beck J, Gerlach R et al (2003) Near-infrared indocyanine green video angiography: a new method for intraoperative assessment of vascular flow. Neurosurgery 52:132–139
16. Raabe A, Beck J, Seifert V (2005) Technique and image quality of intraoperative indocyanine green angiography during aneurysm surgery using surgical microscope integrated near-infrared video technology. Zentralbl Neurochir 66:1–6
17. Raabe A, Nakaji P, Beck J et al (2005) Prospective evaluation of surgical microscope-integrated intraoperative near-infrared indocyanine green videoangiography during aneurysm surgery. J Neurosurg 103:982–989
18. Takagi Y, Kikuta K, Nozaki K, Sawamura K, Hashimoto N (2007) Detection of a residual nidus by surgical microscope integrated intraoperative near-infrared indocyanine green videoangiography in a child with a cerebral arteriovenous malformation. J Neurosurg 107(5 suppl):416–418
19. Woitzik J, Horn P, Vajkoczy P et al (2005) Intraoperative control of extracranial-intracranial bypass patency by near-infrared indocyanine green videoangiography. J Neurosurg 102:692–698
20. Xu BN, Sun ZH, Romani R, Jiang JL, Wu C, Zhou DB, Yu XG, Hernesniemi J, Li BM (2009) Microsurgical management of large and giant paraclinoid aneurysms. Surg Neurol Oct 13 [Epub ahead of print]
21. Kleihues P, Cavenee WK (eds) (2000) World Health Organization classification of tumours. Pathology and genetics of tumours of the nervous system, 2nd edn. IARC Press, Lyon, ISBN 92 83 22409 4
22. Krayenbuhl H, Yasargil MG (1967) Diagnosi strutturale dei tumori intracranici. In: Krayenbuhl H, Yasargil MG (eds) L'angiografia cerebrale, 1st edn. Piccin, Padova, pp 263–314

23. Louis DN, Ohgaki H, Wiestler OD, Cavenee WK, Burger PC, Jouvet A et al (2007) The 2007 WHO classification of tumours of the central nervous system. Acta Neuropathol 114:97–109
24. Mariani L, Schroth G, Wielepp JP, Haldemann A, Seiler RW (2001) Intratumoral arteriovenous shunting in malignant gliomas. Neurosurgery 48(2):353–357
25. Moniz E (1927) L'encéphalograpie artérielle, son imporance dans la localisation des tumeurs cérébrales. Rev Neurol 34:72–89
26. Moniz E (1931) Diagnostic des tumeurs cérébrals et épreuve de l'encephalographie artérielle. Masson & Cie, Paris
27. Moniz E (1934) L'angiographie cérébrale. Masson & Cie, Paris
28. Newton TH, Potts DG (eds) (1971) Radiology of the skull and brain, vol 2. C.V. Mosby, St. Louis
29. Panzini A, Conte P (1983) Diagnostica angiografica dei tumori cerebrali sopratentoriali. Piccin, Padova
30. Gallingioni F (1980) Semeiologia angiografica nella patologia vascolare in Neuroradiologia Piccin, Padova, pp 398–401
31. Zachrisson L (1963) Angiography of cerebral metastases. Acta Radiol 1:521–527
32. Al-Mefty O (1998) Operative atlas of meningiomas. Lippincott-Raven, Philadelphia
33. Cushing H (1922) The meningiomas (dural endotheliomas): their source and favore seats of origin. Brain 45:282
34. Cushing H, Eisenhardt L (1938) Meningiomas: their classification, regional behaviour, life history and surgical end results. Charles C Thomas, Springfield, IL
35. Standard SC, Ahuja A, Livingston K et al (1994) Endovascular embolization and surgical excision for the treatment of cerebellar and brain stem Hemangioblastomas. Surg Neurol 41:405–410
36. Tampieri D, Leblanc R, TerBrugge K (1993) Preoperative embolization of brain and spinal hemangioblastomas. Neurosurgery 33:502–505
37. Feiring EH, Shapiro JH, Lubetsky HW (1963) The ring-like vascular pattern in cerebral angiography. Am J Roentgenol 89:385–390
38. Tonnis W, Walter W (1959) Das glioblastoma multiforme. Bericht über 2611 Fälle. Acta Neurochir Suppl 6:40–62
39. Scheithauer BW, Fuller GN, VandenBerg SR (2008) The 2007 WHO classification of tumors of the nervous system: controversies in surgical neuropathology. Brain Pathol 18:307–316
40. Auque J (1996) Neurochirurgie 42(suppl 1):88–108
41. Jaeger R (1951) Observation on resection of the superior longitudinal sinus at and posterior to the rolandic and venous inflow. J Neurosurg 8:103–109

A Technical Description of the Brain Tumor Window Model: An In Vivo Model for the Evaluation of Intraoperative Contrast Agents

Daniel A. Orringer, Thomas Chen, Dah-Luen Huang, Martin Philbert, Raoul Kopelman, and Oren Sagher

Abstract The evaluation of candidate optical contrast agents for brain tumor delineation in ex vivo models may not accurately predict their activity in vivo. This study describes an in vivo model system designed to assess optical contrast agents for brain tumor delineation. The brain tumor window (BTW) model was created by performing biparietal craniectomies on 8-week-old Sprague-Dawley rats, injecting 9L glioma cells into the cortex and bonding a cover slip to the cranial defect with cyanoacrylate glue. Tumor growth was followed serially and occurred in an exponential fashion. Once tumors on the cortical surface achieved a 1 mm radius, intravenous contrast agents were injected while the appearance of the cortical surface was recorded. Computerized image analysis was used to quantitatively evaluate visible differences between tumor and normal brain. Tumor margins became readily apparent following contrast administration in the BTW model. Based on red component intensity, tumor delineation improved fourfold at 50 min post-contrast administration in the BTW model ($P < 0.002$). In summary, window placement overlying an implanted glioma is technically possible and well tolerated in the rat. The BTW model is a valid system for assessing the in vivo activity of optical contrast agents.

Keywords Brain tumor · Cranial window · Intraoperative imaging

D.A. Orringer, D.-L. Huang, and O. Sagher (✉)
Department of Neurosurgery, University of Michigan Health System, 1500 E. Medical Center Drive, Ann Arbor, MI 48109-5338, USA
e-mail: osagher@umich.edu

T. Chen
University of Michigan, Ann Arbor, MI USA

M. Philbert
Department of Toxicology, University of Michigan, Ann Arbor, MI USA

R. Kopelman
Department of Chemistry, University of Michigan, Ann Arbor, MI USA

Increasingly robust evidence suggests that the extent of surgical resection correlates with patient outcome for all types of brain tumors [1]. Stereotactic navigation, intraoperative ultrasound and intraoperative MRI have been developed been developed to improve the extent of resection. However, these technologies are limited by generating data that physically separated from the operative field, requiring the surgeon to correlate an image with the reality of the appearance of the operative field. To bridge the gap between diagnostic images and the operating field, investigators have long proposed the use of dyes to optically delineate tumor margins [2–9].

Experimental evaluation of tumor-delineating dyes has been carried out exclusively in ex vivo models. However, due to the visual differences between perfused and non-perfused tissue, we suggest that the properties of candidate optical contrast agents could be best characterized using in vivo, rather than ex vivo models. Therefore, we aimed to create an animal model to allow dynamic, in vivo visualization of the tumor brain interface. We describe a combination of the conventional 9L implanted glioma model with the chronic closed cranial window model to create the brain tumor window (BTW) model, a new system for evaluating the visual appearance of experimental brain tumors in vivo.

Materials and Methods

The 9L gliosarcoma cell line was cultured under standard cell culture conditions in RPMI media with 10% fetal bovine serum (InVitrogen, Carlsbad CA).

Approval from the University Committee on Use and Care of Animals at the University of Michigan was obtained prior to all experiments. Sprague-Dawley rats weighing 250–350 g were premedicated with buprenorphine 0.1 mg/kg and anesthetized with inhaled isoflurane delivered through a 16 gauge endotracheal tube. Vancomycin (25 mg/kg) was administered intraperitoneally prior to incision.

DOI 10.1007/978-3-211-99651-5_41,

After fixation in a stereotactic head holder, a midline incision was carried out over the skull from the frontal region to the occipito-cervical junction. Sutures were placed 2 mm from the apex of the superior and inferior apices of the incision and placed on tension to retract the scalp (Fig. 1a). The periosteum was detached from the skull through blunt dissection and removed using bipolar electrocautery. The periosteum, in continuity with fascial layers overlying the muscles of mastication, was removed to expose a sagitally-oriented ridge of bone. The bregma and lambda were identified as landmarks for placement of a craniectomy (Fig. 1a). Bleeding during exposure was controlled with bone wax, bipolar electrocautery and retraction. A high-speed drill was used to perform a nearly full thickness craniectomy of the medial aspect of the parietal bones bilaterally leaving an egg-shell thickness of bone overlying the dura (Fig. 1a). Minimal drilling was carried out of the bone overlying the superior sagittal sinus. The residual layer of bone was removed with a fine forceps and curved Penfield dissector. A linear rent in the dura in the coronal plane, towards the caudal end of the craniectomy was created using a bent 30-gauge needle. The caudal-most dura was then incised in a radial fashion along the base of the cranial defect and reflected cranially so that it could be removed in a single flap. Care was taken to avoid disrupting the large cortical veins entering the superior sagittal sinus in the midline which are continuous with the dura that must be removed medially. A dissecting forcep with curved tines was helpful in dissecting the dura without causing damage to the underlying structures. Once the dura was removed (Fig. 1b), the brain was irrigated with sterile normal saline. 10^5 9L cells were injected at a depth of 1mm into the right or left frontal portion of the exposed brain in an area lacking large blood vessels (Fig. 1c). A thin round glass microscope cover slip (10 mm diameter) was placed over the cranial defect (Fig. 1d). The edges of the cover slip were covered with two layers of cyanoacrylate glue (Fig. 1d) and a custom cut plastic ring was sown to the scalp with 3-0 nylon suture to enable continuous in vivo visualization of the implanted window (data not shown).

Animals were weighed and monitored daily. The surface of the cortex was inspected for signs of tumor growth in the region of the injection. Signs of tumor growth observed

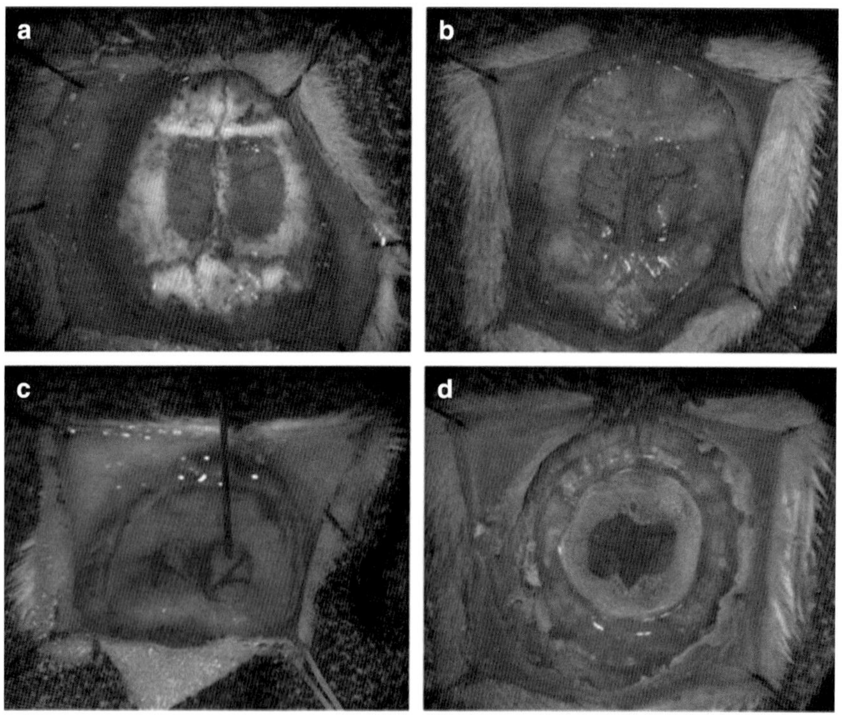

Fig. 1 Essential stages in the creation of a brain tumor window model: After reflecting the scalp edges laterally, a nearly full thickness craniectomy is performed, sparing the bone over the superior sagittal sinus (**a**). Once the remaining bone overlying the dura has been removed, a small durotomy at the base of the craniectomy is created to create a larger linear dural rent which is used to peel the dura forward, ideally in a single flap. Once the dural flap has been removed, the shiny arachnoidal surface of the brain is appreciated (**b**). Under microscopic guidance, a 10 μL, 26 gauge Hamilton syringe mounted to a steretactic injector is lowered through the meninges, 1 mm deep into an avasacular region of cortex (**c**). After injection, the surface of the brain is irrigated to remove residual tumor cells. A 10 mm glass cover slip is carefully placed on the surface of the brain and a confluent circumferential layer of cyanoacrylate glue, overlapping the edge of the coverslip and the craniectomy margin is applied (**d**). Glue is usually dry within 45 min at which time a plastic ring stenting the scalp open for continuous observation is applied

include hypervascularity, pinkish color change in the region of tumor injection and elevated cell mass at the site of injection. The size of the cortical region showing signs of tumor growth was measured serially to generate a tumor growth curve. Animals were imaged by MRI using previously published protocols to confirm the presence of tumors [10].

When the radius of tumors reached 1 mm, and the tumors were clearly visible adjacent to normal brain tissue, they were used for evaluation of optical contrast agents. A cut-down was performed to establish femoral venous access. PE50 surgical tubing was placed (0.25″ inner diameter, Dow Corning, Midland, Michigan) into the right femoral vein. Animals were then placed into a stereotactic head holder and continuous video recording with a high-definition camcorder under visible was then initiated. Coomassie blue (CB), an optical contrast agent was administered intravenously over 5 min using a Medfusion 3500 syringe pump (Medex, Dublin, OH) infusion syringe pump.

Video collected during the experiment was examined qualitatively to evaluate the difference in appearance between normal cortex and tumor tissue. Still images were generated from the video and analyzed colorimetrically with Image J as previously described to quantify the degree of color change in the tumor [11]. The difference in red hue was found to be the best method to reflect the visual difference between tumor and normal brain.

Brain tissue was examined ex vivo following each experiment on both a macroscopic and microscopic level. At the conclusion of each experiment, the brain was removed and photographed digitally on a standard white background. Gross coronal sections were photographed digitally then immersed in 4% paraformaldehyde for 15 min followed by 40% sucrose solution for 24 h. The sections were frozen in Tissue-Tek O.C.T. Compound (Sakura Finetek, The Netherlands). Routine hematoxylin and eosin staining was performed on 15 mm coronal sections created with a cryotome.

Results

Technique Development

The BTW model was refined using 50 animals. 49/50 animals demonstrated a 2–3 day period of approximately 7% body weight loss, but did not show any behavioral abnormalities. Among the complications encountered in the initial model development were, failure to thrive (resulting in death on the 2nd post-operative day), infection underlying the window (8/50), no tumor growth (6/50), diffuse tumor growth (3/50) and extensive hemorrhage under the window (3/50). One animal failed to thrive, possibly due to stroke. All other animals returned to their preoperative weight, baseline neurological status and to the expected rate of growth for rats of their age by the 5th post-operative day.

Tumor growth was evaluated serially whenever possible. The progression of tumor growth observed is demonstrated in Fig. 2. Assuming a spherical growth pattern, tumor growth followed an exponential curve (data not shown). Roughly spherical tumor geometry was confirmed by MRI (data not shown). On average, tumor became visible after four days and achieved a radius of 1 mm by 12.8 days. Tumor tissue appeared slightly redder than the normal cortical surface and has vascular markings that are distinct from normal cortex.

BTW Model Characterization

After the BTW model could be reliably and consistently created, 6 BTW animals possessing optimal imaging characteristics were used to evaluate the ability of contrast agents to delineate neoplastic tissue in the BTW model. Prior to contrast administration, it was difficult to visibly delineate the margins or implanted tumor in comparison to adjacent

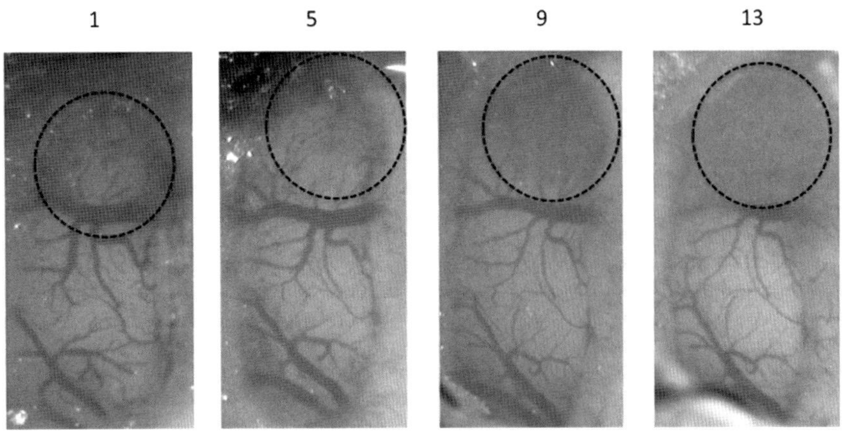

Fig. 2 Progression of tumor growth in the brain tumor window model. Tumor expands radially and can be tracked following implantation. A representative brain tumor window model is shown 1, 5, 9, and 13 days post-implantation

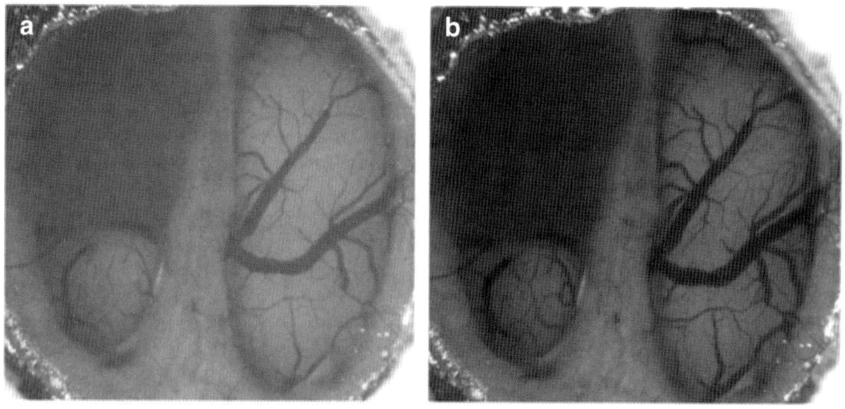

Fig. 3 Images of a brain tumor window model 12-days post-implantation before (**a**) and 50 min after Coomassie blue administration (**b**). Note the relatively subtle difference in the color of the tumor prior to contrast administration and the clear difference between the appearance of tumor and normal brain post-contrast

normal cortex (Fig. 3). Following contrast administration, there was a marked improvement in our ability to distinguish tumor from normal brain (Fig. 3). The calculated difference in red hue, reflecting the degree of color difference between tumor and normal brain, improved from 47.3 pre-contrast to 141.6 post-contrast ($P<0.0002$). Maximal delineation was achieved within 50 min of contrast administration and persisted throughout the entire 2-h experiment.

Whole brains harvested from animals following experiments were evaluated histologically. Grossly, there was a spherical superficial tissue mass at the site of the injection. Microscopic examination of specimens confirmed evidence of a spherical implanted glioma adjacent to normal cortex. Glioma tissue appeared hypercellular in comparison to normal brain. The nuclear to cytoplasmic ratio in the neoplastic appearing tissue was much greater than that of cells identified in the normal cortical tissue. The nuclei of the implanted tumor appeared highly polymorphic. Mitotic figures were easily identified. Fronds of tumor cells could be observed infiltrating into normal cortex adjacent to tumor (data not shown).

Delineation of tumor was compared in the BTW and the conventional implanted 9L glioma model (data not shown). The conventional ex vivo model overestimated the degree of delineation by CB ($P<0.03$). There was a sharp change in red hue at the visually apparent and MRI-defined tumor margin in both the BTW and conventional models.

Discussion

Achieving gross total resection is a key component of current treatment of gliomas [1]. Visible contrast agents such as fluorescein, [7] indocyanine-green [2] and bromophenol blue [6] hold promise in assisting in the delineation of neoplastic tissue within the operative field [3]. Fluorescent contrast agents such as, 5-aminolevulinic acid [8] and 5-aminofluorescein labeled albumin [12] have been demonstrated to be useful in delineating glioma tissue intraoperatively with fluorescent microscopy. We have recently suggested that dye-loaded nanoparticles may hold promise as visible contrast agents for brain tumor delineation [13].

We felt that the best way to evaluate candidate contrast agents was through a model system that would recreate the common difficulty surgeons face in distinguishing glioma from normal brain. We combined a common model for studying gliomas (9L gliosarcoma) with one primarily used to study the cerebral vasculature (cranial window model) to create the brain tumor window model. The initial complications encountered in the development of the model (superficial cortical hemorrhage, infection, failure or tumor growth, excessive tumor growth and stroke) subsided with experience. The result of our efforts was a model that allows direct observation of a proliferating tumor in vivo with subtly visible margins. From a qualitative and quantitative perspective tumor margins in the BTW model are dramatically clearer following the administration of contrast agents.

Our data suggests that conventional ex vivo 9L glioma models may overestimate the degree of delineation afforded by candidate contrast agents. We feel this observation arises from the lack of perfusion in ex vivo specimens. Both models have tumor margins that are well delineated by contrast and correspond to MRI-defined tumor margins. Since human tumors margins are rarely as regular as those of implanted gliomas, the utility of the BTW model might be improved if it were performed with a more infiltrative type of tumor.

In addition, there are a number of potential applications of the brain tumor window model that may not relate to studying visible contrast agents. First, the BTW model might be used for evaluating fluorescent and near-IR agents for tumor delineation. Since the BTW allows direct observation of tumor tissue in situ, it is possible that it could be used to track the response of tumor to anti-cancer therapies. In summary, while we have demonstrated the utility of the

BTW model for evaluating visible contrast agents, it is possible that the BTW model may assist be useful in a variety of in vivo glioma studies.

Disclosures This work was supported by grants from the National Institute of Biomedical Imaging and Bioengineering (1R01EB007977-01, to RK), the National Cancer Institute (1R21CA125297-01A1, to RK, and 1F32CA126295-01A1, to DAO), and the 2007 CNS Basic/Translational Resident Research Fellowship (to DAO). The authors have no personal financial or institutional interest in any of the drugs, materials, or devices described in this article.

Conflict of interest statement We declare that we have no conflict of interest.

References

1. Sanai N, Berger MS (2008) Glioma extent of resection and its impact on patient outcome. Neurosurgery 62:753–764, discussion 264–266
2. Britz GW, Ghatan S, Spence AM, Berger MS (2002) Intracarotid RMP-7 enhanced indocyanine green staining of tumors in a rat glioma model. J Neurooncol 56:227–232
3. Hansen DA, Spence AM, Carski T, Berger MS (1993) Indocyanine green (ICG) staining and demarcation of tumor margins in a rat glioma model. Surg Neurol 40:451–456
4. Moore GE (1947) Fluorescein as an agent in the differentiation of normal and malignant tissues. Science 106:130–131
5. Moore GE, Peyton WT et al (1948) The clinical use of fluorescein in neurosurgery; the localization of brain tumors. J Neurosurg 5:392–398
6. Ozawa T, Britz GW, Kinder DH, Spence AM, VandenBerg S, Lamborn KR, Deen DF, Berger MS (2005) Bromophenol blue staining of tumors in a rat glioma model. Neurosurgery 57:1041–1047, discussion 1041–1047
7. Shinoda J, Yano H, Yoshimura S, Okumura A, Kaku Y, Iwama T, Sakai N (2003) Fluorescence-guided resection of glioblastoma multiforme by using high-dose fluorescein sodium. Technical note. J Neurosurg 99:597–603
8. Stummer W, Pichlmeier U, Meinel T, Wiestler OD, Zanella F, Reulen HJ (2006) Fluorescence-guided surgery with 5-aminolevulinic acid for resection of malignant glioma: a randomised controlled multicentre phase III trial. Lancet Oncol 7:392–401
9. Veiseh M, Gabikian P, Bahrami SB, Veiseh O, Zhang M, Hackman RC, Ravanpay AC, Stroud MR, Kusuma Y, Hansen SJ, Kwok D, Munoz NM, Sze RW, Grady WM, Greenberg NM, Ellenbogen RG, Olson JM (2007) Tumor paint: a chlorotoxin: Cy5.5 bioconjugate for intraoperative visualization of cancer foci. Cancer Res 67:6882–6888
10. Reddy GR, Bhojani MS, McConville P, Moody J, Moffat BA, Hall DE, Kim G, Koo YE, Woolliscroft MJ, Sugai JV, Johnson TD, Philbert MA, Kopelman R, Rehemtulla A, Ross BD (2006) Vascular targeted nanoparticles for imaging and treatment of brain tumors. Clin Cancer Res 12:6677–6686
11. Orringer DA, Koo YE, Chen T, Kim G, Hah HJ, Xu H, Wang S, Keep R, Philbert MA, Kopelman R, Sagher O (2009) In vitro characterization of a targeted, dye-loaded nanodevice for intraoperative tumor delineation. Neurosurgery 64:965–971, discussion 971–972
12. Kremer P, Mahmoudreza F, Ding R, Pritsch M, Zoubaa S, Frei E (2009) Intraoperative fluorescence staining of malignant brain tumors using 5-aminofluorescein-labeled albumin. Neurosurgery 64:53–60, discussion 60–61
13. Orringer DA, Koo YE, Chen T, Kopelman R, Sagher O, Philbert MA (2009) Small solutions for big problems: the application of nanoparticles to brain tumor diagnosis and therapy. Clin Pharmacol Ther 85:531–534

Author Index

Subject Index

Printing: Ten Brink, Meppel, The Netherlands
Binding: Stürtz, Würzburg, Germany